ABDOMINAL
ULTRASOUND

Study Guide
&
Exam Review

ABDOMINAL ULTRASOUND

Study Guide & Exam Review

Sandra L. Hagen-Ansert
B.A., RDMS, RDCS

Program Director of Diagnostic Ultrasound,
Baptist Memorial College of Health Services,
Memphis, Tennessee

Former Program Director of Diagnostic Ultrasound,
Department of Radiology
Clinical and Research Echocardiographic Sonographer,
Pediatric Cardiology Division
Clinical Neonatal Echoencephalographic Sonographer,
Neonatal Support Center

University of California, San Diego Medical Center,
San Diego, California

With 288 illustrations

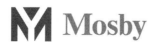 Mosby

St. Louis Baltimore Boston Carlsbad Chicago Naples New York Philadelphia Portland
London Madrid Mexico City Singapore Sydney Tokyo Toronto Wiesbaden

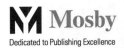

Dedicated to Publishing Excellence

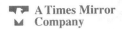

A Times Mirror
Company

Editor: Jeanne Rowland
Developmental Editor: Lisa Potts
Project Manager: Linda McKinley
Production Editor: Julie Zipfel
Production Management: Graphic World Publishing Services
Manufacturing Supervisor: Linda Ierardi

Printed in the United States of America
Composition by Graphic World, Inc.
Printing/binding by Maple/Vail Book Mfg. Group

Mosby-Year Book, Inc.
11830 Westline Industrial Drive
St. Louis, Missouri 63146

Library of Congress Cataloging in Publication Data
Hagen-Ansert, Sandra L.
　　Abdominal ultrasound study giude and exam review / Sandra L.
Hagen-Ansert.—1st ed.
　　　　p.　　cm.
　　Companion v. to: Textbook of diagnostic ultrasonagraphy / Sandra
L. Hagen-Ansert. 4th ed. c1995.
　　Includes bibliographical references.
　　ISBN 0-8151-4176-9
　　1. Diagnosis, Ultrasonic—Examinations, questions, etc.
2. Echocardiography—Examinations, questions, etc.　3. Abdomen—
Ultrasonic imaging—Examinations, questions, etc.　I. Hagen
-Ansert, Sandra L.　Textbook of diagnostic ultrasonagraphy.
II. Title
　　[DNLM: 1. Abdomen—ultrasonography—examination questions.　WE
18.2 H143a 1996]
RC78.7.U4H33　1995 Suppl.
617.5′507543—dc20
DNLM/DLC
for Library of Congress　　　　　　　　　　　　95-40123
　　　　　　　　　　　　　　　　　　　　　　　　　　CIP

96　97　98　99　00　/　9　8　7　6　5　4　3　2　1

Preface

This practical resource serves two purposes. First, as a study guide, it is organized to complement the fourth edition of the *Textbook of Diagnostic Ultrasonography* by Sandra L. Hagen-Ansert. Second, as an examination review, it serves as a complete guide for preparation of the abdomen examination administered by the American Registry of Diagnostic Medical Sonographers (ARDMS).

The most effective way to use this resource is to read the chapters in the textbook and then complete the review exercises, self-tests, and case reviews in this workbook. Each section is organized to follow the format of the *Textbook of Diagnostic Ultrasonography;* therefore, the student may elect to read a short segment of the chapter and then complete the review exercise before moving to the next section. The instructor may want to recommend this format as a way of reinforcing comprehension of assigned reading material.

All 12 chapters have an equivalent chapter in the *Textbook of Diagnostic Ultrasonography.* Each chapter is divided into six sections: course objectives, normal anatomic illustrations and descriptions, review notes, review exercises, self-tests, and case reviews, along with answers that correspond with all questions.

Objectives

As a student, it is important to be familiar with the list of objectives at the beginning of each chapter. These objectives not only emphasize the important elements in each chapter but also help to define the diagnostic sonographer's role.

Anatomy

Anatomic illustrations with descriptions are included in each chapter. To enhance the learning process, students may use marking pens to color the various structures within the illustrations. Frequent reference of the section in chapter 1 on abdominal cross-section and sagittal anatomy will be particularly helpful in understanding sectional anatomy.

Review Notes

Outline notes from the corresponding chapter in the *Textbook of Diagnostic Ultrasonography* are provided to help review the information presented in the textbook. These notes will also serve as useful study outlines in preparation for the abdomen Registry examination.

Review Exercises

The review exercises are the focal point of this study guide and examination review. They will help to reinforce the concepts and the material presented. It is suggested that students first study the corresponding chapter in the *Textbook of Diagnostic Ultrasonography,* and then study the general anatomy section and review notes before completing the review exercises. Once students have completed the worksheets, they should check their answers with those found at the end of the chapter. Careful review of sections that correspond to missed questions will prepare the student for the next step: taking the self-test.

Self-Tests

Students are advised to take the self-test as if they were taking a real test in the classroom. A score of less than 90% indicates that a second review of the material may be helpful. This section should prove very useful in preparation for the Registry examination.

Case Review

Each case review includes a short history and laboratory data to help students arrive at a differential diagnosis. Before answering the case review questions, students should review the figure illustrations in the corresponding chapter from the *Textbook of Diagnostic Ultrasonography.* A clear understanding of differential diagnosis will be reinforced by paying particular attention to sonographic findings with specific disease processes. If students miss a case, they should go back to the chapter to review the discussion of the pathology presented and pay particular attention to the anatomy, pathology, and differential diagnosis.

Practice Exam

The appendix contains a practice examination that is designed to simulate the real abdomen Registry examination. It includes 200 questions that are written in a style that is similar to that of the Registry. In addition, answers are provided so that students can assess their preparedness before taking the real examination.

With all of the combined elements—chapter objectives, anatomic illustrations and descriptions, review notes, review questions, self-tests, and the practice Registry examination—students will find this resource invaluable to reinforce concepts presented in the fourth edition of the *Textbook of Diagnostic Ultrasonography*. Furthermore, all of the information provided combined with the numerous test-taking elements should guarantee success on the Registry examination.

Sandra L. Hagen-Ansert

Contents

1 Anatomic and Physiologic Relationships Within the Abdominal Cavity   1

2 The Muscular System   47

3 The Vascular System   67

4 The Liver   113

5 The Biliary System   173

6 The Pancreas   207

7 The Gastrointestinal Tract   243

8 The Urinary System   265

9 The Spleen   325

10 Retroperitoneal Structures   345

11 The Peritoneal Cavity and Abdominal Wall   362

12 Superficial Structures   385
    The Thyroid   385
    The Breast   405
    The Scrotum   426

APPENDIX Practice Registry Exam   446

References   465

ABDOMINAL ULTRASOUND

Study Guide
&
Exam Review

Anatomic and Physiologic Relationships within the Abdominal Cavity

OBJECTIVES

At the completion of this chapter, students will show orally, in writing, or by demonstration that they will be able to:

1. Describe the anatomic nomenclature.
2. Describe the abdominal regions and body planes.
3. Describe the abdominal viscera as it relates to the abdominal regions.
4. Describe the abdominal wall and its relationships.
5. Illustrate the surface and internal anatomies of the peritoneum, mesentery, and omentum as they relate to the abdominal viscera in cross-section and sagittal planes.

6. Name the peritoneal ligaments, peritoneal fossae, and peritoneal recesses.
7. Describe the true and false pelvis boundary landmarks.
8. Know the cross-sectional anatomy of the abdominal and pelvic cavities.
9. Know the sagittal anatomies of the abdominal and pelvic cavities.

To further enhance learning, students should use marking pens to color the anatomic illustrations that follow.

ANATOMIC TERMS AND DESCRIPTIONS

FIGURE 1-1
Anterior View of the Body in the Anatomic Position

anatomic position (Figure 1-1) Standing erect, with the arms by the side and the face and palms directed forward

median sagittal plane (Figure 1-1) A vertical plane passing through the center of the body, dividing it into right and left halves

paramedian plane (Figure 1-1) The plane situated on each side of the median plane

coronal plane (Figure 1-2) An imaginary vertical plane at right angles to the median plane that divides the body into front and back parts (The terms *ante-rior* and *posterior* relate to this plane.)

transverse (horizontal) plane (Figure 1-1) The plane at right angles to both the median and the coronal planes

supine Lying face up

prone Lying face down

anterior (ventral) (Figure 1-2) The front of the body, or in front of another structure

posterior (dorsal) (Figure 1-2) The back of the body, or in back of another structure

proximal (limb reference only) (Figure 1-1) Location of a structure closer to the median plane or root of the limb than is another structure

distal (limb reference only) (Figure 1-1) Location of a structure farther from the median plane or root of the limb than is another structure

superficial/deep Relative distance of a structure from the surface of the body

superior (cranial)/inferior (caudal) (Figure 1-2) Levels relatively high or low, with respect to the upper and lower ends of the body

medial (Figure 1-1) Situated close to the median plane

lateral (Figure 1-1) Lying far from the median plane

internal/external Relative distance of a structure from the center of an organ or cavity

ipsilateral Located on the same side of the body

contralateral Located on the opposite side of the body

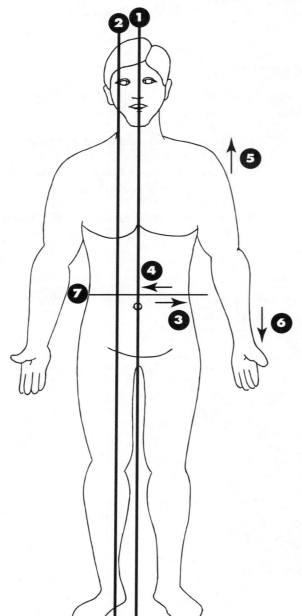

1	median sagittal plane
2	paramedian plane
3	lateral
4	medial
5	proximal
6	distal
7	transverse plane

FIGURE 1-2
Lateral View of the Body

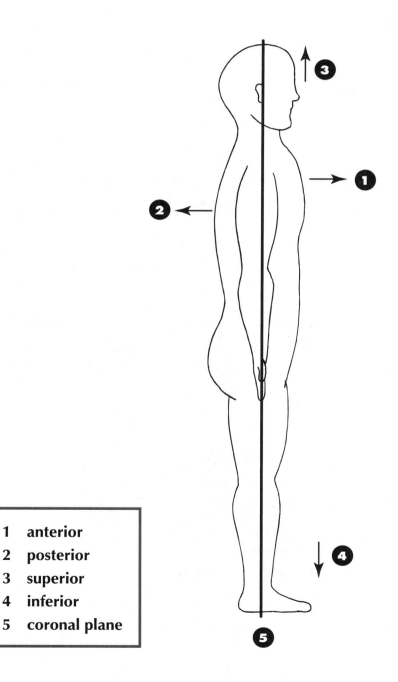

1	anterior
2	posterior
3	superior
4	inferior
5	coronal plane

THE ABDOMEN IN GENERAL

FIGURE 1-3

Surface Landmarks of the Anterior Abdominal Wall

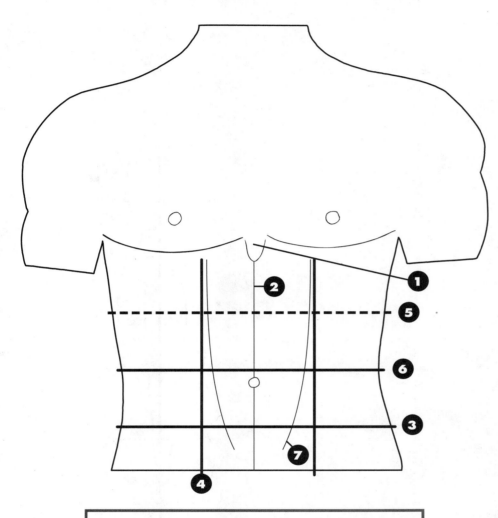

1. xyphoid process
2. median groove
3. tubercle of crest (intertubercular plane)
4. right lateral plane
5. transpyloric plane
6. subcostal plane
7. linea semilunaris

Surface Landmarks

xyphoid process (Figure 1-3) Half as thick as the sternum and easily palpated in the depression where the costal margins meet at the infrasternal angle

costal margin The curved lower margin of the thoracic wall; it is formed anteriorly by the cartilages of the seventh, eighth, ninth, and tenth ribs and posteriorly by the eleventh and twelfth ribs; its lowest level is at the tenth rib, which lies opposite the body of the third lumbar vertebra

iliac crest May be easily palpated and ends in front at the anterior iliac spine and behind at the posterior iliac spine; its highest point lies opposite the body of the fourth lumbar vertebra

inguinal ligament The rolled inferior margin of the aponeurosis of the external oblique muscle; it is attached laterally to the anterior superior iliac spine and curves downward and medial to the pubic tubercle

pubic tubercle A small protuberance along the superior surface of the pubis

pubic symphysis A cartilaginous joint that lies in the midline between the bodies of the pubic bones

midinguinal point A point that lies on the inguinal ligament halfway between the pubic symphysis and the anterior superior iliac spine

superficial inguinal ring A triangular aperture in the aponeurosis of the external oblique muscle situated above and medial to the pubic tubercle

linea alba A midline fibrous band that extends from the pubic symphysis to the xyphoid process; it is formed by the fusion of the aponeuroses of the anterior abdominal wall muscles and is revealed on the surface by a slight median groove

umbilicus The remnant of the fetal umbilical cord; it lies in the linea alba and varies in position

linea semilunaris (Figure 1-3) The lateral edge of the rectus abdominis muscle

FIGURE 1-4
Regions of the Abdominal Wall

Abdominal Regions

The abdomen can be divided into nine regions by two vertical and two horizontal lines (Figure 1-4). Each vertical line passes through the midinguinal point. The subcostal plane (of the upper horizontal line) joins the lowest point of the costal margin at the tenth costal cartilage and lies opposite the third lumbar vertebra. The intertubercular plane (of the lowest horizontal line) joins the tubercles on the iliac crests at the body of the fifth lumbar vertebra.

Upper abdomen
Right hypochondrium
Epigastrium
Left hypochondrium
Middle abdomen
Right lumbar
Umbilical
Left lumbar
Lower abdomen
Right iliac fossa
Hypogastrium
Left iliac fossa

The transpyloric plane passes through the tips of the ninth costal cartilages on both sides. This is the point where the lateral edge of the rectus abdominis (linea semilunaris) crosses the costal margin. This plane passes through the renal hila, the neck of the pancreas, the duodenojejunal junction, and the pylorus.

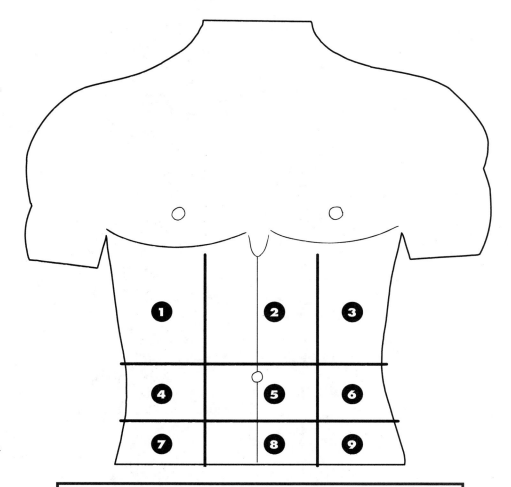

1	right hypochondrium	6	left lumbar region
2	epigastrium	7	right iliac fossa
3	left hypochondrium	8	hypogastrium
4	right lumbar region	9	left iliac fossa
5	umbilical region		

FIGURE 1-5
Basic Abdominal Landmarks and Viscera

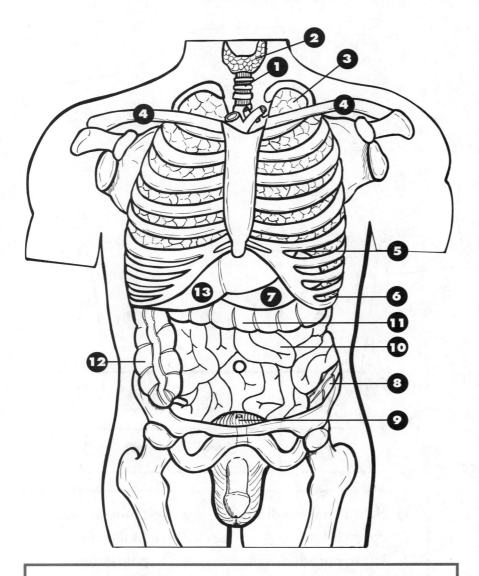

Abdominal Cavity (FIGURE 1-6)

The abdominal cavity (excluding the retroperitoneum and pelvis) is bounded superiorly by the diaphragm; anteriorly by the abdominal wall muscles; posteriorly by the vertebral column, ribs, and iliac fossa; and inferiorly by the pelvis.

Peritoneum

The peritoneum is a thin, translucent, serous membrane that lines the walls of the abdominal cavity and covers the abdominal viscera. It has two layers: the parietal layer and the visceral layer. The parietal layer lines the walls of the abdominal cavity; the visceral layer covers the abdominal organs. Between the two layers is the peritoneal cavity, which contains a small amount of lubricating serous fluid to permit free movement between the viscera. In the male this cavity is closed, but in the female there is a communication with the exterior through the fallopian tubes, the uterus, and the vagina.

The peritoneal cavity may be divided into two parts: the greater sac and the lesser sac. The greater sac is the larger of the two and extends across the abdomen from the diaphragm to the pelvis. The lesser sac lies posterior to the stomach; as a small diverticulum from the greater sac, it opens through a window called the epiploic foramen.

The mesentery is a two-layered fold of peritoneum that attaches part of the intestine to the posterior abdominal wall, including the small intestine, the transverse colon, and the sigmoid colon.

1	trachea	8	descending colon
2	thyroid	9	bladder
3	pulmonary apex	10	intestine
4	clavicle	11	transverse colon
5	diaphragm	12	ascending colon
6	costodiaphragmatic recess	13	liver
7	stomach		

FIGURE 1-6
Abdominal Cavity

Greater Omentum (FIGURE 1-6)

The omentum is a two-layered fold of peritoneum that attaches the stomach to another viscera. The greater omentum is often referred to as an apron hanging between the small intestine and the anterior abdominal wall. It is attached to the greater curvature of the stomach. The lesser omentum attaches the lesser curvature of the stomach to the undersurface of the liver. The gastrosplenic omentum attaches the stomach to the spleen.

There are several peritoneal ligaments that attach the less mobile solid viscera to the abdominal walls:

falciform ligament attaches the liver to the abdominal wall and the diaphragm (Figure 1-6)

median umbilical ligament (urachus) passes from the apex of the bladder to the umbilicus

lateral umbilical ligament obliterated umbilical arteries; passes from the internal iliac artery to the umbilicus

ligamentum teres obliterated umbilical fetal vein; passes upward to enter the groove between the quadrate lobe and the left lobe of the liver

lienorenal ligament a peritoneal layer from the kidney to the hilum of the spleen

gastrosplenic ligament passes from the hilus of the spleen to the greater curvature of the stomach

The mesenteries, omenta, and peritoneal ligaments allow the blood vessels, lymphatics, and nerves to reach the other viscera in the abdomen.

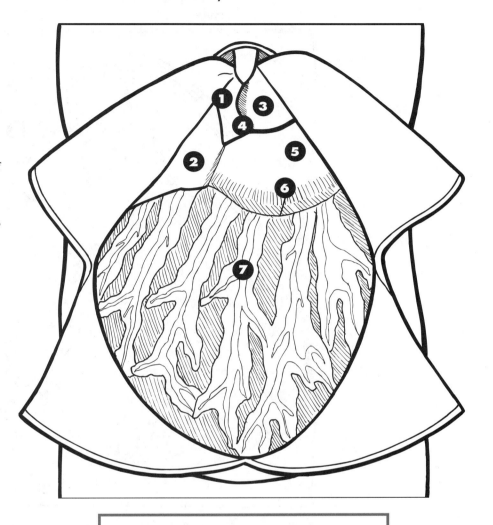

1	falciform ligament
2	right lobe of the liver
3	left lobe of the liver
4	ligamentum teres
5	stomach
6	greater curvature of the stomach
7	greater omentum

FIGURE 1-7

Abdominal Cavity (Greater Omentum Removed)

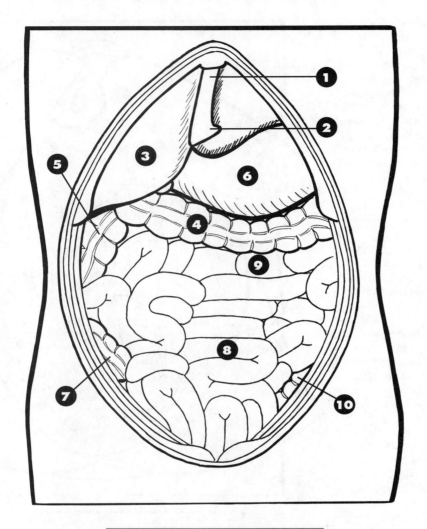

1	falciform ligament
2	ligamentum teres
3	right lobe of the liver
4	transverse colon
5	ascending colon
6	stomach
7	cecum
8	ileum
9	jejunum
10	descending colon

FIGURE 1-8
Abdominal Cross Section, Level 1

Abdomen, Level 1 (FIGURE 1-8)

This cross section is made at the level of the tenth intervertebral disc. The lower portion of the pericardial sac is seen in this section. The splenic artery enters the spleen, and the splenic vein emerges from the splenic hilum. The abdominal portion of the esophagus lies to the left of the midline and opens into the stomach through the orifice. The liver extends to the left mammillary line. The coronary ligament is shown. The falciform liga- ment extends into the section above this. The upper border of the tail of the pan- creas and the body of this structure are shown. The spleen is seen to lie alongside the ninth rib. The upper pole of the left kidney is seen posterior to the spleen.

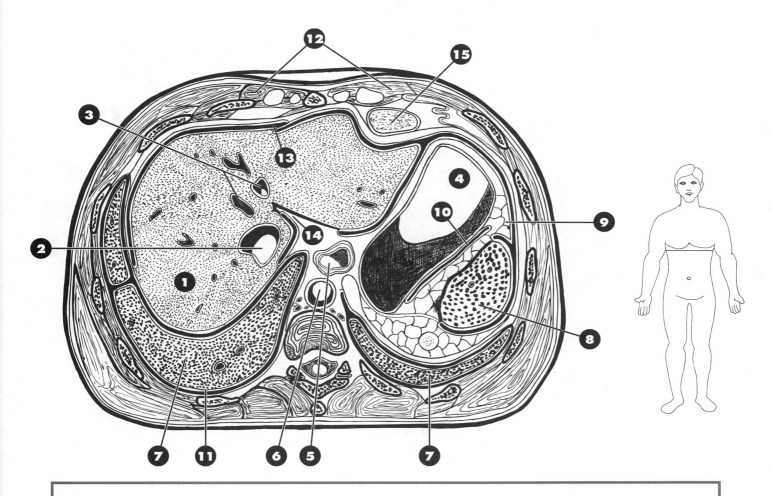

1	right lobe of the liver	6	abdominal aorta	11	pleural sac
2	inferior vena cava	7	inferior lobe of the lung	12	rectus abdominis muscle
3	hepatic veins	8	spleen	13	falciform ligament
4	stomach	9	gastrosplenic ligament	14	ligamentum venosum
5	esophagus	10	omental bursa	15	pericardial sac

FIGURE 1-9
Abdominal Cross Section, Level 2

Abdomen, Level 2 (FIGURE 1-9)

This section is taken at the level of the eleventh thoracic disc and the superior portion of the twelfth thoracic vertebra. The hepatic vein is shown to enter the inferior vena cava. The renal artery and the vein of the left kidney are shown. The left branch of the portal vein is seen to arch upward to enter the left lobe of the liver. The upper part of the stomach is shown with the hepatogastric and gastrocolic ligaments. The lesser omental cavity is behind the stomach. The upper border of the splenic flexture of the colon is seen. The falciform and coronary ligaments of the liver can be seen. The caudate lobe of the liver is seen in this section and in Level 1. The tail and body of the pancreas are seen. The spleen is shown along the left lateral border. The adrenal glands are shown lateral to the crus of the diaphragm.

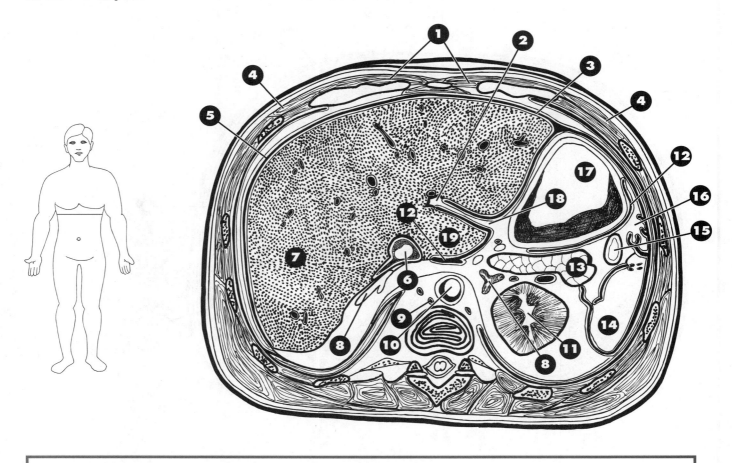

1 **rectus abdominis muscle**	6 **inferior vena cava**	13 **pancreas**
2 **ligamentum venosum**	7 **right lobe of the liver**	14 **spleen**
3 **diaphragm**	8 **suprarenal glands**	15 **colic flexure**
4 **external oblique muscle**	9 **azygos vein**	16 **gastric ligament**
	10 **aorta**	17 **stomach**
5 **peritoneal cavity**	11 **kidney**	18 **hepatogastric ligament**
	12 **omental bursa**	19 **caudate lobe of the liver**

FIGURE 1-10
Abdominal Cross Section, Level 3

Abdomen, Level 3 (FIGURE 1-10)

This section is taken at the level of the twelfth thoracic vertebra, slightly above the intervertebral disc. The celiac axis (not shown) arises in the middle of this section from the anterior abdominal aorta. The right renal artery originates in this section. Again, one of the hepatic veins is shown to enter the inferior vena cava. The section cuts through the mid portion of the greater curvature of the stomach and includes part of the pylorus of the stomach. A small portion of the superior portion of the duodenum is found in the lower part of this section. The ligament of Treitz is shown. The transverse and descending colon are shown below the splenic flexure. (The descending colon is a retroperitoneal structure.) The transverse mesocolon is shown. The falciform ligament, right triangular ligament, and gastrohepatic omentum are shown. The caudate lobe of the liver is well seen. The body of the pancreas, both kidneys, and the lower portions of the adrenal glands are shown.

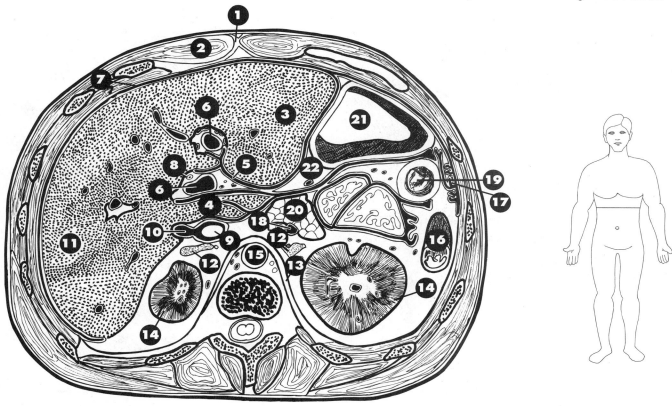

1	**linea alba**	**9**	**inferior vena cava**	**17**	**peritoneal cavity**
2	**rectus abdominis muscle**	**10**	**hepatic vein**	**18**	**splenic vein**
3	**left lobe of the liver**	**11**	**right lobe of the liver**	**19**	**transverse colon**
4	**caudate lobe of the liver**	**12**	**suprarenal gland**	**20**	**pancreas**
5	**hepatic artery**	**13**	**crus of the diaphragm**	**21**	**stomach**
6	**portal vein**	**14**	**kidney**	**22**	**omental bursa**
7	**diaphragm**	**15**	**aorta**		
8	**hepatic duct**	**16**	**descending colon**		

FIGURE 1-11
Abdominal Cross Section, Level 4

Abdomen, Level 4 (FIGURE 1-11)

This section is taken at the level of the first lumbar vertebra. The psoas major muscle is seen. The crura of the diaphragm are shown on each side of the vertebra. The right renal artery is shown. The left renal artery arises from the lateral wall of the aorta. Both renal veins enter the inferior vena cava. The portal vein is seen to be formed by the union of the splenic vein and the superior mesenteric vein. The lower portion of the stomach and the pyloric orifice are seen, as is the superior portion of the duodenum. The duodenojejunal flexure and descending and transverse colon are shown. The greater omentum is very prominent. The small, nonperitoneal area of the liver is shown anterior to the right kidney. The round ligament of the liver and the umbilical fissure, which separates the right and left lobes of the liver, are seen. The neck of the gallbladder (not shown) is found just inferior to this section, between the quadrate and caudate lobes of the liver. The cystic duct is cut in two places. The hepatic duct lies just anterior to the cystic duct. The cystic and hepatic ducts unite in the lower part of the section to form the common bile duct. The pancreatic duct is found within the pancreas at this level. Both kidneys are seen just lateral to the psoas muscles.

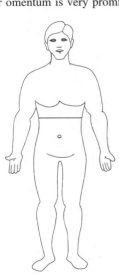

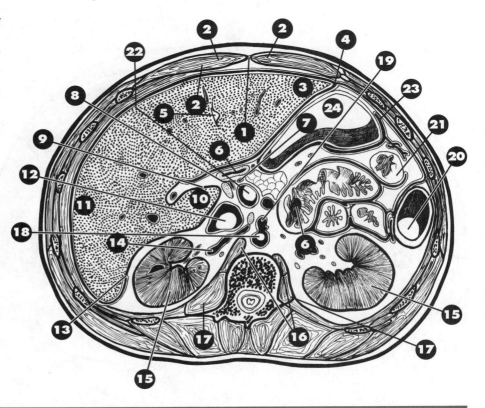

1	**linea alba**	**9**	**epiploic foramen (foramen of Winslow)**	
2	**rectus abdominis muscle**	**10**	**caudate lobe of the liver**	
3	**left lobe of the liver**	**11**	**right lobe of the liver**	
4	**peritoneal cavity**	**12**	**inferior vena cava**	
5	**ligamentum teres**	**13**	**hepatorenal ligament**	
6	**duodenum**	**14**	**renal artery**	
7	**gastroduodenal artery**	**15**	**kidney**	
8	**hepatic duct**	**16**	**crus of the diaphragm**	

17	**psoas major muscle**
18	**aorta**
19	**superior mesenteric artery**
20	**descending colon**
21	**transverse colon**
22	**splenic vein**
23	**omental bursa**
24	**stomach**

FIGURE 1-12
Abdominal Cross Section, Level 5

Abdomen, Level 5 (FIGURE 1-12)

This section is taken at the level of the second lumbar vertebra. The superior pancreaticoduodenal artery originates in Level 4 and shows some of its branches on this section. The lower portion of the stomach is found in this section, and the hepatic flexure of the colon is seen. The lobes of the liver are separated by the round ligament. The left lobe of the liver ends at this level. The head and neck of the pancreas drape around the superior mesenteric vein. Both kidneys and the psoas muscles are shown.

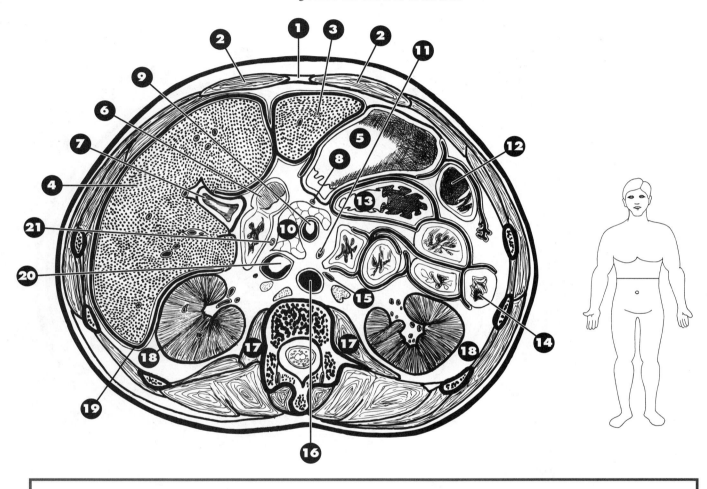

1	linea alba	8	gastroduodenal artery
2	rectus abdominis muscle	9	superior mesenteric vein
3	left lobe of the liver	10	pancreas
4	right lobe of the liver	11	superior mesenteric artery
5	stomach	12	transverse colon
6	duodenum	13	jejunum
7	gallbladder		

14	descending colon
15	left renal vein
16	aorta
17	psoas major muscle
18	kidney
19	peritoneal cavity
20	inferior vena cava
21	common bile duct

FIGURE 1-13
Abdominal Cross Section, Level 6

Abdomen, Level 6 (FIGURE 1-13)

This section is taken at the level of the third lumbar vertebra. The inferior mesenteric artery originates from the abdominal aorta at this level. The greater omentum is shown mostly on the left side of the abdomen. The descending and ascending portions of the duodenum, which lie between the aorta and the superior mesenteric artery and vein, are shown. The fundus of the gallbladder lies in the lower portion of this section. The lower poles of both kidneys lie lateral to the psoas muscles.

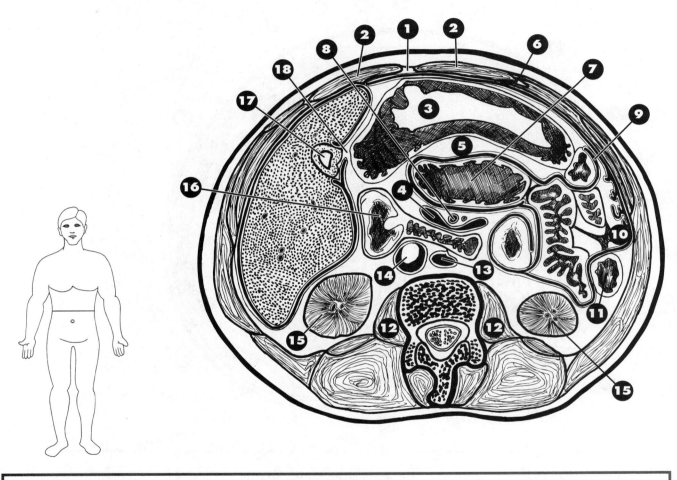

1	**linea alba**	**8**	**superior mesenteric artery**	**14**	**inferior vena cava**
2	**rectus abdominis muscle**			**15**	**kidney**
3	**transverse colon**	**9**	**peritoneal cavity**	**16**	**duodenum**
4	**superior mesenteric vein**	**10**	**greater omentum**	**17**	**gallbladder**
5	**transverse mesocolon**	**11**	**descending colon**	**18**	**hepatocolic ligament**
6	**parietal peritoneum**	**12**	**psoas major muscle**		
7	**jejunum**	**13**	**aorta**		

FIGURE 1-14
Abdominal Cross Section, Level 7

Abdomen, Level 7 (FIGURE 1-14)

This section is taken through the third lumbar disc. The lower portion of the duodenum is shown. The section passes through many loops of jejunum and ileum. The lower margin of the right lobe of the liver is shown along the right lateral border.

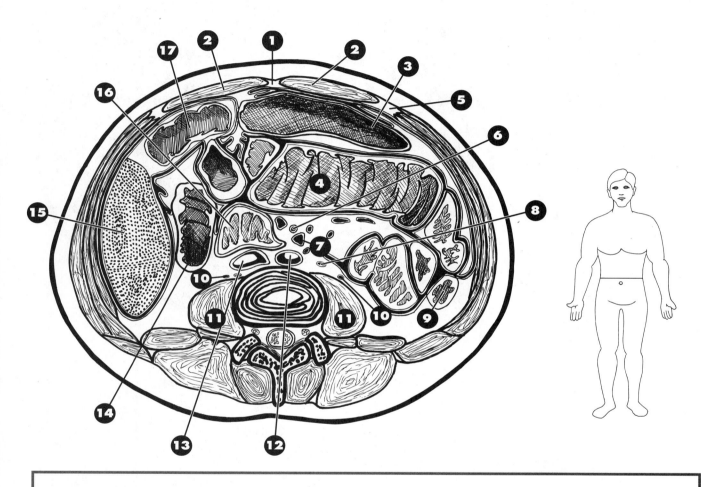

1 linea alba	7 superior mesenteric vein	12 aorta
2 rectus abdominis muscle	8 inferior mesenteric artery	13 inferior vena cava
3 transverse colon	9 descending colon	14 ascending colon
4 jejunum	10 ureter	15 right lobe of the liver
5 linea semilunaris	11 psoas major muscle	16 duodenum
6 superior mesenteric artery		17 ileum

FIGURE 1-15
Abdominal Cross Section, Level 8

Abdomen, Level 8 (FIGURE 1-15)

This section is taken through the lower portion of the fourth lumbar vertebra. The aorta bifurcates into the common iliac arteries in this section, and coils of small intestine are seen throughout. The coils on the left side are through the jejunal portion; those on the right side are through the ileal portion. The ascending and descending colons are shown. The greater omentum is still prominent on the left side.

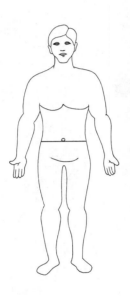

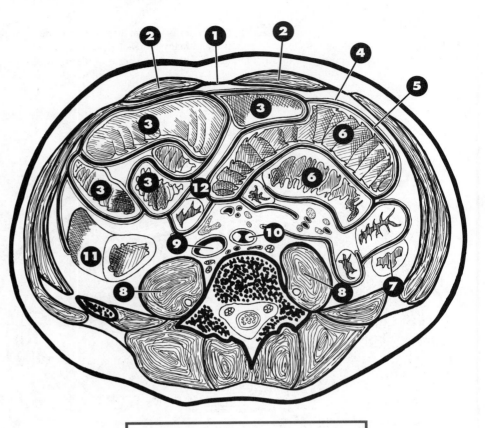

1	**linea alba**
2	**rectus abdominis muscle**
3	**ileum**
4	**parietal peritoneum**
5	**peritoneal cavity**
6	**jejunum**
7	**descending colon**
8	**psoas muscle**
9	**inferior vena cava**
10	**aortic bifurcation**
11	**ascending colon**
12	**mesentery**

Serial Sagittal Sections (FIGURES 1-16 THROUGH 1-27)

FIGURE 1-16

Abdominal Sagittal Section, Level 1

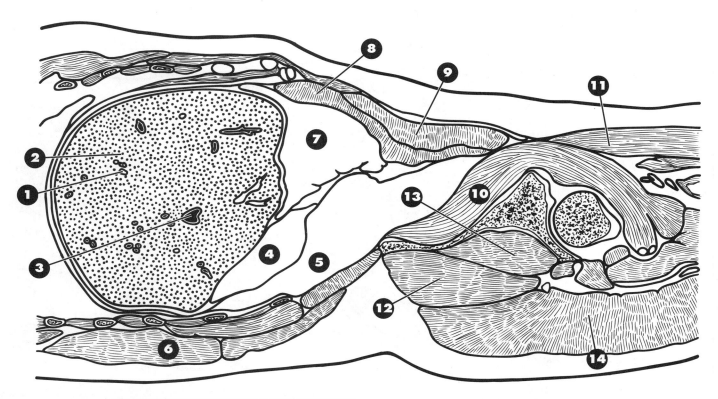

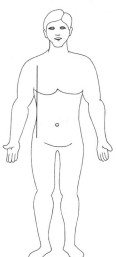

1	portal vein
2	right lobe of the liver
3	hepatic vein
4	perirenal fat
5	retroperitoneal fat
6	latissimus dorsi muscle
7	omentum
8	internal oblique muscle
9	external oblique muscle
10	iliacus muscle
11	psoas major muscle
12	gluteus medius muscle
13	gluteus minimus muscle
14	gluteus maximus muscle

FIGURE 1-17
Abdominal Sagittal Section, Level 2

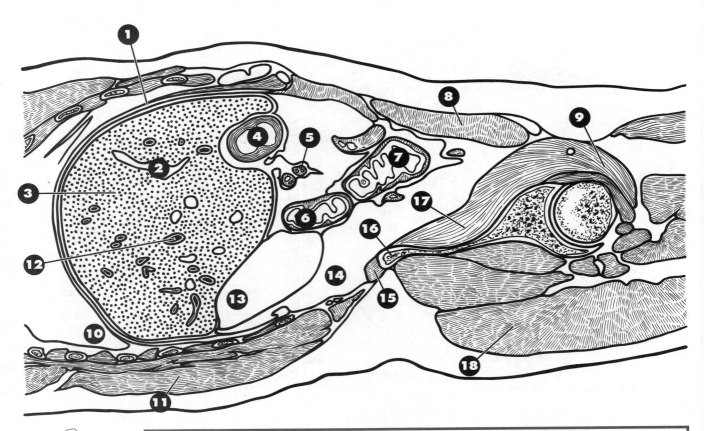

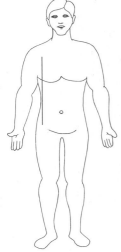

1	diaphragm	10	costodiaphragmatic recess
2	portal vein	11	latissimus dorsi muscle
3	liver	12	hepatic vein
4	gallbladder	13	perirenal fat
5	hepatic flexure	14	retroperitoneal fat
6	ascending colon	15	quadratus lumborum muscle
7	cecum	16	ilium
8	internal oblique muscle	17	iliacus muscle
9	psoas major muscle	18	gluteus maximus muscle

FIGURE 1-18
Abdominal Sagittal Section, Level 3

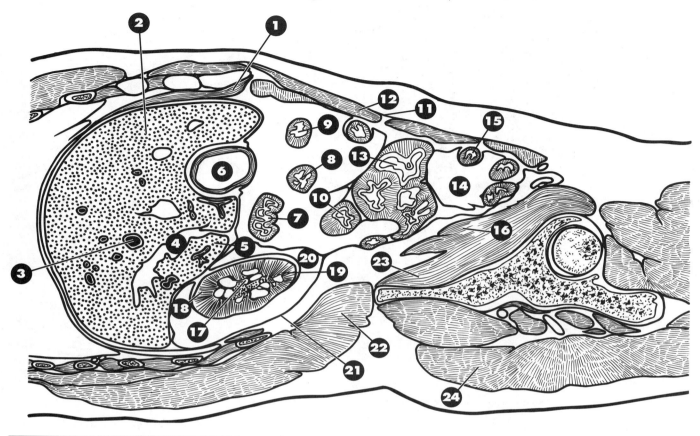

1	**diaphragm**	**13**	**cecum**
2	**liver**	**14**	**mesentery**
3	**hepatic vein**	**15**	**small bowel**
4	**portal vein**	**16**	**psoas major muscle**
5	**caudate lobe of the liver**	**17**	**renal medulla**
6	**gallbladder**	**18**	**right kidney**
7	**hepatic flexure**	**19**	**renal cortex**
8	**transverse colon**	**20**	**perirenal fat**
9	**small bowel**	**21**	**perirenal fascia**
10	**ascending colon**	**22**	**quadratus lumborum muscle**
11	**rectus sheath**	**23**	**iliacus muscle**
12	**rectus abdominis muscle**	**24**	**gluteus maximus muscle**

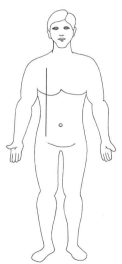

FIGURE 1-19
Abdominal Sagittal Section, Level 4

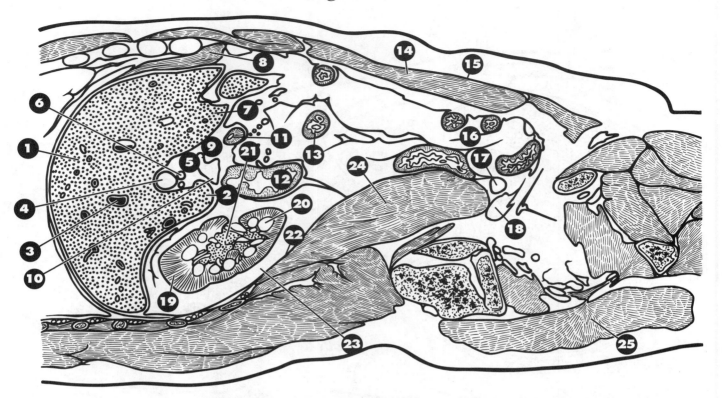

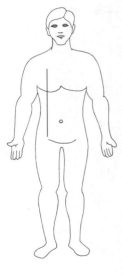

1	liver	13	transverse colon
2	caudate lobe of the liver	14	rectus abdominis muscle
3	hepatic vein	15	anterior rectus sheath
4	portal vein	16	mesentery
5	porta hepatis	17	right external iliac artery
6	hepatic artery	18	right external iliac vein
7	medial segment, left lobe	19	kidney
8	diaphragm	20	renal pyramid
9	neck of the gallbladder	21	renal sinus
10	Hartmann's pouch	22	perirenal fascia
11	superior part of the duodenum	23	perirenal fat
12	descending part of the duodenum	24	psoas major muscle
		25	gluteus maximus muscle

FIGURE 1-20
Abdominal Sagittal Section, Level 5

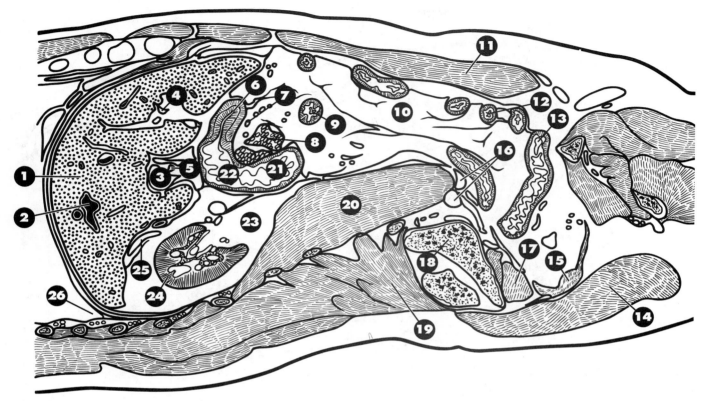

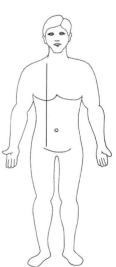

1	right lobe of the liver	14	gluteus maximus muscle
2	hepatic vein	15	levator ani muscle
3	portal vein	16	right external iliac artery
4	left branch of the portal vein	17	piriformis muscle
5	cystic duct	18	sacrum
6	pyloric sphincter	19	erector spinae muscle
7	gastroduodenal artery	20	psoas major muscle
8	head of the pancreas	21	descending duodenum
9	transverse colon	22	superior duodenum
10	mesentery	23	perirenal fat
11	rectus abdominis muscle	24	right kidney
12	small bowel	25	right suprarenal gland
13	ileum	26	costodiaphragmatic recess

FIGURE 1-21
Abdominal Sagittal Section, Level 6

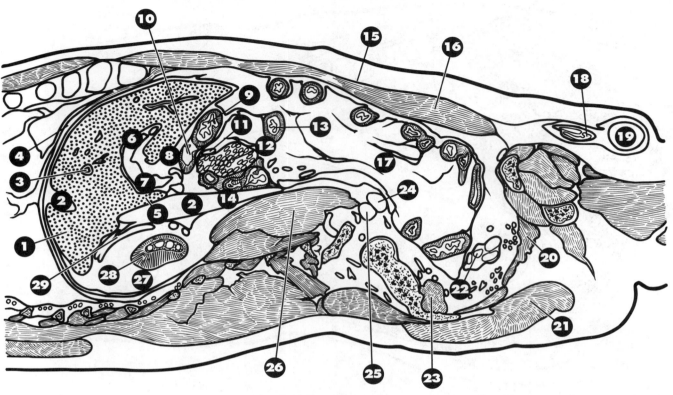

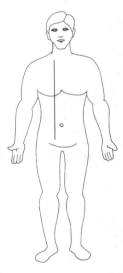

1	right lobe of the liver	16	rectus abdominis muscle
2	inferior vena cava	17	mesenteric fat
3	hepatic vein	18	spermatic cord
4	diaphragm	19	testis
5	caudate lobe of the liver	20	levator ani muscle
6	left portal vein	21	gluteus maximus muscle
7	hepatic artery	22	seminal vesicles
8	cystic duct	23	piriformis muscle
9	pylorus	24	right common iliac artery
10	descending part of the duodenum	25	right common iliac vein
11	gastroduodenal artery	26	psoas major muscle
12	head of the pancreas	27	perirenal fat
13	transverse colon	28	right kidney
14	superior part of the duodenum	29	right suprarenal gland
15	anterior rectus sheath		

FIGURE 1-22
Abdominal Sagittal Section, Level 7

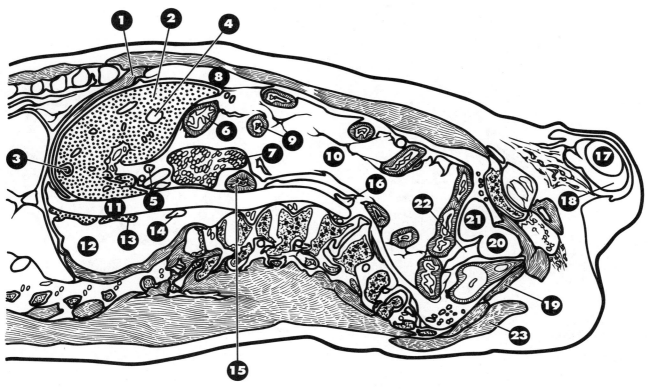

1 diaphragm	**13** right suprarenal gland
2 left lobe of the liver	**14** right renal artery
3 hepatic vein	**15** horizontal part of the duodenum
4 portal vein	**16** right common iliac artery
5 hepatic artery	**17** testis
6 pyloric antrum	**18** scrotum
7 head of the pancreas	**19** levator ani muscle
8 falciform ligament	**20** prostate
9 transverse colon	**21** bladder
10 mesenteric fat	**22** seminal vesicles
11 inferior vena cava	**23** gluteus maximus muscle
12 perirenal fat	

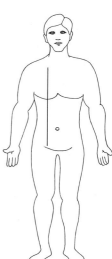

FIGURE 1-23

Abdominal Sagittal Section, Level 8

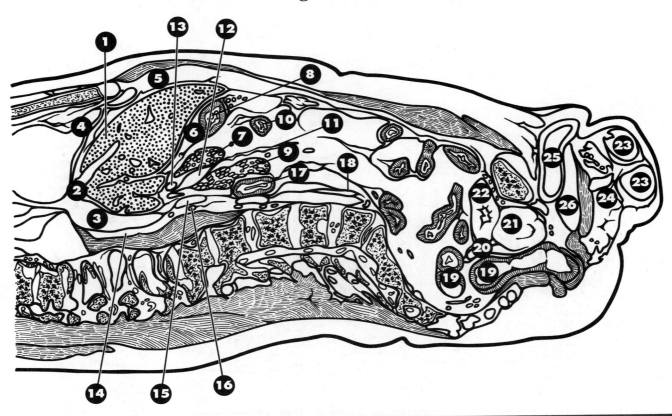

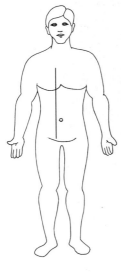

1 left lobe of the liver	15 left renal vein
2 hepatic vein	16 right renal artery
3 inferior vena cava	17 horizontal part of the duodenum
4 diaphragm	
5 falciform ligament	18 right common iliac artery
6 lesser omentum	19 rectum
7 pancreas	20 seminal vesicles
8 pyloric antrum	21 prostate
9 uncinate process of the pancreas	22 bladder
10 transverse colon	23 testis
11 superior mesenteric vein	24 scrotum
12 portal vein	25 corpus cavernosum penis
13 hepatic artery	26 corpus spongiosum penis
14 crus of the diaphragm	

FIGURE 1-24
Abdominal Sagittal Section, Level 9

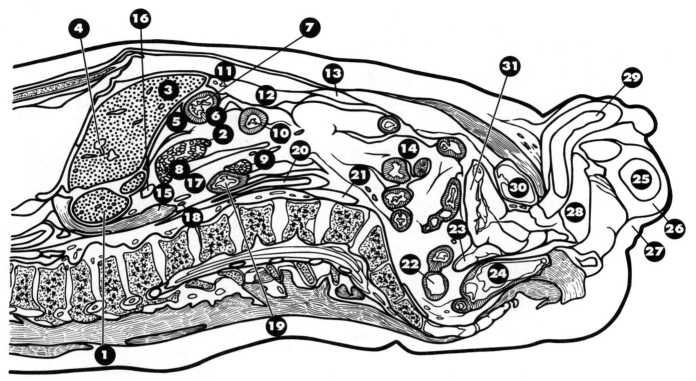

#		#	
1	caudate lobe of the liver	16	hepatic artery
2	body of the pancreas	17	left renal vein
3	left lobe of the liver	18	right renal artery
4	portal vein	19	horizontal part of the duodenum
5	lesser omentum	20	aorta
6	lesser sac	21	left common iliac vein
7	pyloric antrum	22	rectum
8	superior mesenteric vein	23	seminal vesicles
9	uncinate process of the pancreas	24	rectum
		25	testis
10	transverse colon	26	epididymis
11	falciform ligament	27	scrotum
12	greater omentum	28	corpus spongiosum penis
13	linea alba	29	corpus cavernosum penis
14	mesenteric fat	30	symphysis pubis
15	crus of the diaphragm	31	bladder

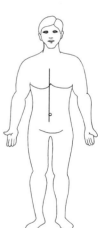

FIGURE 1-25

Abdominal Sagittal Section, Level 10

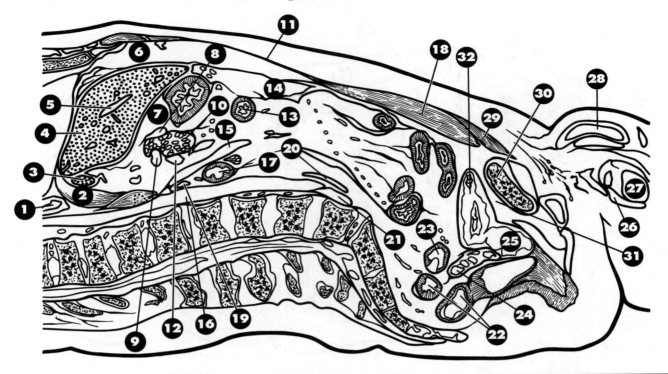

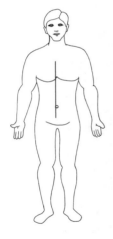

1	esophagus	17	horizontal part of the duodenum
2	crus of the diaphragm	18	rectus abdominis muscle
3	caudate lobe of the liver	19	left renal vein
4	left lobe of the liver	20	inferior mesenteric artery
5	portal vein	21	left common iliac vein
6	falciform ligament	22	rectum
7	lesser omentum	23	sigmoid colon
8	lesser sac	24	seminal vesicles
9	splenic artery	25	prostate
10	pancreas	26	head of the epididymis
11	linea alba	27	testis
12	splenic vein	28	corpus cavernosum penis
13	transverse colon	29	pyramidalis muscle
14	greater omentum	30	symphysis pubis
15	superior mesenteric artery	31	retropubic space
16	aorta	32	bladder

FIGURE 1-26
Abdominal Sagittal Section, Level 11

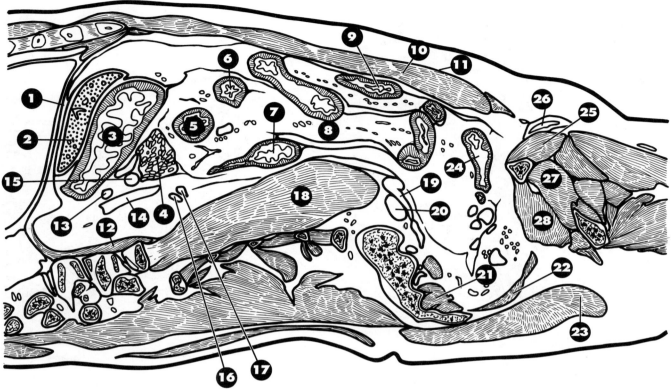

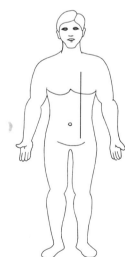

1	diaphragm	15	splenic vein
2	left lobe of the liver	16	left renal artery
3	body of the stomach	17	left renal vein
4	pancreas	18	psoas major muscle
5	ascending part of the duodenum	19	left common iliac artery
6	transverse colon	20	left common iliac vein
7	jejunum	21	piriformis muscle
8	mesentery	22	levator ani muscle
9	small bowel	23	gluteus maximus muscle
10	rectus abdominis muscle	24	sigmoid colon
11	rectus sheath	25	pectineus muscle
12	crus of the diaphragm	26	spermatic cord
13	splenic artery	27	obturator externus muscle
14	left suprarenal gland	28	obturator internus muscle

FIGURE 1-27
Abdominal Sagittal Section, Level 12

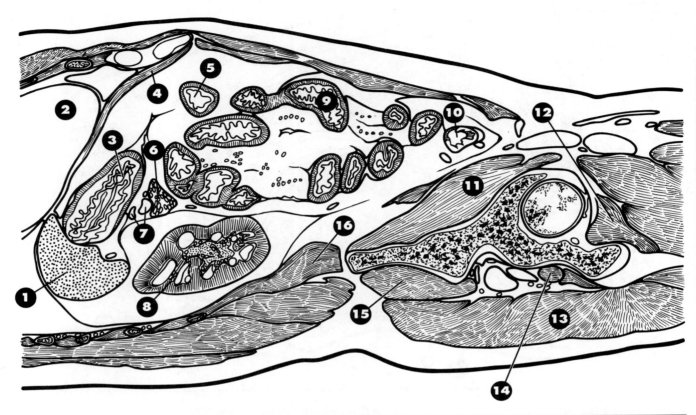

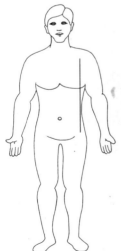

1	spleen	9	small bowel
2	heart	10	sigmoid colon
3	fundus of the stomach	11	iliacus muscle
4	diaphragm	12	obturator externus muscle
5	transverse colon	13	gluteus maximus muscle
6	pancreas	14	obturator internus muscle
7	splenic artery and vein	15	gluteus medius muscle
8	left kidney	16	quadratus lumborum muscle

Abdominal Review Notes

Abdominal Regions

- The abdomen is commonly divided into nine regions by two vertical and two horizontal lines.
- Each vertical line passes through the midinguinal point, which is the point that lies on the inguinal ligament halfway between the pubic symphysis and anterior superior iliac spine.
- The upper horizontal line, referred to as the *subcostal plane,* joins the lowest point of the costal margin on each side of the body.
- The lowest horizontal line, the intertubercular plane, joins the tubercles on the iliac crests.
- The nine abdominal regions are the upper abdomen—right hypochondrium, epigastrium, and left hypochondrium; middle abdomen—right lumbar, umbilical, and left lumbar; and lower abdomen—right iliac fossa, hypogastrium, and left iliac fossa.

Transpyloric Plane

- The transpyloric plane is horizontal and passes through the pylorus, duodenal junction, neck of the pancreas, and hilum of the kidneys.

Abdominal Viscera

- Variations in abdominal viscera occur among patients, from a change in position, or from a change in respiration.

Liver

- The liver lies under the lower ribs, with most of its structure in the right hypochrondrium and epigastrium.

Gallbladder

- The fundus of the gallbladder lies opposite the tip of the right ninth costal cartilage.

Spleen

- The spleen lies in the left hypochondrium under cover of the ninth, tenth, and eleventh ribs.
- The long axis of the spleen corresponds to the tenth rib and in adults, usually does not project forward of the midaxillary line.

Pancreas

- The pancreas lies across the transpyloric plane.
- The head lies below and to the right, the neck lies on the plane, and the body and tail lie above and to the left.

Kidneys

- The right kidney lies slightly lower than the left.
- Each kidney moves about 1 inch vertically during full respiratory movement of the diaphragm.

- The hilus of the kidney lies on the transpyloric plane, about a three-finger width from the midline.

Aorta and Inferior Vena Cava

- The aorta lies in the midline, slightly to the left of the abdomen, and bifurcates into the right and left common iliac arteries opposite the fourth lumbar vertebra on the intercristal plane.
- The inferior vena cava lies in the midline, slightly to the right of the abdomen, and bifurcates into the right and left common iliac veins.

Bladder and Uterus

- The bladder and uterus lie in the lower pelvis in the hypogastric plane.

The Abdominal Wall

- Superiorly, the abdominal wall is formed by the diaphragm.
- Inferiorly, the wall is continuous with the pelvic cavity through the pelvic inlet.
- Anteriorly, the wall is formed above by the lower part of the thoracic cage and below by several muscle layers.

Abdominus Muscles

- Posteriorly, the abdominal wall is formed in the midline by five lumbar vertebrae and their disks and laterally by the twelfth ribs, upper part of the bony pelvis, psoas muscles, quadratus lumborum muscles, and aponeuroses of origin of the transversus abdominis muscles.
- Laterally, the wall is formed above by the lower part of the thoracic wall, including the lungs and pleura, and below by the external and internal oblique muscles and transversus abdominis muscles.

Peritoneal Cavity

- The peritoneal cavity may be divided into two parts, the greater and lesser sacs.
- The greater sac, the primary compartment of the peritoneal cavity, extends across the anterior abdomen and from the diaphragm to the pelvis.
- The lesser sac is the smaller compartment and lies posterior to the stomach.
- The lesser sac is a diverticulum from the greater sac as it opens through a small opening, the epiploic foramen.

Mesentery

- A mesentery is a two-layered fold of peritoneum that attaches part of the intestines to the posterior abdominal wall and includes the mesentery of the small intestine, the transverse mesocolon, and the sigmoid mesocolon.

Omentum

- The omentum is a two-layered fold of peritoneum that attaches the stomach to another viscus organ.
- The greater omentum is attached to the greater curvature of the stomach and hangs down like an apron in the space between the small intestine and anterior abdominal wall.
- The greater omentum is folded back on itself and is attached to the inferior border of the transverse colon.
- The lesser omentum slings the lesser curvature of the stomach to the undersurface of the liver.
- The gastrosplenic omentum ligament connects the stomach to the spleen.

Ligament

- The peritoneal ligaments are two-layered folds of peritoneum that attach the lesser mobile solid viscera to the abdominal walls.
- For example, the liver is attached by the falciform ligament to the anterior abdominal wall and to the undersurface of the diaphragm.
- The ligamentum teres lies in the free borders of this ligament.
- The peritoneum leaves the kidney and passes to the hilus of the spleen as the posterior layer of the lienorenal ligament.
- The visceral peritoneum covers the spleen and is reflected onto the greater curvature of the stomach as the anterior layer of the gastrosplenic ligament.

Peritoneal Fossae

Lesser Sac

- The lesser sac is an extensive peritoneal pouch located behind the lesser omentum and stomach.
- This sac extends upward to the diaphragm and lies inferior between the layers of the greater omentum.
- The left margin is formed by the spleen and gastrosplenic and lienorenal ligaments.
- The right margin of the lesser sac opens into the greater sac through the epiploic foramen.
- The epiploic foramen is bounded anteriorly by the free border of the lesser omentum containing the common bile duct, hepatic artery, and portal vein; posteriorly by the inferior vena cava; superiorly by the caudate process of the caudate lobe of the liver; and inferiorly by the first part of the duodenum.

Subphrenic Spaces

- The subphrenic spaces result from the complicated arrangement of the peritoneum in the region of the liver.
- The right and left anterior subphrenic spaces lie between the diaphragm and the liver, one on each side of the falciform ligament.

- The right posterior subphrenic space lies among the right lobe of the liver, right kidney, and right colic flexure. This is also called *Morison's pouch.*

Paracolic Gutters

- The arrangement of the ascending and descending colon, the attachments of the transverse mesocolon, and the mesentery of the small intestine to the posterior abdominal wall results in the formation of four paracolic gutters.
- The clinical significance of these gutters is their ability to conduct fluid materials from one part of the body to another.
- Materials such as abscesses, ascites, blood, pus, bile, and metastases may be spread through this network.
- The gutters lie on the lateral and medial sides of the ascending and descending colon.
- The right medial paracolic gutter is closed from the pelvic cavity inferiorly by the mesentery of the small intestine.
- The other gutters are in free communication with the pelvic cavity.
- The right lateral paracolic gutter is in communication with the right posterior subphrenic space.
- The left lateral gutter is separated from the area around the spleen by the phrenocolic ligament.

Inguinal Canal

- The inguinal canal is an oblique passage through the lower part of the anterior abdominal wall.
- In males the inguinal canal allows structures to pass to and from the testes to the abdomen.
- In females the inguinal canal permits the passage of the round ligament of the uterus from the uterus to the labium majus.

Abdominal Herniae

- A hernia is the protrusion of part of the abdominal contents beyond the normal confines of the abdominal wall.
- A hernia has three parts: the sac, the contents of the sac, and the coverings of the sac.
- The hernial sac is a diverticulum of the peritoneum and has a neck and a body.
- The hernial contents may consist of any structure found within the abdominal cavity and may vary from a small piece of omentum to a large viscus organ.
- The hernial coverings are formed from the layers of the abdominal wall through which the hernial sac passes.
- Abdominal herniae are one of the following types: inguinal, femoral, umbilical, epigastric, or abdominis rectus.

Pelvis

False Pelvis

- The false pelvis is bounded posteriorly by the lumbar vertebrae, laterally by the iliac fossae and iliacus muscles, and anteriorly by the lower anterior abdominal wall.

True Pelvis

- The true pelvis protects and contains the lower parts of the intestinal and urinary tracts and the reproductive organs.
- The true pelvis has an inlet, an outlet, and a cavity.
- The walls of the pelvis are formed by bones and ligaments that are partly lined with muscles covered with fascia and parietal peritoneum.
- The true pelvis has anterior, posterior, and lateral walls and an inferior floor.
- The piriformis muscles form the posterior pelvic wall.
- The obturator internus muscle lines the lateral pelvic wall.
- The pelvic floor stretches across the pelvis and divides it into the main pelvic cavity, which contains the pelvic viscera, and the perineum below.
- The pelvic diaphragm is formed by the levatores ani muscles and coccygeus muscles.

Recommended Terminology for Ultrasound by the American Institute of Ultrasound in Medicine

A mode A method of echo signal display in which time is represented along one axis, and the echo amplitude is displayed along a perpendicular axis

acoustic attenuation the reduction of intensity of an acoustic signal as it propagates through a material

acoustic enhancement a manifestation of increased acoustic signal amplitude returning from regions lying beyond an object that causes little or no attenuation of the sound beam

acoustic impedance the resistance that a material offers to the passage of a sound wave

aliasing the introduction of artifactual frequency components as a result of sampling a signal at a rate that is lower than twice the highest frequency component in that signal

amplitude the strength or height of the wave measured in decibels

anechoic the property of appearing echo free (without echoes) on a sonographic image

artifact an echo feature present or absent in a sonogram that does not correspond to the presence or absence of a real target

attenuation the decrease in intensity as sound travels through a material resulting from three factors: absorption, scattering, and beam divergence

B mode a method of image display in which the amplitude of the echo signal is represented by modulation of the brightness of the corresponding image point

B scan scanning with B mode display

color flow Doppler the two-dimensional presentation of Doppler shift information superimposed on a real-time, gray-scale anatomic cross-sectional image; flow directions toward and away from the transducer are presented as different colors on the display

complex structure in the body that contains a few echoes (solid) and also has cystic properties

continuous-wave ultrasound a wave of constant or nearly constant amplitude that persists for a large number of cycles

cycle the number of times the wave is repeated per second as measured in hertz (Hz)

cystic any fluid-filled structure in the body

decibel a unit representing a ratio used to express how much larger or smaller a quantity is with respect to a reference quantity

Doppler frequency shift the difference between the frequencies of transmitted and received waves, which is proportional to the velocity of relative motion between the transducer and reflector

duplex scanner an ultrasound instrument that has real-time imaging capability and Doppler capability, with either the imaging transducer or a separate transducer used to collect continuous-wave or pulsed Doppler signals, either simultaneously with imaging or sequentially

echogenic a structure or medium that is capable of producing echoes

frequency the number of cycles of a periodic process per unit of time, usually expressed in hertz or multiples such as megahertz (MHz)

heterogeneous a structure that has an uneven texture (hypoechoic and hyperechoic echoes throughout)

homogeneous a structure that has a smooth, uniform composition

hyperechoic a region in a sonographic image where the echoes are brighter than normal or brighter than surrounding structures

hypoechoic a region in a sonographic image where the echoes are not as bright as normal or are less bright than surrounding structures

megahertz one million cycles per second

M mode a method of display in which tissue interface position is displayed along one axis, and time is displayed along the second axis

real-time the scanning and display of ultrasonic images at a sufficiently rapid rate so that moving structures can be "seen" to move at their natural rate; frame rates of 15 frames per second or greater are considered real-time

shadowing a reduction in echo amplitudes distal to a strongly attenuating or reflecting structure

solid a structure in the body that produces echoes

sonolucent the result of an unattenuated sound traveling through a fluid-filled structure

speckle the granular appearance of an ultrasound image resulting from the coherent addition (i.e., constructive and destructive interference) of detected echo signals arising from randomly distributed scatterers within a sample volume

texture the speckle pattern arising from an area of interest in the body, which depends primarily on the transducer frequency and beam characteristics and secondarily on the structure of the scattering tissues

transducer a device capable of converting energy from one form to another

transducer array a group of transducers working together to form a functional unit; arrays may be of several types depending on the transducer configuration: linear, annular, rectangular, and so on

ultrasound sound at frequencies above the range of human hearing (conventionally, above 20 kilohertz [kHz])

Artifact Terminology

acoustic shadow the sonographic appearance of reduced echo amplitude from regions lying beyond an attenuating object

artifact an echo feature present or absent in a sonogram that does not correspond to the presence or absence of a real target

backscatter sound that is scattered by small reflecting objects in all directions; that part of the scattered sound traveling back to the source transducer

comet tail a reverberation type of sonographic artifact that appears as a dense tapering trail of echoes just distal to strongly reflecting structures

grating artifacts a curvilinear artifact often seen in front of or behind a strong interface with linear array transducers

lateral beam spread the widening of the transducer focus as the beam passes through tissue depth

main bang a high-level echo at the skin's surface resulting partly from the skin and partly from the transducer surface

mirror image a multiple path reflection artifact in which the sonographic image of a structure is duplicated in a different location and appears as a mirror image of the original

noise spurious echoes throughout the image, including areas such as the bladder, that are known to be echo-free

reververation artifactual linear echoes parallel to a strong interface; sound is returned to the transducer and then into the tissues repeatedly

ring down a particular type of reverberation artifact in which numerous parallel echoes are seen for a considerable distance

side lobes secondary off-axis concentrations of energy not parallel to the beam axis; degrades lateral resolution

Review Exercise A • Abdominal Cavity

Adult derivatives of fetal vessels and structures:

1. The intraabdominal portion of the umbilical vein forms the _____ . This structure passes

from the umbilicus to the _____ , where it attaches to the left branch of the portal vein.

2. The _____ becomes the ligamentum venosum. This structure passes through the liver from

the _____ to the _____ .

3. Name the surface landmarks of the anterior abdominal wall
   seen in Figure 1-28.

   1.

   2.

   3.

   4.

   5.

   6.

   7.

4. Name the regions of the abdominal cavity seen in Figure 1-29.

   1.

   2.

   3.

   4.

   5.

   6.

   7.

   8.

   9.

5. The _____ is a thin, translucent, serous membrane that lines the walls of the abdominal cavity and covers the abdominal viscera. It has two layers: _____ and

   _____ .

6. The _____ lines the walls of the abdominal cavity.

7. The _____ covers the abdominal organs.

8. The abdominal cavity may be divided into two parts: _____ and

   _____ .

9. The _____ lies posterior to the stomach; it opens through a window called the *epiploic foramen.*

10. The greater omentum is often referred to as the _____ hanging between the small intestine and the _____ .

11. The lesser omentum attaches the lesser curvature of the stomach to the under surface of the

    _____ .

12. Match the following ligaments:

    a. falciform

    b. ligamentum teres

    c. lienorenal

    d. gastrosplenic

    _____ Passes from the hilus of the spleen to the greater curvature of the stomach

    _____ Attaches the liver to the abdominal wall and the diaphragm

    _____ Peritoneal layer from the kidney to the hilum of the spleen

    _____ Obliterated umbilical fetal vein

13. Name the abdominal cavity structures seen in Figure 1-30.

    1.

    2.

    3.

    4.

    5.

    6.

    7.

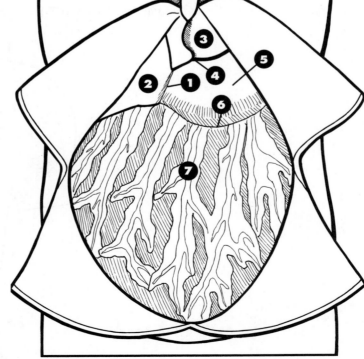

14. The lesser omentum has a free border on the right where it folds around the _____ , _____ , and _____ .

15. This free border forms the anterior margin of the opening into the _____ .

Review Exercise B • Abdominal Anatomy

1. Name the abdominal regions of the body. _____
_____
_____
_____
_____

2. What is the transpyloric plane? _____
_____

3. Describe the location of the liver. _____
_____

4. What is the location of the gallbladder? _____
_____

5. Describe the location of the spleen. _____
_____
_____

6. What is the location of the pancreas? _____
_____

7. Describe the location of the kidneys. _____
_____
_____

8. Describe the location of the great vessels. _____
_____
_____

9. Name the components of the abdominal wall and their locations. _____
_____
_____

10. Name the two parts into which the peritoneal cavity is divided. _____
_____
_____

11. Describe the function of the mesentery. _____
_____
_____
_____

12. What is the purpose of the omentum? _____

_____

_____

_____

13. What are the peritoneal ligaments and to what are they attached? _____

_____

_____

_____

14. Describe the location and purpose of the lesser sac. _____

_____

_____

_____

_____

15. Describe the boundaries of the epiploic foramen. _____

_____

_____

_____

_____

16. What forms the subphrenic spaces? _____

_____

_____

_____

17. Describe the paracolic gutters and their function. _____

_____

_____

_____

18. What is the inguinal canal? _____

_____

19. What are the boundaries of the false pelvis? _____

_____

_____

_____

20. What are the boundaries of the true pelvis? _____

_____

_____

_____

21. Name the muscles of the posterior and lateral pelvic wall. _____

_____

_____

_____

Review Exercise C • Ultrasound Terminology Quiz

Fill in the blanks using the terms from the list below.

cystic	hyperechoic	megahertz
solid	hypoechoic	transducer
complex	shadowing	A mode
homogeneous	sonolucent	B mode
heterogeneous	texture	real-time
echogenic	amplitude	Doppler
anechoic	attenuation	color
fluid-fluid level	cycle	curved-linear transducer
echolucent	decibel	phased array
enhancement	frequency	transvaginal transducer

1. _____ ultrasound term for a structure that produces echoes

2. _____ interface between two fluids with different acoustic characteristics

3. _____ without internal echoes; not necessarily cystic

4. _____ result of attenuated sound traveling through a fluid-filled structure

5. _____ any fluid-filled structure in the body

6. _____ of uniform composition

7. _____ structure that produces echoes

8. _____ a few echoes within a structure; less echogenic

9. _____ failure of the sound beam to pass through an object

10. _____ a mass or organ that contains uniform low-level echoes because the cellular tissues are acoustically very similar

11. _____ a mixture of cystic and solid components

12. _____ without echoes

13. _____ the echo pattern within an organ such as the liver or kidney

14. _____ a one-dimensional image displaying the amplitude strength of the returning echo signals along the vertical axis and the time (the distance from the transducer) along the horizontal axis

15. _____ a method of displaying the intensity (amplitude) of an echo by varying the brightness of a dot to correspond to the echo strength

16. _____ electronically steered system in which many small transducers are electronically coordinated to produce a focus wave front

17. _____ type of imaging in which the image is created so many times per second that a cinematic view of the tissues is obtained

18. _____ strength or height of the wave measured in decibels

19. _____ per second frequency at which the crystal vibrates

20. _____ a unit used to express the intensity of amplitude of sound waves; does not specify voltage

21. _____ number of times the wave is repeated per second as measured in hertz

22. _____ refers to the absorption and reflection of the sound beam

Self-Test • Basic Abdominal Anatomy

1. Which statement is *not* correct?

   a. The umbilical vein may remain patent for some time after birth.

   b. The ductus venosus becomes the ligamentum venosum.

   c. The abdominal portions of the umbilical arteries form the lateral umbilical ligaments.

   d. The foramen ovale usually opens shortly after birth.

2. The abdominal regions of the upper abdomen include all but the:

   a. umbilical

   b. right hypochondrium

   c. epigastrium

   d. left hypochondrium

3. What structure is a thin, translucent serous membrane that lines the walls of the abdominal cavity and covers the abdominal viscera?

   a. the mesentery

   b. the peritoneum

   c. the omentum

   d. the epiploic foramen

4. This structure is referred as the "apron":

   a. the greater omentum

   b. the peritoneum

   c. the mesentery

   d. the visceral peritoneum

5. What ligament attaches the liver to the abdominal wall and the diaphragm?

   a. the median umbilical ligament

   b. the lateral umbilical ligament

   c. the lienorenal ligament

   d. the falciform ligament

6. What is the obliterated umbilical fetal vein?

   a. the ligamentum teres

   b. the falciform ligament

   c. the gastrosplenic ligament

   d. the umbilical ligament

7. What forms the anterior layer of the lesser omentum?

   a. the pancreas

   b. the lesser curvature of stomach

   c. the greater curvature of stomach

   d. the spleen

8. The _____ peritoneum along the anterior abdominal wall may be traced from the falciform ligament to the diaphragm.

   a. visceral

   b. parietal

   c. falciformis

   d. omental

9. In females the peritoneum reflects onto the posterior vagina to form the:

   a. rectovesical pouch

   b. posterovesical pouch

   c. rectovaginal pouch

   d. rectouterine pouch

10. Another name for the answer in question #9 is:

    a. Morison's pouch

    b. Levethal's pouch

    c. Douglas' pouch

    d. Randall's pouch

11. Most of the digestion and absorption of food takes place in the duodenum (true or false).

12. The inferior and posterior surfaces of the liver are *not* marked by the fossae of the:

    a. porta hepatis

    b. gallbladder

    c. caudate

    d. inferior vena cava

13. The portal veins carry blood from the _____ to the liver.

    a. duodenum

    b. bowel

    c. splenic artery

    d. peripheral venous system

14. The quadrate lobe is part of the lateral segment of the left lobe (true or false).

15. The right functional lobe includes everything to the right of a plane through the:

    a. falciform ligament

    b. ligamentum teres

    c. gallbladder fossa, IVC

    d. caudate lobe

16. The _____ area of the liver is where the peritoneal reflections from the liver onto the diaphragm leave an irregular triangle of liver without peritoneal covering.

a. visceral

b. bare

c. hepato

d. diaphragmatic

17. The area bounded by the liver, kidney, colon, and duodenum is:

a. Douglas' pouch

b. Morison's pouch

c. hepatocolonic

d. hepatoadrenal

18. What ligaments divide the medial segment of the left lobe?

a. the ductus arteriosus and venosus

b. the falciform ligament, ligamentum teres

c. the ligamentum venosum, ligamentum teres

d. the inferior ligament, medial ligament

19. After the age of 60 years, the common bile duct increases _____ each decade.

a. 0.5 mm

b. 1 mm

c. 1.5 mm

d. 2 mm

20. The proximal portion of the CBD is medial to the hepatic artery (true or false).

21. The portal triad is composed of:

a. right and left portal veins, CBD

b. right and left hepatic ducts, portal vein

c. portal vein, CBD, hepatic artery

d. right and left hepatic artery, CBD

22. The arterial supply to the gallbladder is via the:

a. hepatic artery

b. superior mesenteric artery

c. cystic artery

d. gastroduodenal artery

23. The portal vein does not drain blood:

a. out of the gastrointestinal tract from the lower end of the esophagus to the upper end of the anal canal

b. from the pancreas, gallbladder, and bile ducts

c. from the spleen

d. from the kidneys

24. The head of the pancreas, the duodenum, and parts of the stomach are supplied by the:

    a. hepatic artery

    b. gastroduodenal artery

    c. splenic artery

    d. superior mesenteric artery

25. The _____ runs posterior to the neck of the pancreas.

    a. superior mesenteric artery

    b. splenic artery

    c. hepatic artery

    d. gastroduodenal artery

26. What vessel passes anterior to the uncinate process of the pancreas?

    a. the hepatic artery

    b. the portal vein

    c. the left renal vein

    d. the superior mesenteric vein

27. The right renal artery passes anterior to the IVC and vertebral column (true or false).

28. The left renal artery passes posterior to the aorta (true or false).

29. The uncinate process is posterior to the superior mesenteric vessels (true or false).

30. The _____ is the anterolateral border of the pancreas.

    a. common bile duct

    b. gastroduodenal artery

    c. cystic artery

    d. pancreaticoduodenal artery

31. The spleen is considered a retroperitoneal structure (true or false).

32. The retroperitoneal space is the area between the posterior portion of the parietal peritoneum and the posterior abdominal wall muscles (true or false).

33. The retroperitoneal space is subdivided into three spaces. Which is the incorrect space?

    a. the perinephris space (fascia of Gerota)

    b. the external paranephric space

    c. the anterior paranephric space

    d. the posterior paranephric space

34. The kidney is surrounded by a fibrous capsule called the *true capsule,* which is closely applied to the renal cortex (true or false).

35. Outside this capsule is a covering of:

    a. peritoneum

    b. peranephric fat

    c. retroperitoneal fascia

    d. paranephric fascia

36. In the portion of the kidney between the cortex and medulla, these arteries are called:

    a. interlobar

    b. pyramidal

    c. renal

    d. arcuate

Answers to Review Exercise A

1. ligamentum teres; porta hepatis
2. ductus venosus; left branch of the PV; IVC
3. (Figure 1-28)
   1. xyphoid process
   2. median groove
   3. tubercle crest
   4. right lateral plane
   5. transpyloric plane subcostal
   6. subcostal plane
   7. linea semilunaris
4. (Figure1-29)
   1. right hypochrondrium
   2. epigastrium
   3. left hypocondrium
   4. right lumbar region
   5. umbilical region
   6. left lumbar region
   7. right iliac fossa
   8. hypogastrium
   9. left iliac fossa

5. peritoneum; parietal; visceral
6. peritoneum
7. viscera
8. lesser sac; greater sac
9. lesser sac
10. apron; anterior abdominal wall
11. liver
12. d; a; c; b
13. (Figure 1-30)
    1. falciform ligament
    2. right lobe of the liver
    3. left lower lobe of the liver
    4. ligamentum teres
    5. stomach
    6. greater curvature of the stomach
    7. greater omentum
14. CBO; HA; PV
15. lesser sac

Answers to Review Exercise B

1. The nine abdominal regions are the upper abdomen—right hypochondrium, epigastrium, and left hypochondrium; middle abdomen—right lumbar, umbilical, and left lumbar; and lower abdomen—right iliac fossa, hypogastrium, and left iliac fossa.
2. The transpyloric plane is horizontal and passes through the pylorus, duodenal junction, neck of the pancreas, and hilum of the kidneys.
3. The liver lies under the lower ribs, with most of its structure in the right hypochrondrium and epigastrium.
4. The fundus of the gallbladder lies opposite the tip of the right ninth costal cartilage.
5. The spleen lies in the left hypochondrium under cover of the ninth, tenth, and eleventh ribs. Its long axis corresponds to the tenth rib, and in adults it usually does not project forward of the midaxillary line.
6. The pancreas lies across the transpyloric plane. The head lies below and to the right, the neck lies on the plane, and the body and tail lie above and to the left.
7. The right kidney lies slightly lower than the left. Each kidney moves about 1 inch vertically during full respiratory movement of the diaphragm. The hilus of the kidney lies on the transpyloric plane, about a 3-finger width from the midline.
8. The aorta and inferior vena cava are the great vessels. The aorta lies in the midline, slightly to the left of the abdomen, and bifurcates into the right and left common iliac arteries opposite the fourth lumbar vertebra on the intercristal plane. The inferior vena cava lies in the midline, slightly to the right of the abdomen, and bifurcates into the right and left common iliac veins.
9. Superiorly, the abdominal wall is formed by the diaphragm. Inferiorly, it is continuous with the pelvic cavity through the pelvic inlet. Anteriorly, the wall is formed above by the lower part of the thoracic cage and below by several muscle layers. Posteriorly, the abdominal wall is formed in the midline by five lumbar vertebrae and their disks and laterally by the twelfth ribs, upper part of the bony pelvis, psoas muscles, quadratus lumborum muscles, and aponeuroses of origin of the transversus abdominis muscles. Laterally, the wall is formed above by the lower part of the thoracic wall, including the lungs and pleura, and below by the external and internal oblique muscles and transversus abdominis muscles.
10. The peritoneal cavity may be divided into two parts, the greater and lesser sacs. The greater sac, the primary compartment of the peritoneal cavity, extends across the anterior abdomen and from the diaphragm to the pelvis. The lesser sac is the smaller compartment and lies posterior to the stomach. The lesser sac is a diverticulum from the greater sac as it opens through a small opening, the epiploic foramen.

11. The mesentery is a two-layered fold of peritoneum that attaches part of the intestines to the posterior abdominal wall and includes the mesentery of the small intestine, the transverse mesocolon, and the sigmoid mesocolon.

12. The omentum is a two-layered fold of peritoneum that attaches the stomach to another viscus organ. The greater omentum is attached to the greater curvature of the stomach and hangs down like an apron in the space between the small intestine and anterior abdominal wall. The greater omentum is folded back on itself and is attached to the inferior border of the transverse colon. The lesser omentum slings the lesser curvature of the stomach to the undersurface of the liver. The gastrosplenic omentum ligament connects the stomach to the spleen.

13. The peritoneal ligaments are two-layered folds of peritoneum that attach the lesser mobile solid viscera to the abdominal walls. For example, the liver is attached by the falciform ligament to the anterior abdominal wall and to the undersurface of the diaphragm. The ligamentum teres lies in the free borders of this ligament. The peritoneum leaves the kidney and passes to the hilus of the spleen as the posterior layer of the lienorenal ligament. The visceral peritoneum covers the spleen and is reflected onto the greater curvature of the stomach as the anterior layer of the gastrosplenic ligament.

14. The lesser sac is an extensive peritoneal pouch located behind the lesser omentum and stomach. It extends upward to the diaphragm and lies inferior between the layers of the greater omentum. The left margin is formed by the spleen and gastrosplenic and lienorenal ligaments. The right margin of the lesser sac opens into the greater sac through the epiploic foramen.

15. The epiploic foramen is bounded anteriorly by the free border of the lesser omentum containing the common bile duct, hepatic artery, and portal vein; posteriorly but the inferior vena cava; superiorly but the caudate process of the caudate lobe of the liver; and inferiorly by the first part of the duodenum.

16. The subphrenic spaces result from the complicated arrangement of the peritoneum in the region of the liver. The right and left anterior subphrenic spaces lie between the diaphragm and the liver, one on each side of the falciform ligament. The right posterior subphrenic space lies among the right lobe of the liver, right kidney, and right colic flexure. This is also called *Morison's pouch.*

17. The arrangement of the ascending and descending colon, the attachments of the transverse mesocolon, and the mesentery of the small intestine to the posterior abdominal wall results in the formation of four paracolic gutters. The clinical significance of these gutters is their ability to conduct fluid materials from one part of the body to another. Materials such as abscesses, ascites, blood, pus, bile, and metastases may be spread through this network. The gutters lie on the lateral and medial sides of the ascending and descending colon. The right medial paracolic gutter is closed from the pelvic cavity inferiorly by the mesentery of the small intestine. The other gutters are in free communication with the pelvic cavity. The right lateral paracolic gutter is in communication with the right posterior subphrenic space. The left lateral gutter is separated from the area around the spleen by the phrenicolic ligament.

18. The inguinal canal is an oblique passage through the lower part of the anterior abdominal wall. In males it allows structures to pass to and from the testes to the abdomen. In females it permits the passage of the round ligament of the uterus from the uterus to the labium majus.

19. The false pelvis is bounded posteriorly by the lumbar vertebrae, laterally by the iliac fossae and iliacus muscles, and anteriorly by the lower anterior abdominal wall.

20. The true pelvis protects and contains the lower parts of the intestinal and urinary tracts and the reproductive organs. The true pelvis has an inlet, an outlet, and a cavity.

21. The piriformis muscles form the posterior pelvic wall. The obturator internus muscle lines the lateral pelvic wall. The pelvic floor stretches across the pelvis and divides it into the main pelvic cavity, which contains the pelvic viscera, and the perineum below. The pelvic diaphragm is formed by the levatores ani muscles and coccygeus muscles.

Answers to Review Exercise C

1. echogenic
2. fluid-fluid level
3. echolucent
4. enhancement
5. cystic
6. homogeneous
7. hyperechoic
8. hypoechoic
9. shadowing

10. solid
11. complex
12. sonlucent
13. texture
14. A mode

15. B mode
16. phased array
17. real-time
18. amplitude

19. cycle
20. decibel
21. frequency
22. attenuation

Answers to Self-Test

1. d
2. a
3. b
4. a
5. d
6. a
7. b
8. b
9. d
10. c
11. false
12. a

13. b
14. c
15. c
16. b
17. b
18. b
19. b
20. false
21. c
22. c
23. d
24. b

25. a
26. d
27. false
28. false
29. false
30. b
31. false
32. true
33. b
34. true
35. b
36. d

2

The Muscular System

OBJECTIVES

At the completion of this chapter, students will show orally, in writing, or by demonstration that they will be able to:

1. Describe the types of muscle in the body.
2. Describe the anterior and posterior triangles of the neck.
3. Describe the anterior abdominal wall muscles and their relationships to one another.
4. Describe the abdominal muscles (external oblique, internal oblique, transversus, diaphragm, and back muscles).

5. Describe the true and false pelvis muscles.
6. Know the surface relationships of the perineum.
7. Know the cross-sectional muscular anatomy of the abdominal and pelvic cavity.
8. Know the sagittal muscular anatomy of the abdominal and pelvic cavity.

To further enhance learning, students should use marking pens to color the anatomic illustrations that follow.

MUSCULAR SYSTEM

FIGURE 2-1
Muscle Groups

Types of Muscles (FIGURE 2-1)

There are three types of muscles that can be identified by their structure, function, and location in the body: skeletal, smooth, and cardiac.

Skeletal Muscle

The skeletal muscles produce movements of the skeleton and are sometimes called voluntary muscles. Skeletal muscles are made up of striped muscle fibers and have two or more attachments. The ends of the muscles are attached to bones, cartilage, or ligaments by cords of tough fibrous tissue called *tendons*.

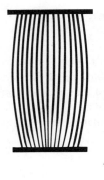

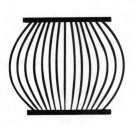

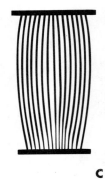

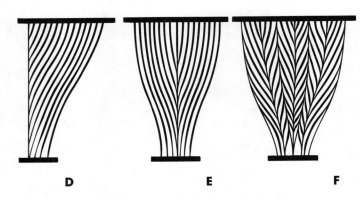

There are four basic forms of dense connective tissue: tendons, which attach muscle to bone; ligaments, which connect the bones that form joints; aponeuroses, which are thin, tendinous sheets attached to flat muscles; and fasciae, the thin sheets of tissue that cover muscles and hold them in place.

The individual fibers of a muscle are arranged either parallel or oblique to the long axis of the muscle. With contraction, the muscle shortens to one half or one third its resting length. Examples of such muscles are the rectus abdominis and the sternocleidomastoid.

Pennate muscles have fibers that run oblique to the line of pull, resembling a feather. A unipennate muscle is one in which the tendon lies along one side of the muscle and the muscle fibers pass oblique to it. A bipennate muscle has a tendon in the center, and the muscle fibers pass to it from two sides. The rectus femoris is a bipennate muscle. A multipennate muscle may have a series of bipennate muscles lying alongside one another (e.g., the deltoid), or it may have the tendon lying within its center and the fibers converging into it from all sides.

Smooth Muscle

Smooth muscle is composed of long, spindle-shaped cells closely arranged in bundles or sheets. Its action—propelling material through vessels or the gastrointestinal tract—is known as peristalsis. In storage organs such as the bladder and uterus, the fibers are arranged irregularly and interlaced with one another. In such organs, contraction is slower and more sustained to expel contents.

Cardiac Muscle

Cardiac muscle consists of striated fibers that branch and unite with one another. As its name indicates, it is found only in the myocardium of the heart and in the muscle layer of the base of the great blood vessels. Cardiac muscle fibers tend to be arranged in spirals and have the ability to contract spontaneously and rhythmically. Specialized cardiac muscle fibers form the conducting system of the heart.

A resting muscle

B contracted muscle

Various Forms of the Internal Structure of Skeletal Muscle

C parallel

D unipennate

E bipennate

F multipennate

FIGURE 2-2
Muscular System of the Neck

Muscles of the Neck
(FIGURE 2-2)

The neck is a very complex structure, with multiple muscle groups, vascular structures, and fascia interwoven throughout. Only the larger, more superficial muscle groups will be presented here; these will later serve as landmarks for internal structures, such as the thyroid, and vascular structures found within the neck.

Triangles of the Neck
The neck is divided into anterior and posterior triangles by the sternocleidomastoid muscle; the anterior triangle lies in front of the muscle, and the posterior triangle lies behind.

Anterior Triangle
The anterior triangle contains several important nerves and vessels and is bordered by the mandible above, the sternocleidomastoid muscle laterally, and the median plane of the neck.

Posterior Triangle
The posterior triangle is bounded anteriorly by the posterior border of the sternocleidomastoid, posteriorly by the anterior border of the trapezius, and inferiorly by the middle third of the clavicle. The muscles of this region arise from the skull, the cervical vertebrae, the head of the ribs (scalene), the scapula (omohyoid and levator scapulae), and the cervical and thoracic vertebral spines.

Suprahyoid Muscles
The suprahyoid muscle group consists of the stylohyoid, digastric, mylohyoid, and hypoglossus muscles. The suprahyoid muscles attach the hyoid bone to the floor of the tongue and the mandible. Vessels and nerves to the tongue are found in this region.

Hyoid Bone
The hyoid bone is suspended from the styloid processes of the skull by the stylohyoid ligaments and is stabilized by the suprahyoid and infrahyoid muscle groups.

Infrahyoid Muscles
The infrahyoid muscle group consists of the sternohyoid, omohyoid, thyrohyoid, and sternothyroid muscles. The infrahyoid muscles arise from the sternum, the thyroid cartilage of the larynx, or the scapula and insert on the hyoid bone. Many vessels and nerves traverse this area.

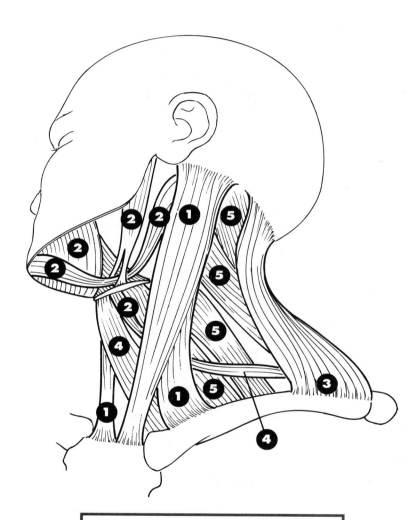

1	**sternocleidomastoid muscles**
2	**suprahyoid muscles***
3	**trapezius muscles**
4	**infrahyoid muscles***
5	**posterior triangle of the neck**

Anterior triangle of the neck

FIGURE 2-3
Posterior View of the Torso

Back Muscles of the Torso
(FIGURE 2-3)

The deep muscles of the back help to stabilize the vertebral column. They also have an influence on the posture and curvature of the spine. The muscles have the ability to extend, flex laterally, and rotate all or part of the vertebral column.

Actions of the Various Muscles

erector spinae extend and laterally flex the spine

gemellus superior and inferior lateral rotator of the thigh at the hip joint

gluteus maximus extends and laterally rotates the hip joint; through the iliotibial tract, it helps to maintain the knee joint in extension

gluteus medius acts with the gluteus minimus and the tensor fasciae latae to abduct the thigh at the hip joint (important in walking or running)

gluteus minimus helps to abduct the thigh at the hip joint; its anterior fibers medially rotate the thigh

infraspinatus laterally rotates the arm

latissimus dorsi extends, adducts, and medially rotates the arm

levator scapulae raises the medial border of the scapula

obturator internus lateral rotator of the thigh at the hip joint

piriformis lateral rotator of the thigh at the hip joint

quadratus femoris lateral rotator of the thigh at the hip joint

rhomboid with the rhomboid minor (and major) and the levator scapulae, elevates the medial border of the scapula and pulls it medially

serratus posterior inferior plays a minor role in pulling down the ribs in respiration

splenius capitis extends and rotates the head

supraspinatus assist the deltoid muscle in abducting the arm at the shoulder joint by fixing the head of the humerus against the glenoid cavity

teres major medially rotates and adducts the arm

trapezius the upper fibers elevate the scapula, the middle fibers pull the scapula medially, and the lower fibers pull the medial border of the scapula downward.

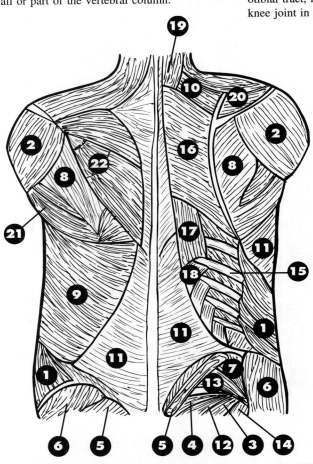

1	external oblique muscle	9	latissimus dorsi muscle	16	rhomboid muscle
2	deltoid muscle	10	levator scapulae muscle	17	erector spinae muscle
3	gemellus inferior muscle	11	lumbodorsal fascia	18	serratus posterior inferior muscle
4	gemellus superior muscle	12	obturator internus muscle	19	splenius capitis muscle
5	gluteus maximus muscle	13	piriformis muscle	20	supraspinatus muscle
6	gluteus medius muscle	14	quadratus femoris muscle	21	teres major muscle
7	gluteus minimus muscle	15	ribs (7-12)	22	trapezius muscle
8	infraspinatus muscle				

FIGURE 2-4
Anterior View of the Abdominal Muscles

Muscles of the Anterior and Lateral Abdominal Walls

The muscles of the anterior and lateral abdominal walls include the external oblique, the internal oblique, the transversus, the rectus abdominis, and the pyramidalis muscles (Figures 2-4 and 2-5).

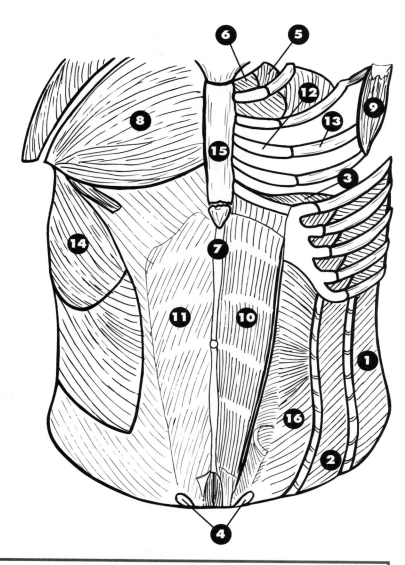

1	**external oblique muscle**	**9**	**pectoralis minor muscle**
2	**internal oblique muscle**	**10**	**rectus abdominis muscle**
3	**diaphragm**	**11**	**rectus sheath**
4	**external inguinal ring**	**12**	**costal cartilage**
5	**external intercostal muscle**	**13**	**rib**
6	**internal intercostal muscle**	**14**	**serratus anterior muscle**
7	**linea alba**	**15**	**sternum**
8	**pectoralis major muscle**	**16**	**transversus abdominis muscle**

FIGURE 2-5
Posterior View of the Abdominal Muscles

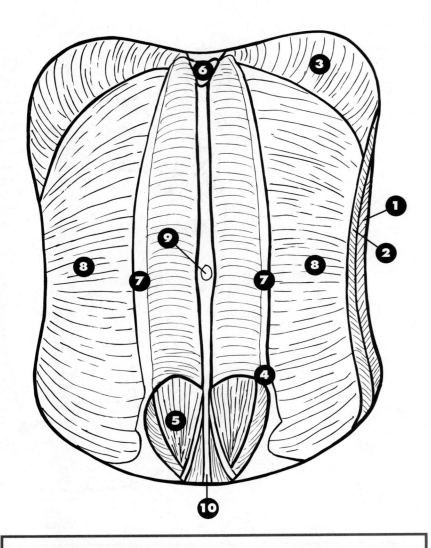

1	external oblique muscle	7	fascia transversalis
2	internal oblique muscle	8	transversus abdominis muscle
3	diaphragm		
4	linea semicircularis	9	umbilicus
5	rectus abdominis muscle	10	umbilical ligaments
6	sternum		

FIGURE 2-6
External Oblique Muscle of the Anterior and Lateral Abdominal Walls

External Oblique

The external oblique muscle arises from the lower eight ribs and fans out to be inserted into the xyphoid process, the linea alba, the pubic crest, the pubic tubercle, and the anterior half of the iliac crest (Figure 2-6).

The superficial inguinal ring is a triangular opening in the external oblique aponeurosis and lies superior and medial to the pubic tubercle. (The spermatic cord or the round ligament of the uterus passes through this opening.)

The inguinal ligament is formed between the anterior superior iliac spine and the pubic tubercle, where the lower border of the aponeurosis is folded backward on itself.

The lateral part of the posterior edge of the inguinal ligament gives origin to part of the internal oblique and transversus abdominal muscles.

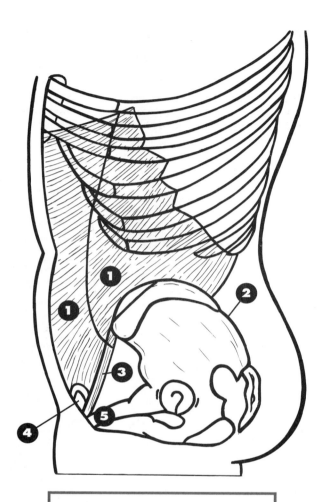

1	external oblique muscle
2	iliac crest
3	inguinal ligament
4	superficial inguinal ring
5	pubic tubercle

FIGURE 2-7

Internal Oblique Muscle of the Anterior and Lateral Abdominal Walls

Internal Oblique

The internal oblique muscle lies deep to the external oblique; the majority of its fibers are aligned at right angles to the external oblique (Figure 2-7). It arises from the lumbar fascia, the anterior two thirds of the iliac crest, and the lateral two thirds of the inguinal ligament. It inserts into the lower borders of the ribs and their costal cartilages, the xyphoid process, the linea alba, and the pubic symphysis. The internal oblique has a lower free border that arches over the spermatic cord or the round ligament of the uterus and then descends behind it to be attached to the pubic crest and the pectineal line. The lowest tendinous fibers are joined by similar fibers from the transversus abdominis to form the conjoint tendon.

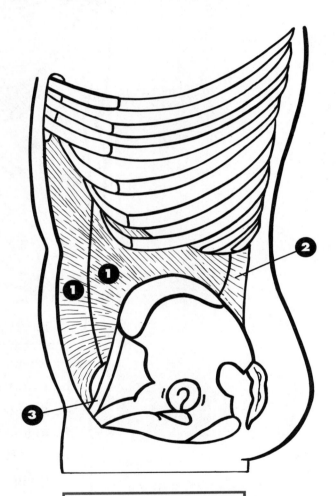

1	**internal oblique muscle**
2	**lumbar fascia**
3	**inguinal ligament**

FIGURE 2-8
Transversus Muscle of the Anterior and Lateral Abdominal Walls

Transversus

The transversus muscle lies deep to the internal oblique, and its fibers run horizontally forward (Figure 2-8). It arises from the deep surface of the lower six costal cartilages (interlacing with the diaphragm), the lumbar fascia, the anterior two thirds of the iliac crest, and the lateral third of the inguinal ligament. It inserts into the xyphoid process, the linea alba, and the pubic symphysis.

It should be noted that the posterior border of the external oblique muscle is unattached, and the posterior borders of the internal oblique and transversus muscles are attached to the lumbar vertebrae by the lumbar fascia.

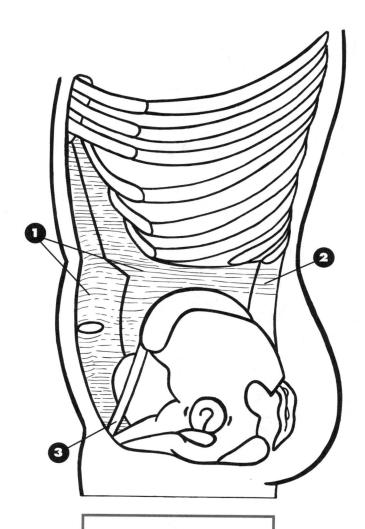

1	**transversus muscle**
2	**lumbar fascia**
3	**inguinal ligament**

FIGURE 2-9
Anterior View of the Rectus Abdominis Muscle and Rectus Sheath

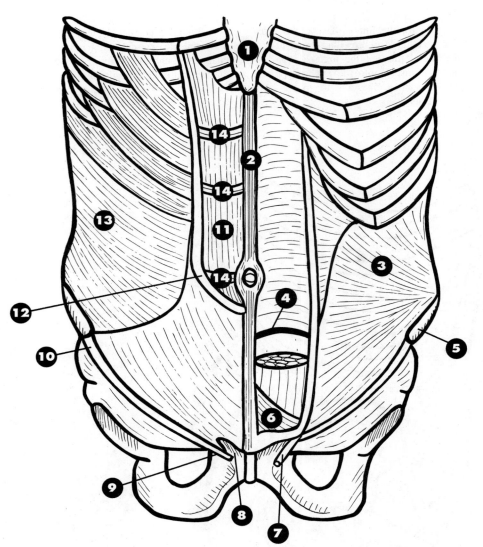

Rectus Abdominis
(FIGURE 2-9)

The rectus abdominis muscle arises from the front of the symphysis pubis and from the pubic crest. It inserts into the fifth, sixth, and seventh costal cartilages and the xyphoid process. On contraction, its lateral margin forms a palpable curved surface, termed the *linea semilunaris,* that extends from the ninth costal cartilage to the pubic tubercle. The anterior surface of the rectus muscle is crossed by three tendinous intersections that are firmly attached to the anterior wall of the rectus sheath.

Pyramidalis (FIGURE 2-9)

Although often absent, the pyramidalis muscle arises by its base from the anterior surface of the pubis and inserts into the linea alba. It lies anterior to the lower part of the rectus abdominis muscle.

1	xyphoid process	8	superficial inguinal ring
2	linea alba	9	pubic tubercle
3	internal oblique muscle	10	inguinal ligament
4	arcuate line	11	rectus muscle
5	anterior superior iliac spine	12	linea semilunaris
6	pyramidalis muscle	13	external oblique muscle
7	spermatic cord	14	tendinous intersections

FIGURE 2-10
Transverse Sections of the Rectus Sheath at Four Levels

Rectus Sheath

The long rectus sheath encloses the rectus abdominis and pyramidalis muscles and contains the anterior rami of the lower six thoracic nerves and the superior and inferior epigastric vessels and lymphatics. It is largely formed by the aponeuroses of the external oblique, internal oblique, and transverse lateral abdominal muscles. It can be divided into four areas:

1. Above the costal margin, the anterior wall is formed by the aponeurosis of the external oblique (Figure 2-10, Level I). The posterior wall is formed by the fifth, sixth, and seventh costal cartilages and intercostal spaces.

2. Between the costal margin and the level of the anterior superior iliac spine (Figure 2-10, Level II), the aponeurosis of the internal oblique splits to enclose the rectus muscle; the aponeurosis of the internal oblique muscle is directed in front of the muscle, and the aponeurosis of the transversus muscle is directed behind the rectus muscle.

3. Between the level of the anterior superior iliac spine and the pubic (Figure 2-10, Level III), the aponeuroses of all three muscles form the anterior wall. The posterior wall is absent, and the rectus muscle lies in contact with the fascia transversalis.

4. In front of the pubis (Figure 2-10, Level IV), the origin of the rectus muscle and the pyramidalis (if present) is covered anteriorly by the aponeuroses of the three muscles. The posterior wall is formed by the body of the pubis.

The arcuate line is the point at which the aponeuroses that form the posterior wall pass in front of the rectus at the level of the anterior superior iliac spine. At this point the inferior epigastric vessels enter the rectus sheath to anastomose with the superior epigastric vessels.

The midline linea alba separates the muscles of the rectus sheath. It is formed by the fusion of the aponeuroses of the lateral muscles and extends from the xyphoid process to the pubis.

The anterior wall of the rectus sheath is firmly attached to the rectus abdominis muscle by tendinous intersections, while its posterior wall remains free.

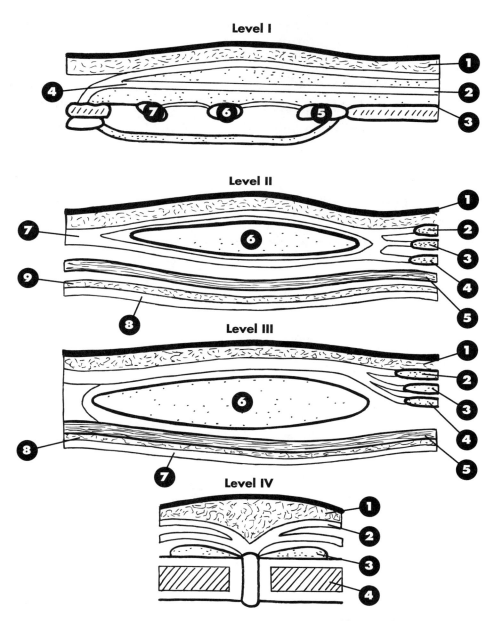

Level I

Level II

Level III

Level IV

(Continued on Page 58)

Level I (above costal margin)

1 superficial fascia
2 pectoralis major muscle
3 rectus muscle
4 aponeurosis of the external oblique muscle
5 external oblique muscle
6 internal oblique muscle
7 transversus muscle

Level II (between the costal margin and the level of the anterior superior iliac spine)

1 superficial fascia
2 external oblique muscle
3 internal oblique muscle
4 transversus muscle
5 fascia transversalis
6 rectus muscle
7 linea alba

8 peritoneum
9 extraperitoneal fat

Level III (below the level of the anterior superior iliac spine and above the pelvis)

1 superficial fascia
2 external oblique muscle
3 internal oblique muscle
4 transversus muscle
5 fascia transversalis
6 rectus muscle
7 peritoneum
8 extraperitoneal fat

Level IV (the level of the pubis)

1 superficial fascia
2 aponeurosis of the external oblique muscle
3 rectus muscle
4 pubis

FIGURE 2-11
Inferior View of the Diaphragm

Diaphragm

The diaphragm is a dome-shaped muscular and tendinous septum that separates the thorax from the abdominal cavity. Its muscular part arises from the margins of the thoracic outlet (Figure 2-11). The right dome may reach as high as the upper border of the fifth rib, and the left dome reaches the lower border of the fifth rib (Figure 2-12).

The right crus arises from the sides of the bodies of the first three lumbar vertebrae; the left crus arises from the sides of the bodies of the first two lumbar vertebrae.

Lateral to the crura, the diaphragm arises from the medial and lateral arcuate ligaments. The medial ligament is the thickened upper margin of the fascia that covers the anterior surface of the psoas muscle. It extends from the side of the body of the second lumbar vertebrae to the tip of the transverse process of the first lumbar vertebrae. The lateral ligament is the thickened upper margin of the fascia that covers the anterior surface of the quadratus lumborum muscle. It extends from the tip of the transverse process of the first lumbar vertebra to the lower border of the twelfth rib.

The median arcuate ligament connects the medial borders of the two crura as they cross anterior to the aorta.

The diaphragm inserts into a central tendon. The superior surface of the tendon is partially fused with the inferior surface of the fibrous pericardium. Fibers of the right crus surround the esophagus to act as a sphincter to prevent regurgitation of the gastric contents into the thoracic part of the esophagus.

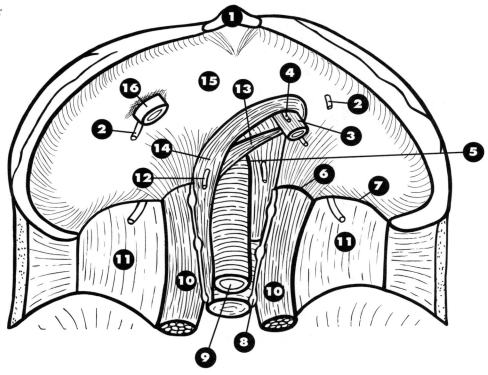

1	xyphoid process	7	lateral arcuate ligament	13	left crus
2	right and left phrenic nerves	8	sympathetic trunk	14	right crus
3	esophagus	9	aorta	15	central tendon
4	vagi	10	psoas muscle	16	inferior vena cava
5	median arcuate ligament	11	quadratus lumborum muscle		
6	medial arcuate ligament	12	splanchnic nerves		

FIGURE 2-12

Muscles of the Posterior Thoracic Wall and Diaphragm

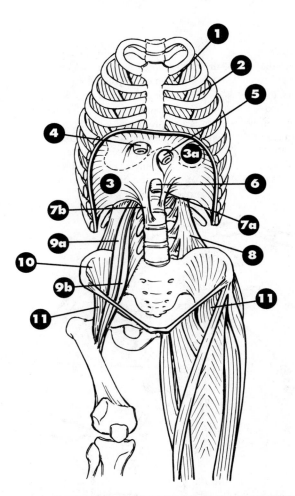

Openings in the Diaphragm

The aortic opening transmits the aorta, thoracic duct, and azygos vein and lies anterior to the body of the twelfth thoracic vertebra between the crura.

The esophageal opening carries the esophagus, the right and left vagus nerves, the esophageal branches of the left gastric vessels, and the lymphatics from the lower third of the esophagus. It lies at the level of the tenth thoracic vertebra in a muscle sling from the right crus.

The caval opening transmits the inferior vena cava and the terminal branches of the right phrenic nerve and lies at the level of the eighth thoracic vertebra within the central tendon.

In addition to these openings, the splanchnic nerves pierce the crura, the sympathetic trunk passes posterior to the medial arcuate ligament on both sides, and the superior epigastric vessels pass between the sternal and costal origins of the diaphragm on each side.

The left phrenic nerve pierces the diaphragm to supply the peritoneum.

1	internal intercostal muscle	7a	left crus
2	external intercostal muscle	7b	right crus
3	diaphragm	8	quadratus lumborum muscle
3a	central tendon	9a	psoas major muscle
4	inferior vena cava	9b	psoas minor muscle
5	esophagus	10	iliacus muscle
6	aorta	11	iliopsoas muscle

Review Exercise • The Muscular System

The basic function of muscle is to produce movement of the body or part of the body. In addition, muscles protect the internal organs, maintain posture, and produce large amounts of body heat.

1. An essential function of the human body is _____ .

2. This function is made possible by the development of the property of _____ in muscle tissue.

3. Name the three types of muscles that can be identified by their structure, function, and location in the body.

   _____

   _____

4. Which muscles are also called voluntary muscles and have attachments of their ends to bones, cartilage, or ligaments by cords of tough fibrous tissue called tendons? _____

5. The ends of these muscles are attached to bones, cartilage, or ligaments by _____ .

6. What are the four basic forms of connective tissue?

7. The tendons attach _____ to _____ .

8. The ligaments connect the _____ that form the _____ .

9. _____ are thin tendinous sheets attached to flat muscles.

10. _____ are thin sheets of tissue that cover muscles and hold them in their place.

11. Individual fibers of muscle are arranged either _____ or _____ to the long axis of the muscle.

12. What happens to the muscle during contraction?

13. What muscle group resembles a feather? Why?

14. A _____ muscle is one in which the tendon lies along one side of the muscle, and the muscle fibers pass oblique to it.

15. A _____ muscle has a tendon in the center, and the muscle fibers pass to it from two sides.
    Example:

16. A _____ muscle may have a series of bipennate muscles lying alongside one another.
    Example:

17. What muscle group is composed of long, spindle-shaped cells closely arranged in bundles or sheets?

18. Examples of the above muscle are:

19. What muscle is found in the myocardium? _____

20. What five pelvic muscles may be useful landmarks in sonography? _____

    _____

    _____

    _____

21. What two neck muscles are identified in the thyroid transverse scans? _____

    _____

22. What anterior and posterior abdominal wall muscles are easily seen on sonography? _____

_____

_____

_____

23. The neck is divided into the anterior and posterior triangles by the _____ muscle.

24. What are the four muscle groups of the anterior abdominal wall? _____

_____

_____

_____

25. The central muscle is the _____ .

26. The _____ is a fibrous band stretching from the xyphoid to the symphysis pubis.

27. Define the origin of the rectus sheath.

28. What is the purpose of the diaphragm?

29. What is the crus of the diaphragm?

30. What are the openings in the diaphragm?

Self-Test • The Muscular System

1. The three types of muscle in the body may be identified by all except:

   a. function

   b. structure

   c. elasticity

   d. location

2. The three types of muscle are known as all of the following except:

   a. skeletal

   b. rough

   c. smooth

   d. cardiac

3. Skeletal muscle produces movements of the skeleton and is sometimes called:

   a. involuntary muscle

   b. responsive muscle

   c. irresponsive muscle

   d. voluntary muscle

4. The four basic forms of dense connective tissue include all except:

   a. tendons

   b. ligaments

   c. aponeuroses

   d. fibers

   e. fasciae

5. What attaches muscle to bone?

   a. ligaments

   b. tendons

   c. fibers

   d. nerves

6. What connects the bones that form joints?

   a. tendons

   b. ligaments

   c. nerves

   d. fibers

7. An example of a smooth muscle is the:

   a. bladder

   b. liver

   c. heart

   d. deltoid

8. The neck is divided into two triangles, anterior and posterior, by the:

   a. infrahyoid muscle

   b. sternocleidomastoid muscle

   c. thyrohyoid muscle

   d. omohyoid

9. The _____ is a fibrous ban stretching from the

   xyphoid to the symphysis pubis.

   a. rectus sheath

   b. aponeuroses

   c. linea semilunaris

   d. linea alba

10. The _____ separates the thorax from the abdominal cavity.

    a. transversus muscle

    b. internal oblique muscle

    c. diaphragm

    d. external oblique muscle

11. The anterior and lateral margins of the true pelvis are formed by all of the following except the:

    a. diaphragm

    b. pubis

    c. ischium

    d. ilium

12. The muscular "sling" is composed of:

    a. pubis and ischium

    b. coccygeus and levator ani

    c. perineum and peritoneum

    d. Douglas' pouch and retrovesical space

13. The anterior compartment of the true pelvis contains:

    a. rectosigmoid muscle

    b. perirectal fat

    c. the bladder and reproductive organs

    d. presacral space

14. The anterior pouch of the uterus is called:

    a. Douglas' pouch

    b. uterovesical space

    c. rectouterine space

    d. broad ligament

15. The fallopian tubes extend laterally from the fundus of the uterus and are enveloped by a fold of peritoneum known as:

   a. broad ligament

   b. round ligament

   c. ovarian ligament

   d. tubal ligament

16. The _____ muscles are symmetrically aligned along the lateral border of the pelvis with a concave medial border.

   a. pubococcygeus

   b. obturator internus

   c. obturator externus

   d. transversus

17. The _____ muscles are rounded, concave muscles that lie more posterior than the obturator internus muscles.

   a. obturator externus

   b. periformis

   c. pubococcygeus

   d. cremaster

18. The posterior border of the _____ lies along the iliopectineal line and may be used as a separation landmark of the true pelvis from the false pelvis.

   a. ilium

   b. ischium

   c. iliac crest

   d. iliopsoas

Answers to Review Exercise

1. movement
2. elasticity
3. skeletal; smooth; cardiac
4. skeletal
5. tendons
6. tendons; ligaments; aponeuroses; fasciae
7. muscle; bone
8. bones; joints
9. Aponeuroses
10. Fasciae
11. parallel; oblique
12. The muscle shortens to one half or one third of its resting length.
13. Pennate muscle has fibers that run oblique to the line of pull.
14. unipennate
15. bipennate; example: rectus femoris
16. multipennate; example: deltoid
17. smooth muscle
18. vessels or gastrointestinal tract
19. cardiac muscle
20. transversus muscle; internal oblique muscle; piriformis muscle; coccygeus; levator ani
21. sternocleidomastoid; suprahyoid
22. diaphragm; crus; rectus sheath; quadratus lumborum
23. sternocleidomastoid
24. external oblique; internal oblique; transversus; rectus abdominis
25. linea alba
26. rectus abdominis
27. The rectus sheath is formed by the aponeuroses of the external oblique, internal oblique, and transverse lateral abdominal muscles.
28. The diaphragm is a muscular and tendinous septum that separates the thorax from the abdominal cavity.
29. The right crus arises from the sides of the bodies of the first three lumbar vertebrae; the left crus arises from the sides of the bodies of the first two lumbar vertebrae.
30. The aorta, thoracic duct, azygos vein lie between the crura; the esophageal, vagus nerves, esophageal branches of the left gastric vessels, and lymphatics lie at the level of the right crus; the IVC and right phrenic nerve lie with the central tendon.

Answers to Self-Test

1. c
2. b
3. d
4. d
5. b
6. b
7. a
8. b
9. d
10. c
11. a
12. b
13. c
14. b
15. a
16. b
17. c
18. d

CHAPTER

3

The Vascular System

OBJECTIVES

At the completion of this chapter, students will show orally, in writing, or by demonstration that they will be able to:

1. Define the origins of the aorta and inferior vena cava.
2. Diagram the paths of the aorta and inferior vena cava in detail.
3. Describe at least four main branches of the aorta and their origins.
4. Describe the main tributaries of the inferior vena cava and their origins.
5. Diagram the distribution of the main arteries to the viscera and mesentery.
6. Diagram the distribution of blood from the structures in the upper and lower abdomen through its major tributaries to the inferior vena cava.
7. Describe the origin and course of each of the following minor arteries:
   a. celiac trunk
   b. superior mesenteric artery
   c. inferior mesenteric artery
   d. renal arteries
   e. gastroduodenal artery
   f. uterine artery
   g. ovarian artery
8. Describe the origin and course of each of the following minor veins:

   a. splenic vein
   b. superior mesenteric vein
   c. inferior mesenteric vein
   d. portal vein
   e. hepatic vein
   f. renal veins
   g. suprarenal veins
9. Differentiate sonographic appearances by explaining the clinical significance of the pathologic processes as related to the vascular system in the following diseases:
   a. atherosclerosis
   b. aneurysm
   c. dissection
   d. calcification
   e. thrombus
10. Create high-quality diagnostic scans to illustrate the appropriate anatomy in all planes pertinent to the vascular system.
11. Select the correct equipment settings appropriate to individual body habitus.
12. Distinguish between the normal and abnormal sonographic appearances of the vascular anatomy.

To further enhance learning, students should use marking pens to color the anatomic illustrations that follow.

VASCULAR STRUCTURES

FIGURE 3-1

Cross Section of a Vein and an Artery

General Composition of Vessels

Blood is carried away from the heart by the arteries and is returned from the tissues to the heart by the veins. Arteries divide into smaller and smaller branches, the smallest of which are the arterioles. These lead into the capillaries, which are minute vessels that branch and form a network where the exchange of materials between blood and tissue fluid takes place. After the blood passes through the capillaries, it is collected into the small veins, or venules. These small vessels unite to form larger vessels that eventually return the blood to the heart for recirculation.

A typical artery in cross section consists of three layers (Figure 3-1):

The **tunica intima** (inner layer), which itself consists of three layers:

A layer of endothelial cells that line the arterial passage (lumen)

A layer of delicate connective tissue

An elastic layer made up of a network of elastic fibers

The **tunica media** (middle layer), which consists of smooth muscle fibers with elastic and collagenous tissue

The **tunica adventitia** (external layer), which is composed of loose connective tissue with bundles of smooth muscle fibers and elastic tissue.

Smaller arteries contain less elastic tissue and more smooth muscle. The elasticity of the large arteries is vital to the maintenance of a steady blood flow.

The veins have the same three layers as the arteries, but they differ in that the tunica media is thinner. They appear collapsed because of the little elastic tissue or muscle in their walls.

Veins have special valves within them that permit blood to flow only in one direction, toward the heart. They have a larger total diameter than do arteries, and the blood moves toward the heart slowly, as compared with the arterial circulation.

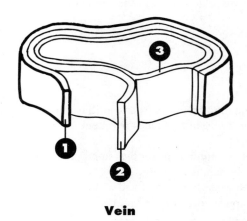

Vein

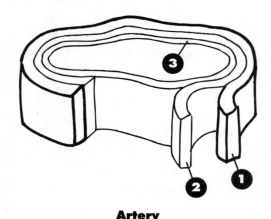

Artery

1	tunica adventitia
2	tunica media
3	tunica intima

FIGURE 3-2
FIGURE 3-2
Inferior Vena Cava and Its Tributaries

Main System Veins
(FIGURES 3-2 AND 3-3)

Inferior Vena Cava

The inferior vena cava is formed by the union of the common iliac veins behind the right common iliac artery. It ascends vertically through the retroperitoneal space on the right side of the aorta posterior to the liver, piercing the central tendon of the diaphragm at the level of the eighth thoracic vertebrae and enters the right atrium of the heart. Its entrance into the lesser sac separates it from the portal vein.

The tributaries of the inferior vena cava are the hepatic veins, the right adrenal veins, the renal veins, the right testicular or ovarian vein, the inferior phrenic vein, the four lumbar veins, the common iliac veins, and the median sacral vein.

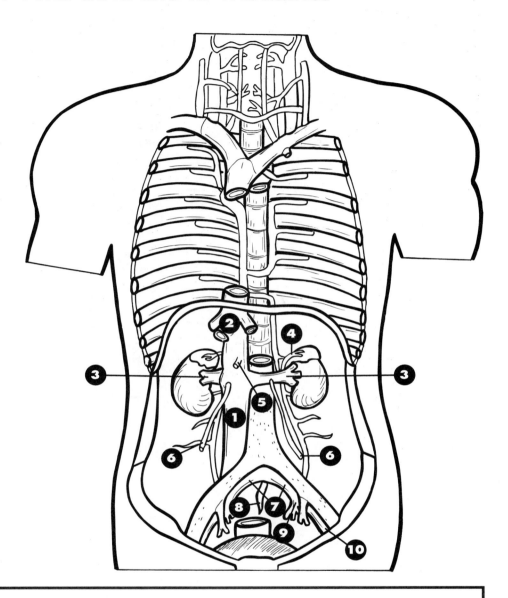

1	**inferior vena cava**	**6**	**testicular or ovarian veins**
2	**hepatic veins**	**7**	**common iliac (right and left) veins**
3	**renal veins**	**8**	**middle sacral vein**
4	**suprarenal vein**	**9**	**internal iliac vein**
5	**phrenic vein**	**10**	**external iliac vein**

FIGURE 3-3
Azygos Vein and Its Tributaries

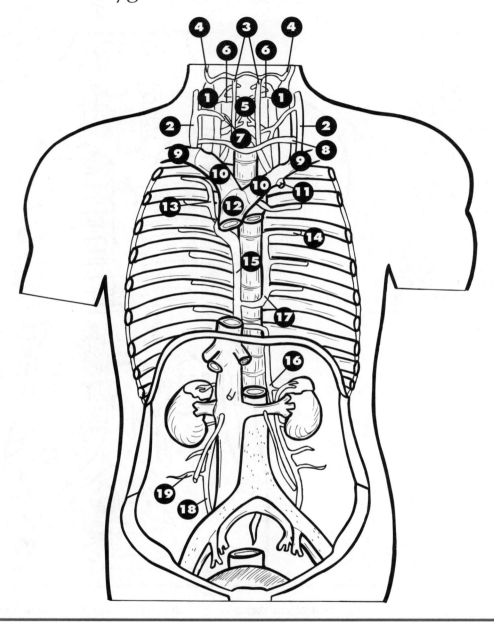

1	internal jugular veins	**9**	subclavian (right and left) veins	**14** posterior intercostal vein
2	external jugular veins			**15** azygos vein
3	anterior jugular veins	**10**	brachiocephalic (right and left) veins	**16** hemiazygos vein
4	facial veins			**17** accessory hemiazygos vein
5	middle thyroid veins	**11**	internal thoracic vein	
6	superior thyroid veins	**12**	superior vena cava	**18** ascending lumbar vein
7	inferior thyroid vein	**13**	superior intercostal vein	**19** lumbar vein
8	jugular venous arch			

FIGURE 3-4
Portal Venous Supply in the Liver

Portal Vein (FIGURE 3-4)

The portal vein is formed posterior to the pancreas by the union of the superior mesenteric and splenic veins. It runs upward and to the right, posterior to the first part of the duodenum, and enters the lesser omentum. It then ascends anterior to the opening into the lesser sac to the porta hepatis, where it divides into right and left terminal branches. It drains blood out of the gastrointestinal tract from the lower end of the esophagus to the upper end of the anal canal, from the pancreas, gallbladder, and bile ducts, and from the spleen. It has an important anastomosis with the esophageal veins, rectal venous plexus, and superficial abdominal veins. The portal venous blood traverses the liver and drains into the inferior vena cava via the hepatic veins.

The portal veins become smaller as they progress from the porta hepatis. Large radicles situated near or approaching the porta hepatis are portal veins, not hepatic veins.

The right and left portal veins course transversely through the liver. Anatomically, any intraparenchymal segment of the portal venous system lying to the right of the lateral aspect of the inferior vena cava is a branch of the right portal system. The left portal vein has a narrow-caliber trunk and may be seen coursing transversely through the left hepatic lobe from posterior to anterior.

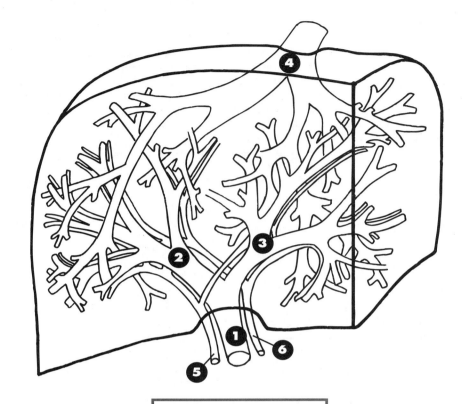

1	**main portal vein**
2	**right portal vein**
3	**left portal vein**
4	**hepatic veins**
5	**bile ducts**
6	**hepatic artery**

FIGURE 3-5
Formation of the Portal Vein

Splenic Vein (FIGURE 3-5)

The splenic vein is a tributary of the portal circulation. It begins at the hilum of the spleen as the union of several veins and is then joined by the short gastric and left gastroepiploic veins. It passes to the right within the lienorenal ligament and runs posterior to the pancreas below the splenic artery. It joins the superior mesenteric vein behind the neck of the pancreas to form the portal vein. It is joined by veins from the pancreas and the inferior mesenteric vein.

Superior Mesenteric Vein

The superior mesenteric vein is a tributary of the portal circulation. It begins at the ileocolic junction and runs upward along the posterior abdominal wall within the root of the mesentery of the small intestine and to the right of the superior mesenteric artery. It passes anterior to the third part of the duodenum and posterior to the neck of the pancreas, where it joins the splenic vein to form the portal vein. It also receives tributaries that correspond to the branches of the superior mesenteric artery, joined by the inferior pancreaticoduodenal vein to the right and the right gastroepiploic vein from the right aspect of the greater curvature of the stomach to the left.

Inferior Mesenteric Vein

The inferior mesenteric vein is a tributary of the portal circulation. It begins midway down the anal canal as the superior rectal vein. It runs up the posterior abdominal wall on the left side of the inferior mesenteric artery and the duodenojejunal junction and joins the splenic vein behind the pancreas. It receives many tributaries along its way, including the left colic vein.

Hepatic Veins

The hepatic veins are the largest visceral tributaries of the inferior vena cava. They originate in the liver, and as they increase in caliber, they drain into the inferior vena cava at the level of the diaphragm. The hepatic veins return blood from the liver that was brought to it by the hepatic artery and the portal vein. The hepatic vein has three branches: the right hepatic vein in the right lobe of the liver, the middle hepatic vein in the caudate lobe, and the left hepatic vein in the left lobe of the liver.

Renal Veins

The right renal vein can be seen to flow directly from the renal sinus into the posterolateral aspect of the inferior vena cava. The left renal vein exits the renal sinus and follows a course anterior to the abdominal aorta and posterior to the superior mesenteric artery to enter the medial aspect of the inferior vena cava. Above the entry of the renal veins, the inferior vena cava enlarges to accommodate the increased volume of blood returning from the kidneys.

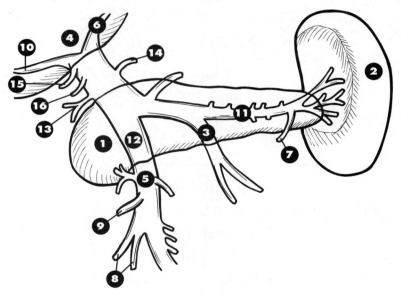

1	pancreas	9	right gastroepiploic vein
2	spleen	10	right branch of the portal vein
3	inferior mesenteric vein	11	splenic vein
4	liver	12	superior mesenteric vein
5	inferior pancreaticoduodenal vein	13	superior pancreaticoduodenal vein
6	left branch of the portal vein	14	accessory pancreatic vein
7	left gastroepiploic vein	15	cystic vein
8	right colic vein	16	right gastric vein (pyloric)

FIGURE 3-6
Thoracic Aorta and Its Tributaries

Main System Arteries
(FIGURES 3-6 AND 3-7)

Aorta

The systemic circulation leaves the left ventricle of the heart by way of the aorta, the largest artery in the body. The ascending aorta arises from the left ventricle to form the aortic arch. It then arches to the left and curves downward to form the descending aorta. The descending aorta enters the abdomen through the aortic opening of the diaphragm in front of the twelfth thoracic vertebra in the retroperitoneal space. It descends anteriorly to the bodies of the lumbar vertebrae. At the level of the fourth lumbar vertebra it divides into the two common iliac arteries.

The diameter of the aorta is generally between 2 cm and 4 cm. This diameter is fairly uniform throughout its length, with slight variations in contour as it branches to the visceral organs. The aorta has four main branches that supply other visceral organs and the mesentery: the celiac trunk, the superior and inferior mesenteric arteries, and the renal arteries.

The common iliac arteries arise at the bifurcation of the aorta and run downward and laterally along the medial border of the right and left psoas muscles. At the level of the sacroiliac joint, each iliac artery bifurcates into an external and internal iliac artery.

The external iliac artery runs along the medial border of the psoas, following the pelvic brim. It gives off the inferior epigastric and deep circumflex branches before passing under the inguinal ligament to become the femoral artery.

The internal iliac artery enters the pelvis in front of the sacroiliac joint, at which point it is crossed anteriorly by the ureter. It also divides into anterior and posterior branches to supply the pelvic viscera, peritoneum, buttocks, and sacral canal.

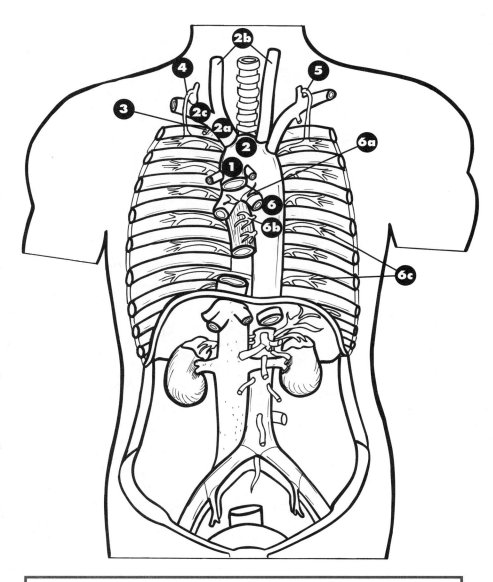

1	**ascending aorta**	**5**	**highest intercostal artery**
2	**aortic arch**		
2a	**brachiocephalic artery**	**6**	**thoracic (descending) aorta**
2b	**common carotid arteries**		
		6a	**bronchial arteries**
2c	**subclavian artery**	**6b**	**esophageal arteries**
3	**internal thoracic artery**	**6c**	**posterior intercostal arteries**
4	**costocervical trunk**		

FIGURE 3-7
Abdominal Aorta and Its Tributaries

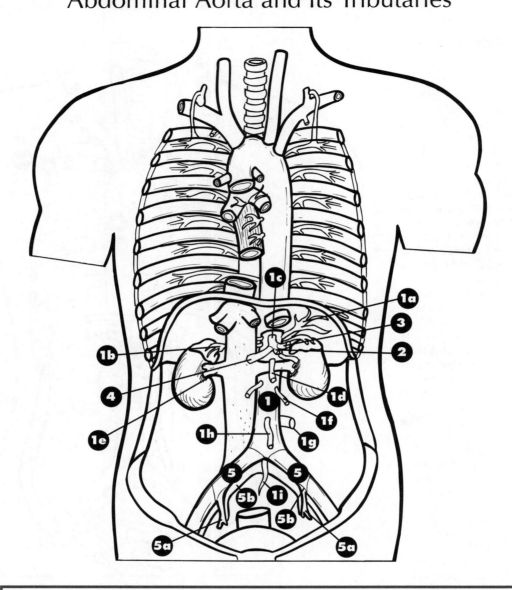

1	abdominal aorta	1h	inferior mesenteric artery
1a	inferior phrenic artery	1i	middle sacral artery
1b	suprarenal artery	2	left gastric artery
1c	celiac trunk	3	splenic artery
1d	superior mesenteric artery	4	hepatic artery
1e	renal vein	5	common iliac arteries
1f	testicular or ovarian artery	5a	internal iliac arteries
1g	lumbar artery	5b	external iliac arteries

FIGURE 3-8
Celiac Artery and Its Branches

Celiac Trunk (FIGURE 3-8)

The celiac trunk, originating within the first 2 cm of the abdominal aorta, is surrounded by the liver, spleen, inferior vena cava, and pancreas. It immediately branches into the left gastric, splenic, and common hepatic arteries.

The splenic artery is the largest of the three branches of the celiac trunk. From its origin, it takes a somewhat tortuous course horizontally to the left along the upper margin of the pancreas (Figure 3-9). Near the splenic hilum, it divides into two branches. The left gastroepiploic artery runs caudally into the greater omentum and toward the right gastroepiploic artery. The other branch runs cephalad and divides into the short gastric artery, which supplies the fundus of the stomach, and a number of splenic branches that supply the spleen. Several small branches originate at the splenic artery as it runs along the upper border of the pancreas: the dorsal pancreatic, the great pancreatic, and the caudal pancreatic, among others.

The dorsal pancreatic, or superior pancreatic, artery usually originates from the beginning of the splenic artery but may also arise from the hepatic artery, celiac trunk, or aorta. It runs behind and in the substance of the pancreas, dividing into right and left branches. The left branch is the transverse pancreatic artery. The right branch constitutes an anastomotic vessel to the anterior pancreatic arch and also a branch to the uncinate process.

The great pancreatic artery originates from the splenic artery farther to the left and passes downward, dividing into branches that anastomose with the transverse or inferior pancreatic artery.

The caudal pancreatic artery supplies the tail of the pancreas and divides into branches that anastomose with terminal branches of the transverse pancreatic artery.

The transverse pancreatic artery courses behind the body and tail of the pancreas close to the lower pancreatic border. It may originate from or communicate with the superior mesenteric artery.

The common hepatic artery comes off the celiac trunk and courses to the right of the aorta at almost a 90° angle. It courses along the upper border of the pancreatic head, behind the posterior layer of the peritoneal omental bursa, to the upper margin of the superior part of the duodenum, which forms the lower boundary of the epiploic foramen. It ascends into the liver with the hepatic ducts and portal vein. It divides into two main branches: the right hepatic branch, which serves the gallbladder via the cystic artery, and the left hepatic branch, which serves the caudate and left lobes of the liver.

Within the liver parenchyma, the hepatic arterial branches further divide repeatedly into progressively smaller vessels that eventually supply the portal triad.

The head of the pancreas, the duodenum, and parts of the stomach are supplied by the gastroduodenal artery, which arises from the common hepatic artery.

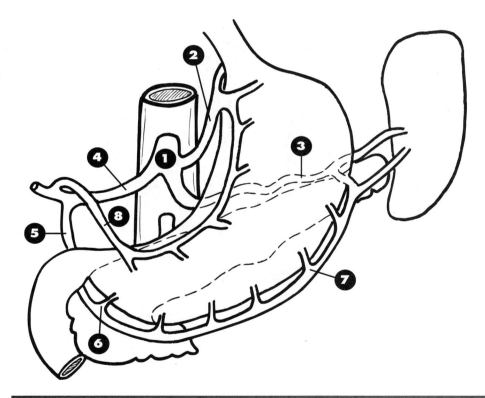

1	celiac artery	5	gastroduodenal artery
2	left gastric artery	6	right gastroepiploic artery
3	splenic artery	7	left gastroepiploic artery
4	common hepatic artery	8	right gastric artery

FIGURE 3-9

Anterior View of the Pancreas and Its Vascular Structures

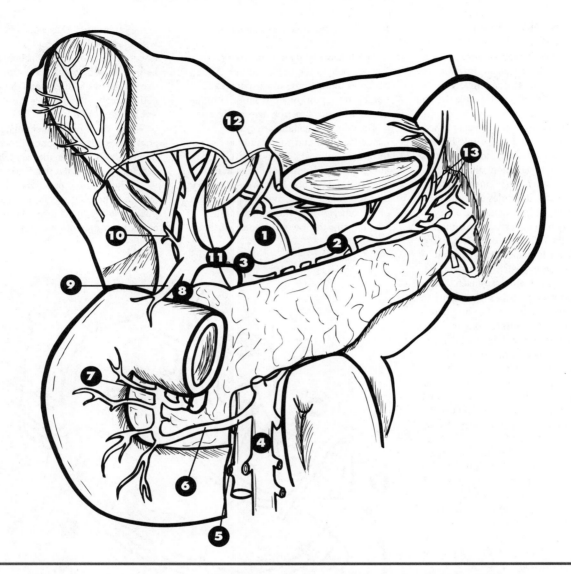

1	aorta	8	gastroduodenal artery
2	splenic artery	9	supraduodenal artery
3	celiac trunk	10	right gastric artery
4	superior mesenteric artery	11	common hepatic artery
5	inferior pancreaticoduodenal artery	12	left gastric artery
6	anterior inferior pancreaticoduodenal artery	13	short gastric arteries
7	anterior superior pancreaticoduodenal artery		

FIGURE 3-10
Blood Supply to the Jejunum and Ileum*

Superior Mesenteric Artery
(FIGURE 3-10)

The superior mesenteric artery arises anteriorly from the abdominal aorta approximately 1 cm below the celiac trunk. It runs posterior to the neck of the pancreas, passing over the uncinate process of the pancreatic head anterior to the third part of the duodenum, where it enters the root of the mesentery and colon. It has five main branches: the inferior pancreatic, duodenal, colic, ileocolic, and intestinal arteries. These branch arteries to the small bowel each consist of 10 to 16 branches arising from the left side of the superior mesenteric trunk. They extend into the mesentery, where adjacent arteries unite to form loops, or arcades. Their distribution is to the proximal half of the colon and small intestine.

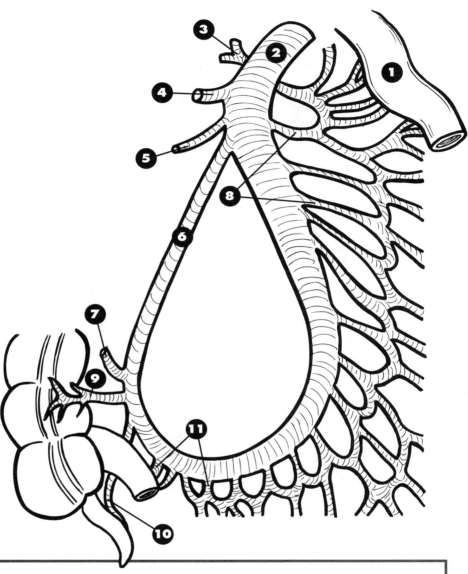

1	duodenojejunal flexure	7	ascending branch of ileocolic artery
2	superior mesenteric artery	8	intestinal arteries
3	inferior pancreaticoduodenal arteries	9	cecal arteries
4	middle colic artery	10	appendicular artery
5	right colic artery	11	ileal branches of the ileocolic artery
6	ileocolic artery		

The ileocolic artery lies at the base of the mesentery of the intestine; the stem of the superior mesenteric artery flows into the mesentery.

FIGURE 3-11
Blood Supply of the Colon

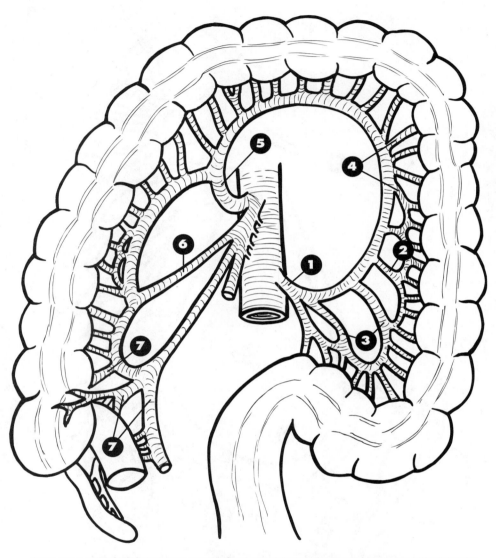

Inferior Mesenteric Artery
(FIGURE 3-11)

The inferior mesenteric artery arises from the anterior abdominal aorta approximately at the level of the third or fourth lumbar vertebrae. It proceeds to the left to distribute arterial blood to the descending colon, sigmoid colon, and rectum. It has three main branches: the left colic, sigmoid, and superior rectal arteries.

Renal Arteries

The right and left renal arteries arise anterior to the first lumbar vertebra and inferior to the superior mesenteric artery from the posterolateral or lateral walls of the aorta. They divide into anterior and inferior suprarenal branches.

The right renal artery passes posterior to the inferior vena cava and anterior to the vertebral column in a posterior and slightly caudal direction. The left renal artery has a direct course from the aorta anterior to the psoas to enter the renal sinus.

1	inferior mesenteric artery	5	middle colic artery
2	left colic artery	6	right colic artery
3	sigmoid artery	7	ileocolic arteries
4	marginal arteries		

Vascular System Review Notes

FUNCTION

As part of the circulatory system, the vascular system and the heart and lymphatics transport gases, nutrient materials, and other essential substances to the tissues and then transport waste products from the cells to the appropriate sites for excretion.

ANATOMIC COMPOSITION

Three layers of arteries and veins comprise the vascular system:

1. *Tunica intima*—the inner layer—single layer of endothelial cells in a longitudinal organization
2. *Tunica media*—the middle layer—smooth muscle and collagenous fiber
3. *Tunica adventitia*—the outer layer—thin fibrous layer that surrounds elastic tissue

Specific differences among arteries, veins, and capillaries are listed as follows:

Arteries

- Hollow elastic tubes
- Carry blood away from heart
- Enclosed within a sheath that includes an accompanying vein and nerve

Arterioles

- Small arteries

Veins

- Hollow, collapsible tubes caused by diminished tunica media
- Carry blood toward the heart
- Venous valves (extension of intimas), semilunar type, which prevent backflow; numerous valves in the extremities, especially the lower extremities, caused by flow against gravity
- Venous return aided by muscle contraction, valves, overflow from capillary beds, force of gravity, and suction from negative thoracic pressure
- Less muscle and elastic components result in ability to passively expand; decrease in exertion of venous pressure

Capillaries

- Minute, hair-size vessels connecting the arterial and venous systems
- One-walled structures
- Nutrients for cells and tissues of the body received from fluids passing through the capillary walls; at the same time, passage of waste products from the cells into the capillaries

- Arteries not always ending in capillary beds; anastomoses (end-to-end grafts between different vessels) providing equalization of pressure over vessel length as well as alternative flow channels

MAJOR VESSELS

Aorta

- Principal artery of the body
- Divided into five sections:
  1. root of the aorta
  2. ascending aorta
  3. descending aorta
  4. abdominal aorta
  5. bifurcation of the aorta into iliac arteries

Root of the Aorta

- The aorta arises from the left ventricular outflow tract in the heart and is comprised of three semilunar cusps that prevent blood from flowing back into the left ventricle. The cusps open with ventricular systole to allow blood to be ejected into the ascending aorta. The cusps are closed during ventricular diastole. The coronary arteries arise superiorly from the right and left coronary cusps to form right and left coronary arteries, respectively; these arteries further bifurcate to supply the vasculature of the cardiac structures.

Ascending Aorta

- The ascending aorta ascends a short distance from the ventricle and arches superiorly to form the *aortic arch.* There are three arterial branches that arise from the superior border of the aortic arch to supply the head, neck, and upper extremities: the right innominate, the left common carotid, and the left subclavian.

Descending Aorta

- From the aortic arch, the descending aorta flows posterior to the heart and through the thoracic cavity, where it pierces the diaphragm.

Abdominal Aorta

- The abdominal aorta then continues to flow anterior to the vertebral column to the level of the fourth lumbar vertebrae, where it bifurcates into the right and left common iliac arteries.

Abdominal Aortic Branches

- Celiac trunk, the first anterior branch arising 1 to 2 cm from the diaphragm, from which three vessels arise:
  1. the splenic artery
  2. the hepatic artery
  3. the left gastric artery

- Superior mesenteric artery, the second anterior branch arising 2 cm from the celiac trunk
- Right and left renal arteries, the lateral branches arising just inferior to the superior mesenteric artery
- Inferior mesenteric artery, the small anterior branch arising near bifurcation

Distribution
- Visceral organs
- Mesentery

Common Iliac Arteries
- The abdominal aorta terminates at the fourth lumbar vertebrae and divides into right and left iliac arteries.
- These vessels divide into internal iliac arteries and external iliac arteries.
- The external iliac artery extends down to the thigh to become the femoral artery.
- The portion of the femoral artery posterior to the knee is the popliteal artery, which divides into the anterior and posterior tibial arteries.

Inferior Vena Cava
- The inferior vena cava ascends retroperitoneally along vertebral bodies toward the right atrium.
- Caudal to renal vein entrance, the inferior vena cava shows posterior "hammocking" through the bare area of the liver.
- Proximal to the caval hiatus (T8), the inferior vena cava accepts hepatic venous drainage from three large hepatic veins.
- At the level of L4, the bifurcation of common iliac veins drains the lower half of the body.

Major Tributaries:
- Hepatic veins: right, middle, left
- Renal veins: right, left

Distribution:
- The inferior vena cava drains blood from all organs and structures into the upper and lower abdomen through its major tributaries.

MINOR ARTERIAL VESSELS
Anterior Branch of the Abdominal Aorta
Celiac Trunk
- Originates with the first 2 cm from the diaphragm
- Surrounded by liver, spleen, IVC, and pancreas
- Immediately branches into the common hepatic artery, the left gastric artery, and the splenic artery
  1. The common hepatic artery passes anterior to the portal vein to enter the liver through the porta hepatis. It consists of the left hepatic artery and right hepatic artery, which is subdivided as follows:

  a. cystic artery
  b. gastroduodenal artery (branches inferiorly, travels anteriorly to pancreatic head)
  c. right gastric artery
  2. The left gastric artery, the smallest of the branches, passes anterior and toward the stomach.
  3. The splenic artery, the largest of the branches, is very tortuous. It usually forms the superior border of the pancreas and divides into several branches to supply splenic tissues.

Distribution:
- Liver
- Spleen
- Stomach
- Duodenum

Superior Mesenteric Artery
- Arises 1 cm below the celiac trunk
- Runs posterior to the neck of the pancreas and anterior to the uncinate process, then branches into the mesentery and colon

Main Branches:
- inferior pancreatic artery
- duodenal artery
- colic artery
- iliocolic artery
- intestinal artery
- right hepatic artery possibly arising from the superior mesenteric artery

Distribution:
- Proximal half of colon (cecum, ascending, transverse)
- Small intestine

Inferior Mesenteric Artery
- Arises at level of L3 to L4 about 3 to 4 cm proximal to aortic bifurcation
- Main branches:
  left colic artery
  sigmoid artery
  superior rectal artery

Distribution:
- Left transverse colon
- Descending colon
- Sigmoid
- Rectum

Lateral Branches of the Abdominal Aorta
Phrenic Artery
- Small vessel clinging under surface of the diaphragm, which it supplies

Right and Left Renal Arteries
- Arise anterior to L1, inferior to SMA
- Both arteries branching into anterior branch and inferior suprarenal arteries
  1. The right renal artery is a longer vessel than the left and courses from the aorta posterior to IVC to RK. The renal artery passes posterior to the renal vein before entering the renal hilus.
  2. The left renal artery courses from the aorta directly to LK.

Gonadal Artery
- Arises inferior to renal arteries
- Courses along psoas muscle to respective gonadal area

Dorsal Aortic Branches
Lumbar Arteries
- Usually four on each side
- Travel lateral to posterior to supply muscle, skin, bone, and spinal cord
- Midsacral artery supplying sacrum and rectum

Terminal Branches
- See iliac artery under abdominal aorta section

MINOR VENOUS VESSELS
Lateral Tributaries to the Inferior Vena Cava
Right and Left Renal Veins
- Originate anterior to the renal arteries at respective sides of the IVC at the level of L2
  1. The left renal vein does the following:
     Arises medial from the hilus
     Flows from the left kidney posterior to SMA and anterior to the aorta to enter the IVC
     Is larger than the right renal vein
     Accepts branches from the left adrenal vein, the left gonadal vein, and the lumbar vein
  2. The right renal vein does the following:
     Flows from right kidney directly into the IVC
     Seldom accepts tributaries because the right adrenal and right gonadal enter IVC directly

Gonadal Veins (Testicular and Ovarian)
- Course anterior to external and internal iliac veins and continue cranially and retroperitoneally along psoas muscle until their terminus
  1. The left gonadal vein usually enters LRV or left adrenal vein, which further enters IVC.
  2. The right gonadal vein enters IVC anterolateral above the entrance of lumbar veins.

Suprarenal Veins
- The right suprarenal vein arises from the suprarenal gland and usually drains directly into the IVC.
- The left suprarenal vein arises from the suprarenal gland and drains into the left renal vein, which drains into the IVC.

Anterior Tributaries to the Inferior Vena Cava
Hepatic Veins
- Originate in the liver and drain into the IVC at the level of the diaphragm
- Collect blood from the following three minor tributaries within the liver: right hepatic vein (RLL), middle hepatic vein (caudate lobe), and left hepatic vein (LLL)

Portal Vein
- Forms posterior to the pancreas at the level of L2 from the junction of SMV and SV
- Courses posterior to the first portion of the duodenum and then flows between the layers of the lesser omentum to the porta hepatis, where it bifurcates into its hepatic branches
- Has a trunk of 7 to 8 cm in length
- Carries blood from the intestinal tract to the liver via its main branches, the right branch and the left branch

Tributaries:
- SMV
- IMV
- SV
- Left gastric vein
- Has **important anastomosis** with esophageal vein, rectal venous plexus, and superficial abdominal vein

Splenic Vein
- Is a large, tortuous vessel that arises from five to six tributaries from the hilus of the spleen
- Courses posterior to the pancreas to meet the SMV (at right angles) to form the main portal vein

Tributaries
- Pancreatic vein
- Left gastroepiploic vein
- Short gastric vein

Distribution
- Drains blood from stomach, spleen, and pancreas

Superior Mesenteric Vein
- Originates at root of mesentery, from distal half of duodenum to left colic flexure
- Courses inferior to right side and drains blood from each of the following:
  - middle colic vein (transverse colon)
  - right colic vein (from ascending colon)
  - pancreatic duodenal vein

• Joins with splenic vein posterior to pancreas to form portal vein

Inferior Mesenteric Vein

• Arises from left third of colon and upper colon and ascends retroperitoneally along left psoas muscle
• Drains several tributaries:
  • left colic vein (from descending colon
  • sigmoid vein (from sigmoid colon)
  • superior rectal vein (from upper rectum)

PATHOPHYSIOLOGY OF VASCULAR DISEASE
Aortic Abnormalities
Aortic Aneurysm
  Definition: a localized abnormal dilation of any vessel
  There are three important factors predisposing to aneurysm formation:
  1. Arteriosclerosis
  2. Syphilis
  3. Cystic medial necrosis

Arteriosclerosis
• Most common cause of aneurysms (97%)
• Usually in persons over 50 years of age
• Ratio of 5:1, men to women
• Involvement of aorta and/or common iliacs
• Sometimes involvement of ascending and descending aorta
• Possibly fusiform, cylindroid, or saccular
• Usual beginning below renal arteries and extension to bifurcation
• Fusiform or saccular dilations of common iliacs common

Classifications of Aneurysms
1. Berry aneurysm—small spherical aneurysm of 1 to 1.5 cm
2. Saccular—spherical and larger (5 to 10 cm)
   • Aneurysm connected to vascular lumen by a mouth that may be as large as aneurysm
   • Partially or completely filled with thrombus
3. Fusiform—most common
   • Gradual dilation of vascular lumen
   • May be eccentric so one aspect of wall more severely affected

Symptoms of Aneurysms
• May vary
• May produce symptoms by impinging on adjacent structures
• May be occlusion of vessel by direct pressure or thrombus
• May result in embolism
• May rupture into peritoneal cavity or retroperitoneum

Growth Patterns
• Normal lumen diameter is under 3 cm
• Ultrasound has 98.8% accuracy in detecting aneurysms
• From 3 to 5.9 cm; annual growth is 0.23 to 0.28 cm
• Under 6 cm—patients are followed at yearly intervals
• 75% of patients have 1 year survival if under 6 cm
• 50% of patients have 1 year survival if over 6 cm
• 25% of patients have 1 year survival if over 7 cm
• 75% risk of fatal rupture is present if over 7 cm
• 1% risk of rupture is present if under 5 cm
• Operative mortality rate before rupture is 5%, but with emergency surgery after rupture, mortality rate increases to 50%

Ultrasound Findings for Aneurysm
• Increased aortic diameter > 3 cm (measure of anterior aortic wall to posterior wall)
• Focal dilation
• Lack of normal tapering distally
  • Usually seen in large aneurysms as high-amplitude linear echo "line" along the surface of the thrombus; internal echoes are fine, very soft.
  • Thrombus usually occurs along anterior or anterolateral wall; old clot easier to see; calcification appears as thick, echogenic echoes, sometimes with shadowing.
• Presence of thrombus
• Occasional *aortic dissection* (Look for dissection "flap" or recent channel with or without frank aneurysmal dilation.)
  • Dissection of blood is along the laminar planes of the aortic media, with formation of a blood-filled channel within the aortic wall.
  • Patients are 40 to 60 years of age.
  • Males are more common than females.
  • Patients are hypertensive.
  • Hemorrhage occurs between the middle and outer thirds of the media.
  • Intimal tear is found in the ascending portion of the arch in 90% of cases, usually within 10 cm of the aortic valve.
  • Dissection extends proximally toward the heart, in addition to distally, sometimes to the iliac and femoral arteries.
  • Some blood may rerupture into the lumen of the aorta, producing a second or distal intimal tear.
  • Site of reentry most often is in the iliac, followed by neck vessels.
  • 5% to 10% of dissections do not have obvious intimal tear.
  • *Extravasation* may completely encircle the aorta or extend along one segment of its circumference, or the aneurysm may rupture into any of the body cavities.

- Types of dissections include the following:
    Type A: involves the ascending and descending aorta
    Type B: involves the level of the left subclavian artery, extending into the descending and abdominal aorta
- The cause may be **cystic medial necrosis, Marfan's syndrome,** and **hypertension.**
- Symptoms include excruciating anterior chest pain, with radiation to back, moving downward, and shock. (Approximately 15% of patients may have no symptoms.)

Pulsatile Abdominal Masses

- Masses other than an aortic aneurysm that can simulate a pulsatile abdominal mass include the following:
    - retroperitoneal tumor
    - fibroid mass
    - paraortic nodes

Other than an aneurysm, the most common cause of a pulsatile abdominal mass is a node, which is usually a result of lymphoma in persons who are 30 to 40 years of age. Symptoms may include fever, weight loss, and malaise. On ultrasound the nodes are seen as homogeneous masses surrounding the aorta. The aortic wall may be poorly defined because of the close acoustic impedance of the nodes and the aorta. The sonographer should also look for splenomegaly.

- Pancreatic carcinoma—appears as hypoechoic mass; may displace normal pancreas, may have biliary dilation.
- Retroperitoneal sarcoma—may initially appear as a pulsatile mass and may extend into root of mesentery and give rise to larger intraperitoneal component; echodensity depends on tissue type that predominates: fatty lesions are more echodense than fibrous or myomatous lesions.

Ruptured Aortic Aneurysms

- Classic symptoms include excruciating abdominal pain, shock, and expanding abdominal mass.
- Operative mortality rate for rupture is 40% to 60%.
- Rupture may be into perirenal space; displacement of renal hilar vessels, effacement of the aortic border, and silhouetting of the lateral psoas border at the level of the kidney may occur.
- The most common site is the lateral wall below the renals.
- Hemorrhage into the posterior pararenal space accounts for loss of lateral psoas that merges inferior to kidney and also may displace kidney. (Perinephric hematoma may displace kidney.)

Other Complications of Aortic Aneurysms

- Large aneurysms may compress neighboring structures (e.g., compression of the common bile duct results in obstruction; compression of the renal artery results in hypertension and renal ischemia; retroperitoneal fibrosis with aneurysm may have ureteral involvement)
- High aneurysm may be initially seen as a chest mass.
- Mycotic aneurysm may produce septic symptoms.

Aortic Grafts

- Sharp demarcation between native vessel and graft
- Ultrasound showing distinct, clearly defined borders
- Normal appearance of aortofemoral graft placed in end-to-end fashion that of a straightened discrete vascular channel with echogenic walls emanating anterior from the distal aorta; proximal anastomosis usually widened

Possible Complications of Prosthetic Grafts.
- Hematoma
- Infection
- Degeneration of graft material
- False aneurysm formation at site (pulsating hematoma connected to arterial lumen possibly seen with false aneurysm or pseudoaneurysm; communication of these hematomas with the lumen)

Aortic Branch Abnormalities

Celiac Artery Aneurysms

- Anechoic and spherical mass anterior to aorta, cephalad to pancreas
- Defined continuity with celiac axis

Superior Mesenteric Artery Aneurysms

- Secondary to pancreatitis

Splenic Artery Aneurysms

- **Caused by** atherosclerosis, infective emboli, infections, congenital factors, or trauma
- Seen in patients with portal hypertension and in females of childbearing age
- Are often seen with no symptoms
- Have **symptoms** that are vague, involving left upper quadrant pain to shoulder and nausea and vomiting
- Have an incidence of rupture of 8% to 46% with a high mortality rate, especially if the rupture is into the stomach
- Differentiate from the following:
    - pancreatic cyst
    - segmental dilation of pancreatic duct
    - ectasia of splenic vein
    - lymphadenopathy
    - gastric varices

Renal Artery Aneurysm

- Uncommon
- True (congenital or acquired) or false (false aneurysms arise from blunt or penetrating trauma)

Iliac Arteries

- **Origin** includes the following:
  - atherosclerotic
  - trauma
  - pregnancy
  - congenital abnormality
  - abdominal or pelvic surgery
  - syphilis
  - bacterial infection
- Approximately 50% of aneurysms in the iliac arteries rupture if untreated.
- Most are extensions of an abdominal aneurysm.
- Aneurysms may be isolated, usually bilateral, and 3 to 8 cm in diameter; they occur more often in men.

Arteriovenous Fistulas

- The majority are acquired secondary to trauma.
- Some may develop as a complication of arteriosclerotic aortic aneurysms.

Clinical Signs:

- Clinical signs include low back and abdominal pain, progressive cardiac decompensation, pulsatile abdominal mass associated with a bruit, and massive swelling of the lower trunk and lower extremities.
- Clinical signs are explained on the basis of the altered hemodynamics produced by a high-velocity shunt leading to increased blood volume, venous pressure, and cardiac output with cardiac failure and cardiomegaly.

Ultrasound Findings. If lower trunk and leg edema and a dilated IVC are present, an AV fistula should be suspected. If the fistula is large, the vein is very distended. A normal IVC is less than 2.5 cm. (Right-sided heart disease or failure may also cause IVC distention.)

Renal Arteriovenous Fistulas

- Can be congenital or acquired
- **Congenital** fistulas may be the crisoid type or the aneurysmal type.
- **Acquired** fistulas are secondary to trauma, surgery, or inflammation or may be associated with neoplasms such as renal cell carcinoma.

Ultrasound Findings. Multiple anechoic tubular structures feed the malformation with an enlarged renal artery and renal vein, confirming increased blood flow to the kidney.

- The fistulas may resemble hydropelvic or parapelvic cyst in association with a dilated IVC.

- **Diagnosis** made by identifying one or more channels entering the mass, suggesting that the lesion is related to renal vasculature.
- The sonographer should look for pulsations.
- Crisoid type of fistula has a characteristic ultrasound appearance of a cluster of tubular anechoic structures within the kidney; the crisoid fistula is supplied by an enlarged renal artery and drained by a dilated renal vein.
- In the aneurysmal type of fistula, a vascular lesion should be suspected when the presence of thrombus is noted in the periphery of a mass with a tubular anechoic lumen with pulsations.
- Occasionally, renal cell CA may be associated with AV shunting caused by invasion of larger arteries and venous structures.

INFERIOR VENA CAVAL ABNORMALITIES
Congenital Abnormalities

- The IVC is formed by three pairs of cardinal veins in the retroperitoneum, which undergo sequential development and regression. The posterior cardinal veins appear at 6 weeks and form no part of the IVC but may be part of the anomalies.
- The subcardinal veins appear at 7 weeks and produce the prerenal segment of the IVC.
- The supracardinal system at 8 weeks produces the postrenal segment of the IVC.
- The supracardinals form the azygos and hemiazygos system above the diaphragm.
- The anastomosis between the subcardinal and supracardinal systems forms the renal veins.
- The normal left cardinal system involutes, and the right is composed of the posterior infrarenal vein, supracardinal vein, renal segment, anterior suprarenal subcardinal vein, and the confluence of hepatic veins.

Double IVC

- The incidence is less than 3%—the size of the two vessels can be the same or may vary depending on the dominant side.
- The most common type is where the left IVC joins the LRV, which crosses the midline at its normal level to join the right IVC. There is no continuation of the left IVC above the LRV.
- Less commonly, the right IVC joins the left IVC to join hemiazygos.

Infrahepatic Interruption of the IVC

- Failure of union of the hepatic veins and the right subcardinal vein occurs and may be accompanied by azygos or, less commonly, hemiazygos continuation.
- Interruption of the IVC is associated with acyanotic and cyanotic CHD, abnormalities of cardiac position, and abdominal situs with asplenia and polysplenia.

- On ultrasound examination, the azygos vein continuation is identical to or larger than the IVC that passes along the aorta medial to the right crus.
- Hepatic veins drain into an independent confluence that passes through the diaphragm to enter the right atrium.
- Membranous obstruction of the IVC may simulate infrahepatic interruption of IVC with azygos continuation.
- A web or membrane obstructs the IVC at the level of the diaphragm and leads to chronic congestion of the liver, with centrilobular and periportal fibrosis.
- Three types of obstruction may be described as follows:
  1. thin membrane at the level of the entrance to the right atrium
  2. absent segment of the IVC without characteristic conical narrowing
  3. complete obstruction secondary to thrombosis
- Clinically, patients are 30 to 40 years of age and have portal hypertension.

Ultrasound Findings. Obstruction at the diaphragm and dilation of azygos system are seen.

Inferior Vena Caval Dilation

- In patients with right ventricular failure, the IVC does not collapse with expiration.
- Dilation may be caused by atherosclerosis, pulmonary hypertension, pericardial tamponade, constrictive pericarditis, or atrial tumor.

Inferior Vena Caval Tumor

- It is important to identify entire IVC; the distal vessel may be difficult to visualize because of bowel gas.

Hepatic Portion of IVC

- Masses posterior to this segment are right adrenal, neurogenic, or hepatic.
- With enlargement of the liver, the IVC is compressed rather than displaced.
- A localized liver mass would produce posterior, lateral, or medial displacement of the IVC.
- A mass in the posterior caudate lobe and right lobe may elevate the IVC.

Middle or Pancreatic Portion of IVC

- Abnormalities of right renal artery, right kidney, lumbar spine, and lymph nodes may elevate this segment.

Lower or Small Bowel Segment

- Lumbar spine abnormalities or lymph nodes would elevate the IVC.

Thrombosis and Tumor

Ultrasound Findings Single or multiple echogenic nodules are seen along the wall. The IVC may be distended and filled with the tumor.

- Most common tumor is renal cell CA, which is usually on the right.
- Wilms' tumor is also seen to extend into IVC.
- In a tumor with AV shunting, the renal vein may be dilated in the absence of venous extension of the tumor.
- Other less common tumors are retroperitoneal liposarcoma, leiomyosarcoma, pheochromocytoma, osteosarcoma, and rhadomyosarcoma.
- Benign tumors such as angiomyolipoma may have venous involvement.

Inferior Vena Caval Thrombosis

- Complete thrombosis is life threatening.

Clinical Signs

- Leg edema, low back pain, pelvic pain, gastrointestinal complaints, and renal and liver abnormalities

Inferior Vena Caval Filters

- Most common origin of pulmonary emboli is venous thrombosis from the lower extremities.
- Placement of transvenous filters into the IVC has been used to prevent recurrent embolization in patients who cannot tolerate anticoagulants.
- The preferred location of the filter is the iliac bifurcation, below the renal veins.
- Some filters can migrate cranially or caudally and can perforate the cava, producing a retroperitoneal bleed.
- Filters can also perforate the duodenum, aorta, ureter, and hepatic vein.

Renal Vein Obstruction

- Seen in dehydrated or septic infant
- May also be seen in adults with multiple renal abnormalities (nephrotic syndrome, shock, renal tumor, kidney transplant, trauma)

Clinical Signs

- Flank pain, hematuria, blank mass, and proteinuria associated with maternal diabetes and transient high blood pressure
- Faint or absent image of affected kidney on IVP

Ultrasound Findings. The ultrasound findings can be used to confirm a palpable mass in the kidney and to exclude hydrocystic and multicystic kidney as a cause of nonfunction.

- In infants, enlarged kidneys without cysts are seen.
- Medium or clumps of echoes randomly scattered within the kidney with surrounding echo-free spaces are present.
- Parenchymal anechoic areas are caused by hemorrhage and infarcts.
- The renal pattern progresses to atrophy over 2 months.
- Late findings include increased parenchymal echoes, loss of corticomedullary junction, and decreased renal size.

- *If the following are present on ultrasound examination, renal vein thrombosis can be diagnosed:*
  1. direct visualization of thrombi in the renal vein and IVC
  2. demonstration of renal vein dilated proximal to point of occlusion
  3. loss of normal renal structure
  4. increased renal size (acute phase)
  5. Doppler showing decreased or no flow

Clinical Signs

- pain, nephromegaly, hematuria, thromboembolic phenomena elsewhere in the body
- a variety of lesions possibly associated with this abnormality

Renal Vein Enlargement

- Left renal vein obstruction may result from spread of such nonrenal malignancies as carcinoma of the pancreas and of the lung and lymphoma.

- Retroperitoneal tumor may occlude the LRV by direct extension into the vein lumen or compression of the lumen by a contiguous mass.
- Renal vein obstruction may occur from thrombosis secondary to hypercoagulable state that accompanies certain malignancies—colon, pancreas, and bronchogenic CA.

Ultrasound Findings. Ultrasound findings include renal vein dilation, increased renal size, and loss of normal renal echopattern.

Superior Mesenteric Vein Aneurysm

- Rare occurrence
- Possibly involving the leg, neck, portal vein, or splenic vein
- If large, possibly compressing surrounding structures

Review Exercise • Vascular System

1. What is the function of the vascular system? _____
_____
_____
_____

2. Define the anatomic composition of the arteries and veins and their differences. _____
_____
_____
_____

3. Illustrate and name the five sections of the aorta. _____
_____
_____
_____
_____

4. Discuss the systolic and diastolic timing of the aortic leaflets. _____
_____
_____

5. Name the three arterial branches that arise from the superior wall of the ascending aorta. _____
_____
_____

6. Describe the course of the abdominal aorta. _____
_____
_____

7. Describe the flow pattern of the abdominal aorta at the following levels:
   Above the renal arteries: _____
   _____
   _____

   Below the renal arteries: _____
   _____
   _____

   At the level of the iliac arteries: _____
   _____
   _____

8. Name the major branches of the abdominal aorta.
   a. _____   c. _____
   b. _____   d. _____

9. What is the distribution of the abdominal aortic branches to the rest of the body? _____

_____

10. The common iliac artery divides into what two branches? _____

_____

11. The external iliac artery extends down the thigh to become: _____

12. What is the artery that extends behind the knee? _____

_____

13. What does the popliteal artery divide into? _____

_____

14. Describe the course of the inferior vena cava. _____

_____

_____

15. What are the major tributaries of the inferior vena cava, and what is their distribution? _____

_____

_____

_____

16. Name the branches of the celiac trunk and their distribution.

_____

_____

_____

_____

_____

_____

_____

17. Describe the Doppler flow pattern of the celiac axis. _____

_____

_____

18. Describe the Doppler flow pattern of the common hepatic and left gastric arteries. _____

_____

19. Describe the Doppler flow pattern of the splenic artery. _____

_____

20. Describe the pattern of the superior mesenteric artery, its branches, and its distribution. _____

_____

_____

21. Describe the Doppler flow pattern of the superior mesenteric artery. _____

_____

_____

22. Describe the flow pattern, branches, and distribution of the inferior mesenteric artery. _____

_____

_____

23. Describe the pathway and Doppler flow patterns of the renal arteries. _____

_____

_____

24. Describe the course of the renal veins. _____

_____

_____

25. What is the course of the gonadal veins? _____

_____

_____

26. Describe the course of the hepatic veins, their distribution, and Doppler flow pattern. _____

_____

_____

_____

_____

27. What is the formation of the portal vein? Name the tributaries, and describe the normal Doppler flow pattern in

the portal system. _____

_____

_____

_____

28. Describe the course, tributaries, and distribution of the splenic vein. _____

_____

_____

_____

_____

29. What is the origin and distribution of the superior mesenteric vein? _____

_____

_____

_____

30. What is the pathway of the inferior mesenteric vein and its tributaries? _____

_____

_____

31. What is the definition of an abdominal aortic aneurysm? _____

_____

_____

32. What are three important factors predisposing to aortic aneurysm formation? _____

_____

_____

33. Discuss the three classifications of aneurysms.

a. _____

b. _____

c. _____

34. Discuss the general symptoms and growth patterns found in patients with an aortic aneurysm. _____

_____

_____

_____

_____

_____

_____

_____

35. Discuss the ultrasound findings for an abdominal aortic aneurysm. _____

_____

_____

_____

_____

_____

36. What are the causes for an aortic dissection, and what are the symptoms and the ultrasound findings? _____

_____

_____

_____

_____

37. What are other abnormalities that may simulate an aortic aneurysm? _____

_____

_____

38. Describe the clinical signs and symptoms of a ruptured aortic aneurysm. _____

_____

_____

_____

_____

39. Discuss the complications of prosthetic aortic grafts. _____

_____

_____

_____

40. How does an arteriovenous fistula develop, and what are the clinical signs? _____

_____

_____

_____

41. What are the ultrasound findings of an arteriovenous fistula? _____

_____

_____

_____

42. Name the three types of obstruction to the inferior vena cava. _____

_____

_____

43. What are the clinical signs and ultrasound findings in a patient with inferior vena cava obstruction? _____

_____

_____

_____

_____

_____

44. What are some of the causes for inferior vena cava dilation? _____

_____

_____

45. Discuss the ultrasound findings seen in a patient with an inferior vena caval tumor at these levels:

Hepatic: _____

_____

_____

_____

Middle or pancreatic portion of IVC: _____

_____

_____

46. What is the most common tumor found in the inferior vena cava, and what is the ultrasound appearance? _____

_____

_____

_____

47. What is the significance of inferior vena caval thrombosis, and what are the clinical signs? _____

_____

_____

_____

48. Discuss the importance and significance of inferior vena caval filters. _____

_____

_____

_____

49. Describe the clinical signs and ultrasound appearance of a renal vein obstruction. _____

_____

_____

_____

50. What are the clinical signs and ultrasound appearance of renal vein thrombosis? _____

_____

_____

_____

Self-Test • The Vascular System

1. Which statement is *not* correct?

a. The umbilical vein may remain patent for some time after birth.

b. The ductus venosus becomes the ligamentum venosum.

c. The abdominal portions of the umbilical arteries form the lateral umbilical ligaments.

d. The foramen ovale usually opens shortly after birth.

2. What is the obliterated umbilical fetal vein?

a. The ligamentum teres

b. The faliciform ligament

c. The gastrosplenic ligament

d. The umbilical ligament

3. The portal veins carry blood from the _____ to the liver.

a. hepatic artery

b. intestine

c. splenic artery

d. peripheral venous system

4. The hepatic veins carry blood from the IVC to the liver (true or false).

5. The hepatic arteries carry oxygenated blood from the aorta to the liver (true or false).

6. Which arterial vessel shows the most turbulent flow pattern?

a. the hepatic artery

b. the cystic artery

c. the gastroduodenal artery

d. the splenic artery

7. The arterial supply to the gallbladder is via the:

a. hepatic artery

b. superior mesenteric artery

c. cystic artery

d. gastroduodenal artery

8. The portal vein does not drain blood:

a. out of the GI tract from the lower end of the esophagus to the upper end of the anal canal

b. from the pancreas, gallbladder, and bile ducts

c. from the spleen

d. from the kidneys

9. The portal veins become larger as they progress cephalad from the porta hepatis (true or false).

10. The portal veins course transversely through the liver (true or false).

11. The splenic vein runs along the superior, anterior margin of the pancreas (true or false).

12. What vessel passes anterior to the third part of the duodenum and posterior to the neck of the pancreas?

    a. the superior mesenteric artery

    b. the superior mesenteric vein

    c. the inferior mesenteric vein

    d. the splenic vein

13. The hepatic artery comes off the celiac trunk and courses to the right of the aorta at almost a 90-degree angle (true or false).

14. The head of the pancreas, the duodenum, and parts of the stomach are supplied by the:

    a. hepatic artery

    b. gastroduodenal artery

    c. splenic artery

    d. superior mesenteric artery

15. What vessel passes anterior to the uncinate process of the pancreas?

    a. the hepatic artery

    b. the portal vein

    c. the left renal vein

    d. the superior mesenteric vein

16. The distribution of the superior mesenteric artery is to the:

    a. distal half of colon, liver

    b. small intestine, proximal half of colon

    c. large intestine, distal half of colon

    d. proximal half of colon, stomach

17. The right renal artery passes anterior to the IVC and vertebral column (true or false).

18. The left renal artery passes posterior to the aorta (true or false).

19. The entrance of the inferior vena cava into the lesser sac separates it from the:

    a. hepatic vein

    b. portal vein

    c. splenic vein

    d. pancreatic vein

20. What vein begins at the hilum of the spleen and is joined by the short gastric and left gastroepiploic vein?

    a. the pancreatic vein

    b. the portal vein

    c. the splenic vein

    d. the superior mesenteric vein

21. Which of these statements are false?

  a. The portal vein is formed anterior to the pancreas.

  b. The portal vein enters the lesser omentum.

  c. The portal vein drains blood out of the GI tract from the lower end of the esophagus to the upper end of the anal canal, and from the pancreas, gallbladder, bile ducts, and the spleen.

  d. The portal vein has an anastomosis with the esophageal veins, rectal venous plexus, and superficial abdominal veins.

22. What vein originates at the root of the mesentery from the distal half of the duodenum to the left colic flexure?

  a. the portal vein

  b. the splenic vein

  c. the superior mesenteric vein

  d. the inferior mesenteric vein

23. What vein arises from the left third of the colon and upper colon and ascends retroperitoneally along the left psoas muscle?

  a. the portal vein

  b. the splenic vein

  c. the superior mesenteric vein

  d. the inferior mesenteric vein

24. Which statements are true regarding the hepatic veins?

  a. They are the largest visceral tributary of the IVC.

  b. They originate in the liver.

  c. They decrease in caliber as they flow into the IVC.

  d. They drain into the porta hepatis.

  e. They return blood from the liver that was brought by the hepatic artery and portal vein.

  f. The hepatic veins have three main branches.

25. The _____ is seen to flow directly from the renal sinus into the posterolateral aspect of the IVC.

  a. right renal vein

  b. left renal vein

  c. right renal artery

  d. left renal artery

26. The _____ leaves the renal sinus and flows _____ to the aorta and _____ to the superior mesenteric artery.

  a. right renal vein; anterior; posterior

  b. right renal vein; posterior; posterior

  c. right renal vein; anterior; anterior

  d. left renal vein; anterior; posterior

27. The normal diameter of the aorta is less than

   a. 2 mm

   b. 5 mm

   c. 3 cm

   d. 8 cm

28. The common iliac arteries arise at the bifurcation of the aorta and run downward

   and laterally along the medial border of the _____ .

   a. psoas muscles

   b. quadratus lumborum muscles

   c. piriformis muscles

   d. rectus sheath

29. The external iliac artery eventually turns into the femoral artery (true or false).

30. The internal iliac artery is crossed _____ by the _____ .

   a. posteriorly; ureter

   b. anteriorly; ureter

   c. anteriorly; iliac vein

   d. anteriorly; inferior mesenteric vein

31. Which are true statements regarding the celiac trunk?

   a. The trunk originates just below the SMA.

   b. The three branches are right gastric, splenic, common hepatic arteries.

   c. The splenic artery is tortuous and runs horizontally along the upper margin
      of the pancreas.

   d. The gastroepiploic artery is a branch of the splenic artery.

   e. The hepatic artery courses the upper border of the pancreatic head.

   f. The hepatic artery forms the lower boundary of the epiploic foramen.

   g. The gastroduodenal artery arises from the hepatic artery.

32. What is the portal triad composed of?

   a. portal artery, common duct, hepatic artery

   b. portal vein, cystic duct, hepatic vein

   c. portal vein, common duct, hepatic artery

   d. portal vein, cystic duct, hepatic artery

33. The superior mesenteric artery runs posterior to the neck of the pancreas, passing over

   the _____ of the pancreatic head anterior to the _____ part of the

   duodenum.

   a. uncinate process; third   c. lateral part; second

   b. medial part; third   d. middle; first

34. (Choose 2 answers) The distribution of the superior mesenteric artery is to the:

    a. distal half of colon, small intestine

    b. proximal half of colon, small intestine

    c. proximal half of colon, large intestine

    d. distal half of colon, large intestine

35. The inferior mesenteric artery distributes blood to the:

    a. left transverse colon, descending colon, sigmoid, rectum

    b. ascending colon, sigmoid, rectum

    c. descending colon

    d. ascending colon, rectum

36. The right renal artery passes _____ to the IVC.

    a. anterior

    b. posterior

    c. lateral

    d. medial

37. What is the difference between the course of the aorta and that of the inferior vena cava on a sagittal ultrasound image?

    a. The inferior vena cava moves _____ at the level of the diaphragm to enter into the right atrium.

    b. The aorta moves _____ at the level of the diaphragm.

    c. The _____ collapses and expands with respiration.

38. What will congestive heart failure do to the vascular system?

    a. decrease the caliber of the inferior vena cava

    b. increase the caliber of the inferior vena cava

    c. dilate the superior mesenteric artery

    d. increase the hepatic artery size

39. The aorta bifurcates at approximately L4 into the:

    a. right and left common carotids

    b. inferior and superior mesenteric

    c. right and left common iliacs

    d. left and right renals

40. At the point of bifurcation of the common iliac arteries and veins, which structure is more anterior?

    a. an artery

    b. a vein

41. The aortic diameter just proximal to the bifurcation of the aorta should be:

    a. 2.0 cm   c. 0.5 cm

    b. 1.0 cm   d. 1.5 cm

42. The superior mesenteric artery is larger in caliber than the superior mesenteric vein (true or false).

43. The vessel that arises from the anterior aortic wall and takes a parallel course to the aorta is the:

    a. hepatic artery

    b. renal artery

    c. superior mesenteric artery

    d. inferior mesenteric artery

44. The following specific "ultrasound signs" are used to describe each of the structures (listed in questions below) that are seen on the transverse scans:

    Mickey Mouse   *seagull*
    Playboy bunny   *white collar worker*
    reindeer

Fill in the next four blanks with the correct ultrasound sign(s).

    a. The common bile duct anterior and lateral to portal vein; hepatic artery anterior and medial:

    _____

    b. Hepatic veins drain into the inferior vena cava: _____

    c. Splenic artery, hepatic artery, celiac trunk arising from the anterior aortic wall: _____

    d. A distinguishing feature of the superior mesenteric artery: _____

45. What vascular structure courses between the aorta and the SMA?

    a. celiac trunk

    b. gastroduodenal artery

    c. left renal vein

    d. left renal artery

46. The middle branch of the left hepatic artery supplies what lobe of the liver?

    a. the right lobe

    b. the left lobe

    c. the caudate lobe

47. Renal arteries branch from the lateral wall of the aorta:

    a. at the level of L4

    b. superior to SMA

    c. inferior to SMA

    d. superior to hepatic arteries

48. The IVC can be found by sonography:

    a. to the left of midline

    b. only by experienced sonography technicians

    c. if there is plenty of overlying gas

    d. to the right of midline

49. The IVC courses anteriorly to enter the:

    a. right ventricle

    b. left atrium

    c. right atrium

    d. right coronary sinus

50. If there is an interruption of the IVC, what vascular structure will "take over" its job?

    a. the superior vena cava

    b. the azygos vein

    c. the lumbar veins

    d. the iliac veins

51. The _____ renal vein crosses anterior to the aorta in the crook formed by the SMA.

52. The _____ renal vein has a much shorter course than the _____ renal vein.

53. Label the following as arterial or venous:

    _____ a. collapsible tube caused by diminished tunica media.

    _____ b. carries blood away from the heart

    _____ c. carries blood toward the heart

    _____ d. has less muscle and elastic components to enable the vessel to expand

    _____ e. elastic tube

    _____ f. enclosed within a sheath

54. What are the three layers of the vascular structures?

55. The femoral artery is a branch of the internal iliac artery (true or false).

56. Which vascular structure passes anterior and toward the stomach?

    a. the superior mesenteric artery

    b. the superior mesenteric vein

    c. the gastroduodenal artery

    d. the left gastric artery

57. Which vascular structure arising from the celiac trunk passes anterior to portal vein to enter liver at porta hepatitis?

    a. the common bile duct

    b. the hepatic artery

    c. the superior mesenteric artery

    d. the gastroduodenal artery

58. Which structure is usually the superior border of the pancreas?

    a. the splenic artery

    b. the hepatic artery

    c. the superior mesenteric artery

    d. the superior mesenteric vein

59. What structure is the medial to inferior border of the pancreas?

   a. the splenic artery

   b. the hepatic artery

   c. the superior mesenteric artery

   d. the splenic vein

60. How can you differentiate thrombus from a reverberation artifact in an abdominal aneurysm?

61. What would an aortic graft look like on ultrasound examination?

62. How would you evaluate a patient for a thoracic aneurysm?

63. What is the rule-of-thumb definition for an abdominal aneurysm?

64. The distribution to the liver, spleen, stomach and duodenum is via the:

   a. portal vein

   b. celiac trunk vessels

   c. gastroduodenal artery

   d. inferior mesenteric artery

65. The gastroduodenal artery is a branch of the:

   a. left gastric artery

   b. splenic artery

   c. right hepatic artery

   d. superior mesenteric artery

66. The distribution of the proximal half of the colon and small intestine is via the:

   a. splenic artery

   b. inferior mesenteric artery

   c. superior mesenteric artery

   d. hepatic artery

67. The most common cause for abdominal aneurysms is:

   a. cystic medial necrosis

   b. syphilis

   c. atheroma

   d. arteriosclerosis

68. An aneurysm that is connected to the vascular lumen by a mouth that may be as large as an aneurysm is:

   a. fusiform

   b. saccular

   c. berry

   d. cylindroid

69. The most common type of aneurysm that has a gradual dilation of the vascular lumen is:

a. saccular

b. fusiform

c. berry

d. cylindroid

70. What percent of patients may survive an abdominal aneurysm under the following conditions?

_____ a. 1 year survival under 6 cm

_____ b. 1 year survival over 6 cm

_____ c. 1 year survival over 7 cm

_____ d. risk of fatal rupture if over 7 cm

71. What ultrasound findings would you search for in an aortic dissection?

72. Masses other than an abdominal aneurysm that can simulate a pulsatile abdominal mass are:

a. retroperitoneal tumor

b. hepatic cyst

c. pancreatitis

d. gas

73. In patients with lower trunk and leg edema and a dilated IVC, a(an) _____ should be suspected.

a. rupture

b. AV fistula

c. retroperitoneal tumor

d. infection

74. In patients with right ventricular failure, the IVC does not collapse with expiration (true or false).

75. With enlargement of the liver, the IVC is:

a. compressed

b. dilated

c. unchanged

d. thrombosed

76. A localized liver mass would produce what type of displacement of the IVC?

a. posterior, lateral, or medial displacement

b. anterior displacement

c. no displacement

d. inferior displacement

77. The most common tumor to fill the IVC is:

    a. islet cell CA

    b. renal cell CA

    c. venous angioma

    d. nephroma

78. The clinical signs of leg edema, low back pain, pelvic pain, gastrointestinal complaints, and renal and liver problems may represent:

    a. abdominal rupture

    b. retroperitoneal tumor

    c. IVC thrombosis

    d. superior mesenteric thrombus

79. The most common origin of pulmonary emboli is venous thrombosis from the lower extremities (true or false).

80. For a patient with renal vein thrombosis, which statement is false?

    a. Direct visualization of thrombi in the renal vein and IVC is possible.

    b. There is loss of normal renal structure.

    c. Renal size increases in the acute phase.

    d. Doppler flow increases.

Clinical Studies

1. Mr. Harry Johansen arrives at the emergency room with back pain that has progressed over the past 4 hours. An ultrasound of the abdomen is ordered. What questions would you ask Mr. Johansen before beginning the ultrasound examination, and what would you look for?

2. Brian Simmonds is a 21-year-old man who arrives at the emergency room with a pulsatile abdominal mass. He is sent to the ultrasound lab to rule out an abdominal aortic aneurysm. What would your differential diagnosis be?

3. Mr. Jack Daniels is a 65-year-old veteran who arrives at the hospital with a distended abdomen and elevated liver enzymes. He hasn't had a drink in 4 hours. What would you expect to find on the abdominal ultrasound examination?

4. Abe Lincoln was diagnosed as having Marfan's syndrome. What is the medical significance of this disease, and what structures would you want to investigate completely?

5. If problems occurred, what clinical symptoms might Abe Lincoln have?

Case Reviews

1. Identify all labeled structures in Figure 3-12.

a.   f.   k.

b.   g.   l.

c.   h.   m.

d.   i.   n.

e.   j.   o.

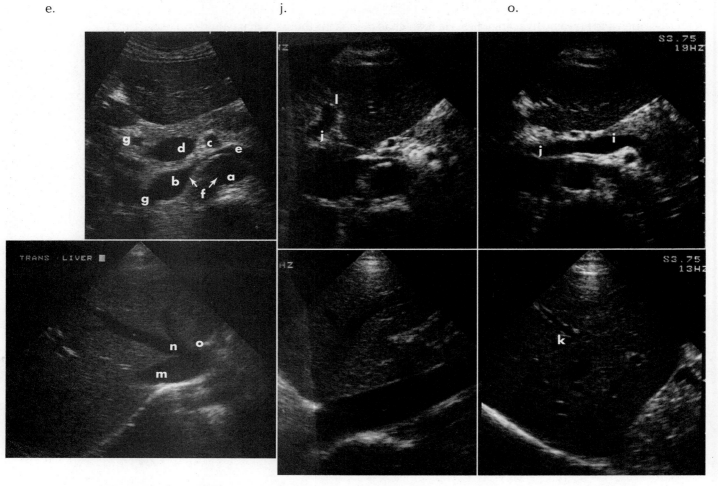

2. Describe the ultrasound findings in this 26-year-old patient who complains of fever, weight loss over the past month, and night sweats (Figure 3-13).

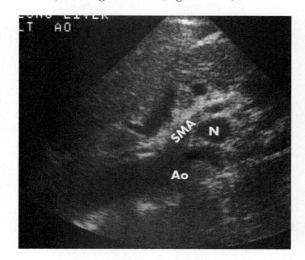

3. A 67-year-old man complains that he has had persistent leg pain over the past several months. He states that his leg pain decreases slightly when he elevates his legs. What significant ultrasound findings may lead you to his diagnosis (Figure 3-14)?

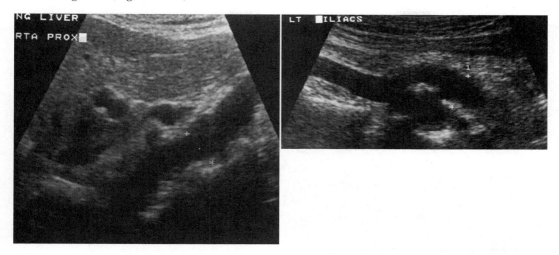

4. Describe this ultrasound view (Figure 3-15). What anatomy is visualized? Why would you attempt to obtain this view?

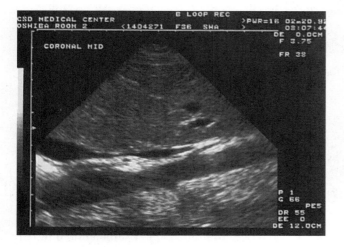

5. An asymptomatic 45-year-old woman comes to the hospital with a pulsatile abdominal mass in the area of the umbilicus. What are your ultrasound findings (Figure 3-16)?

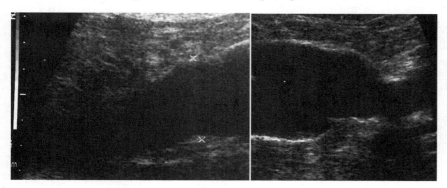

6. A 73-year-old man arrives at the hospital with a pulsatile abdominal mass. He states there is nothing to worry about because this mass has been there for the past 20 years. He is experiencing mild back pain, which is causing him discomfort during his tennis games. What are the ultrasound findings (Figure 3-17)?

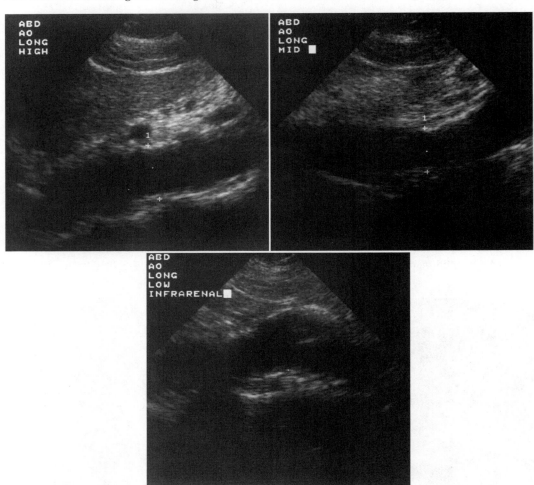

7. A 64-year-old man arrives at the emergency room in shock. He had a previous ultrasound examination 6 months earlier that showed an aneurysm measuring 5.7 cm. What would you look for and what would the ultrasound images show (Figure 3-18)?

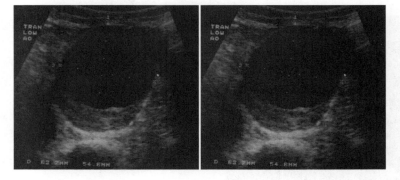

Answers to Review Exercise

1. As part of the circulatory system, the vascular system and the heart and lymphatics, transport gases, nutrient materials, and other essential substances to the tissues, and then transport waste products from the cells to the appropriate sites for excretion.

2. Construction of the three layers of arteries and veins is as follows:

    Tunica intima—the inner layer—single layer of endothelial cells with the longitudinal organization

    Tunica media—the middle layer—smooth muscle and collagenous fiber

    Tunica adventitia—the outer layer—thin fibrous layer surrounding elastic tissue

    Specific differences among arteries, veins, and capillaries are listed as follows:

    Arteries are hollow, elastic tubes that carry blood away from heart. They are enclosed within a sheath that includes an accompanying vein and nerve

    Arterioles are small arteries.

    Veins are hollow, collapsible tubes (caused by diminished tunica media) that carry blood toward the heart. The venous valves (extension of intimas) are semilunar type, which prevent backflow. There are numerous valves in the extremities, especially the lower extremities, caused by the flow against gravity. Venous return is aided by muscle contraction, valves, overflow from capillary beds, force of gravity, and suction from negative thoracic pressure. Veins have less muscle and elastic components, which results in the ability to passively expand; there is also a decrease in exertion of venous pressure.

    Capillaries are minute, hair-size vessels connecting the arterial and venous systems. They have only one wall. Cells and tissues of the body receive their nutrients from fluids passing through the capillary walls. At the same time, waste products from the cells pass into the capillaries. Arteries do not always end in capillary beds; anastomoses (end-to-end grafts between different vessels) provide equalization of pressure over vessel length and also provide alternate flow channels

3. The aorta may be divided into five sections: root of the aorta; ascending aorta; descending aorta; abdominal aorta; bifurcation of the aorta into iliac arteries

4. The root of the aorta arises from the left ventricular outflow tract in the heart and is comprised of three semilunar cusps that prevent blood from flowing back into the left ventricle. The cusps open with ventricular systole to allow blood to be ejected into the ascending aorta. The cusps are closed during ventricular diastole. The coronary arteries arise superiorly from the right and left coronary cusps.

5. There are three arterial branches that arise from the superior border of the aortic arch to supply the head, neck, and upper extremities: the right innominate artery, the left common carotid artery, the left subclavian artery.

6. The abdominal aorta continues to flow anterior to the vertebral column to the level of the fourth lumbar vertebra, where it bifurcates into the right and left common iliac arteries.

7. The flow pattern of the abdominal aorta depends on what level is investigated:

    Above the renal arteries: the aortic flow shows a high systolic peak and low diastolic waveform. There is a "window" in the systolic component. There is little turbulence in the aorta at this level; most blood cells are moving about the same velocity, which is known as "plug flow."

    Below the renal arteries: a small reverse component may be present during diastole. The reversal of flow becomes more obvious as the bifurcation of the iliacs is approached.

    Iliac vessels: show diastolic reversal of flow as a result of the high impedance of the peripheral circulation in the leg, thereby causing flow rebound up the distal aorta.

8. The major abdominal aortic branches are as follows:
    a. The celiac trunk is the first anterior branch and arises 1 to 2 cm from the diaphragm.
    b. The superior mesenteric artery is the second anterior branch and arises 2 cm from the celiac trunk.
    c. The right and left renal arteries are the lateral branches that arise just inferior to the superior mesenteric artery.
    d. The inferior mesenteric artery is the small anterior branch that arises near bifurcation.

9. The abdominal aortic branches distribute to the visceral organs and the mesentry.

10. The common iliac artery divides into internal iliac arteries and external iliac arteries.

11. The external iliac artery extends down to the thigh to become the femoral artery.

12. The portion of the femoral artery posterior to the knee is the popliteal artery.

13. The popliteal artery divides into the anterior and posterior tibial arteries.

14. The inferior vena cava ascends retroperitoneally along vertebral bodies to drain into the right atrium. Caudal to renal vein entrance, the inferior vena cava shows posterior "hammocking" through the bare area of liver. Proximal to the caval hiatus, the inferior vena cava accepts hepatic venous drainage from three large hepatic veins.

15. The major tributaries of the inferior vena cava are the hepatic veins: right, middle, and left; and the renal veins: right and left. The inferior vena cava drains blood from all organs and structures into the upper and lower abdomen through its major tributaries.

16. The common hepatic artery passes anterior to the portal vein to enter the liver through the porta hepatis. The other branches of the celiac trunk include the left hepatic artery; right hepatic artery; cystic artery; gastroduodenal artery, which branches inferiorly and travels anteriorly to the pancreatic head; right gastric artery; left gastric artery, which is the smallest of the branches and passes anterior and toward the stomach; and splenic artery, which is the largest of the branches, is very tortuous, usually forms the superior border of the pancreas, and divides into several branches to supply splenic tissues. Distribution is to the liver, spleen, stomach, and duodenum.

17. With regard to Doppler flow pattern, the celiac axis shows a small window under the systolic component with spectral broadening during diastole.

18. The common hepatic and left gastric arteries show a smaller systolic component than the celiac axis, with more spectral broadening during systole and diastole.

19. The splenic artery shows the most turbulent flow of all branches and may be related to marked tortuosity.

20. The superior mesenteric artery arises 1 cm below the celiac trunk. It runs posterior to the neck of the pancreas and anterior to the uncinate process, then branches into the mesentery and colon.
Main branches include the inferior pancreatic artery, duodenal artery, colic artery, iliocolic artery, intestinal artery, and right hepatic artery, which may arise from the SMA.
   Distribution is to the proximal half of the colon (cecum, ascending, transverse) and the small intestine.

21. The flow of the superior mesenteric artery may be more turbulent than in the celiac axis, but it loses turbulence in the distal segment. In the fasting state, a high impedance pattern of flow with little flow in diastole is seen; sometimes there is reversal of diastolic flow. After eating, a low impedance waveform with enhanced diastolic flow is present.

22. The inferior mesenteric artery arises at the level of L3 to L4 about 3 to 4 cm proximal to aortic bifurcation. Main branches include the left colic artery, sigmoid artery, and superior rectal artery.
   Distribution includes the left transverse colon, descending colon, sigmoid, and rectum.

23. The right and left renal arteries arise anterior to L1, inferior to SMA. Both branch into an anterior branch and inferior suprarenal arteries. The right renal artery is a longer vessel than the left; it courses from the aorta posterior to IVC to RK. The renal artery passes posterior to the renal vein before entering the renal hilus. The left renal artery courses from the aorta directly to the LK.
   With regard to Doppler flow patterns, there is a low impedance waveform with significant diastolic flow. A broad spectrum of velocities is present during systole and diastole. A continuous diastolic flow represents ongoing perfusion of the kidneys.

24. The right and left renal veins originate anterior to the renal arteries at respective sides of the IVC at the level of L2. The left renal vein arises medial from the hilus and flows from the left kidney posterior to the SMA and anterior to the aorta to enter the IVC. It is larger than the right renal vein and accepts branches from the left adrenal, left gonadal, and lumbar veins. The right renal vein flows from the right kidney directly into the IVC and seldom accepts tributaries because the right adrenal and right gonadal veins enter the IVC directly.

25. Gonadal veins course anterior to external and internal iliac veins and continue cranially and retroperitoneally along the psoas muscle until their terminus. The left gonadal vein usually enters the LRV or the left adrenal vein, which further enters the IVC. The right gonadal vein enters the IVC anterolateral above the entrance of the lumbar veins.

26. Hepatic veins originate in the liver and drain into the IVC at the level of the diaphragm. The veins collect blood from the three minor tributaries within the liver: the right hepatic vein (RLL), middle hepatic vein (Caudate lobe), and left hepatic vein (LLL).
   With regard to Doppler flow patterns, in both the IVC and the hepatic veins, the waveform is triphasic. This is caused by the flow of blood to the right atrium during atrial and ventricular filling, plus the reflux of blood from the right atrium during atrial contraction.

27. The portal vein forms posterior to the pancreas at the level of L2 from the junction of the SMV and SV. It courses posterior to the first portion of the duodenum and then flows between the layers of the lesser omentum to the porta hepatis, where it bifurcates into its hepatic branches. The trunk of portal is 7 to 8 cm in length. The portal vein carries blood from the intestinal tract to the liver via its main branches. Tributaries of the portal vein are the SMV, IMV, SV, and left gastric vein.
   There is important anastomosis with the esophageal vein, rectal venous plexus, and superficial abdominal vein.
   (Doppler wave form terms to know:
   hepatopetal = toward the liver; *hepatofungal* = away from the liver). The portal vein flows normally toward

the liver, which is a hepatopetal flow. It has a low velocity, continuous flow that changes slightly with variations in respiration. This change is absent in patients with portal hypertension.

28. The splenic vein is a large, tortuous vessel that arises from 5 to 6 tributaries from the hilus of the spleen. It courses posterior to the pancreas to meet the SMV (at right angles) to form the main portal vein. Tributaries include the pancreatic vein, left gastroepiploic vein, and short gastric vein. The splenic vein drains blood from the stomach, spleen, and pancreas.

29. The superior mesenteric vein originates at the root of the mesentery, from the distal half of the duodenum to the left colic flexure. It courses inferior to the right side and drains blood from the middle colic vein (transverse colon), the right colic vein (from ascending colon), and the pancreatic duodenal vein.

30. The inferior mesenteric vein arises from the left third of the colon and upper colon and ascends retroperitoneally along the left psoas muscle. It drains several tributaries: the left colic vein (from the descending colon), the sigmoid vein (from the sigmoid colon), and the superior rectal vein (from the upper rectum).

31. An aortic aneurysm is a localized abnormal dilation of any vessel.

32. Three important factors predisposing to formation of an aortic aneurysm include arteriosclerosis; syphilis; and cystic medial necrosis.

33. Classifications of aneurysms are listed as follows:
    a. *Berry aneurysm*—small spherical aneurysm of 1 to 1.5 cm.
    b. *Saccular*—spherical and larger (5 to 10 cm). This type of aneurysm is connected to vascular lumen by a mouth that may be as large as the aneurysm. A saccular aneurysm is partially or completely filled with thrombus.
    c. *Fusiform*—most common. This aneurysm is a gradual dilation of vascular lumen and may be eccentric so one aspect of wall is more severely affected.

34. The symptoms may vary. Symptoms may be caused by the aneurysm impinging on adjacent structures. An aneurysm may be caused by an occlusion of a vessel by direct pressure or thrombus. The aneurysm may rupture into the peritoneal cavity or retroperitoneum.

    With regard to growth patterns, the normal lumen diameter is under 3 cm. Aneurysms under 6 cm generally grow less than 3 mm per year. Patients with aneurysms under 6 cm are followed at yearly intervals.

35. Ultrasound findings for an aneurysm include increased aortic diameter > 3 cm (measure the anterior aortic wall to the posterior wall), focal dilation,

and lack of normal tapering distally, which is usually seen in large aneurysms as a high-amplitude linear echo "line" along the surface of the thrombus; internal echoes are fine and very soft. Thrombus usually occurs along the anterior or anterolateral wall; the old clot is easier to see. Calcification appears as thick, echogenic echoes, sometimes with shadowing.

36. The causes of aortic dissection may include cystic medial necrosis, Marfan's syndrome, and/or hypertension. Patients who have aortic dissection usually are 40 to 60 years of age, and may be hypertensive. Males more commonly have aortic dissection.

    Symptoms include excruciating anterior chest pain, with radiation to the back, moving downward; and shock. (15% of patients may have no symptoms). On examination of ultrasound findings, look for dissection "flap" or recent channel with or without frank aneurysmal dilation. Blood is dissected along the laminar planes of the aortic media, with formation of a blood-filled channel within the aortic wall. Hemorrhage occurs between the middle and outer thirds of the media. An intimal tear is found in the ascending portion of the arch in 90% of cases, usually within 10 cm of the aortic valve. Dissection extends proximally toward the heart, in addition to tally, sometimes to the iliac and femoral arteries. Blood may rerupture into the lumen of the aorta, producing another intimal tear.

37. Masses other than an aortic aneurysm that can simulate a pulsatile abdominal mass include the following: retroperitoneal tumor, fibroid mass, or paraortic nodes.

    Beside an aneurysm, the most common cause of a pulsatile abdominal mass is a node, which is usually a result of lymphoma in persons who are 30 to 40 years of age. Symptoms include fever, weight loss, and malaise. On ultrasound the nodes are seen as homogeneous masses surrounding the aorta. The aortic wall may be poorly defined because of the close acoustic impedance of the nodes and the aorta. The ultrasound technician should also look for splenomegaly.

    Pancreatic carcinoma appears as a hypoechoic mass and may displace the normal pancreas and have biliary dilation.

    A retroperitoneal sarcoma may present as a pulsatile mass and may extend into the root of the mesentery and give rise to a larger intraperitoneal component. Echodensity depends on the tissue type that predominates: fatty lesions are more echodense than fibrous or myomatous lesions.

38. The operative mortality for rupture of an aortic aneurysm is 40% to 60%. The rupture may be into perirenal space; there may be displacement of renal hilar

vessels, effacement of the aortic border, and silhouetting of the lateral psoas border at the level of the kidney. The most common site of a ruptured aortic aneurysm is the lateral wall below the renals. Hemorrhage into the posterior pararenal space may cause loss of lateral psoas merging inferior to the kidney and also may displace the kidney.

Classic symptoms of a ruptured aortic aneurysm include excruciating abdominal pain, shock, and expanding abdominal mass.

39. Complications of prosthetic aortic grafts include hematoma, infection, degeneration of graft material, and false aneurysm formation at the site of the graft. (Pulsating hematoma connected to arterial lumen may be seen with false aneurysm or pseudoaneurysm.) These hematomas communicate with the lumen.

40. The majority of arteriovenous fistulas are acquired secondary to trauma, although some may develop as complications of arteriosclerotic aortic aneurysms.

Clinical signs include low back and abdominal pain, progressive cardiac decompensation, pulsatile abdominal mass associated with a bruit, and massive swelling of the lower trunk and lower extremities.

41. On examination of ultrasound, if there is lower trunk and leg edema and a dilated IVC, an AV fistula should be suspected. If the fistula is large, the vein becomes very distended. A normal IVC is less than 2.5 cm. (Right-sided heart disease or failure may also cause IVC distention). Occasionally, renal cell carcinoma may be associated with AV shunting as a result of invasion of larger arteries and venous structures.

42. The three types of inferior vena cava obstruction include a thin membrane at the level of the entrance to the right atrium; an absent segment of the IVC without characteristic conical narrowing; and complete obstruction secondary to thrombosis.

43. Clinically patients with inferior vena cava obstruction are 30 to 40 years of age and have portal hypertension. Ultrasound findings show obstruction at the diaphragm and dilation of the azygos system.

44. In patients with right ventricular failure, the IVC does not collapse with expiration. Dilation may be caused by athersclerosis, pulmonary hypertension, pericardial tamponade, constrictive pericarditis, or atrial tumor.

45. The ultrasound findings seen in a patient with an inferior vena caval tumor at two levels are listed as follows:

Inferior vena cava tumor in the hepatic portion of IVC: Masses posterior to this segment are right adrenal, neurogenic, or hepatic. With enlargement of the liver, the IVC is compressed rather than displaced. A localized liver mass would produce posterior, lateral, or medial displacement of the IVC. A mass in the posterior caudate lobe and right lobe may elevate the IVC.

Middle or pancreatic portion of IVC: Abnormalities of right renal artery, right kidney, lumbar spine, and lymph nodes may elevate this segment.

46. The most common tumor in the IVC is renal cell carcinoma, which is usually on the right. (Wilms' tumor is also seen to extend into the IVC.) The ultrasound appearance includes single or multiple echogenic nodules along the wall. IVC may be distended and filled with tumor.

47. Complete thrombosis is life threatening. Clinical signs include leg edema, low back pain, pelvic pain, gastrointestinal complaints, and renal and liver abnormalities.

48. The most common origin of pulmonary emboli is venous thrombosis from the lower extremities. The placement of transvenous filters into the IVC has been used to prevent recurrent embolization in patients who cannot tolerate anticoagulants. The preferred location of the filter is the iliac bifurcation, below the renal veins. Some filters can migrate cranially or caudally and can perforate the cava, producing a retroperitoneal bleed. They can also perforate the duodenum, aorta, ureter, and hepatic vein.

49. Renal vein obstruction is a complication seen in a dehydrated or septic infant and may also be seen in adults with multiple renal abnormalities, such as nephrotic syndrome, shock, renal tumor, kidney transplant, and trauma.

Clinical findings include flank pain, hematuria, blank mass, and proteinuria associated with maternal diabetes and transient high blood pressure. An ultrasound can be used to confirm a palpable mass in the kidney and to exclude hydrocystic and multicystic kidney as a cause of nonfunction. In infants, enlarged kidneys without cysts are seen. Parenchymal anechoic areas are caused by hemorrhage and infarcts. Renal pattern progresses to atrophy over 2 months. Late findings are increased parenchymal echoes, loss of corticomedullary junction, and decreased renal size.

50. If the following are present on ultrasound examination, the diagnosis of renal vein thrombosis can be made:

Direct visualization of thrombi in the renal vein and IVC; demonstration of renal vein dilated proximal to the point of occlusion; loss of normal renal structure; increased renal size (acute phase); doppler shows decreased on no flow.

Clinical signs include pain, nephromegaly, hematuria, and thromboembolic phenomena elsewhere in body.

Answers to Self-Test

1. d
2. a
3. b
4. false
5. true
6. d
7. c
8. d
9. false
10. true
11. false
12. a
13. true
14. b
15. d
16. d
17. false
18. false
19. b
20. c
21. a
22. c
23. d
24. a, b, e, f
25. a
26. d
27. c
28. a
29. true
30. b
31. b, c, d, e, f, g
32. c
33. a
34. b, d
35. a
36. b
37. anterior; posterior; inferior vena cava

38. b
39. c
40. a
41. a
42. false
43. c
44. a. Mickey Mouse sign
    b. Playboy bunny, reindeer sign
    c. seagull sign
    d. white collar worker
45. c
46. c
47. c
48. d
49. c
50. b
51. left
52. right; left
53. a. venous
    b. arterial
    c. venous
    d. venous
    e. arterial
    f. arterial
54. tunica adventitia; tunica media; tunica intima
55. false
56. d
57. b
58. a
59. d
60. Thrombus within the aorta appears as smooth, homogeneous echoes, usually along the posterior aortic wall; reverberation echoes appear along the anterior

aortic wall as equally spaced linear echo reflections.
61. An aortic graft is very echogenic compared with normal aortic tissue.
62. The patient should be scanned posteriorly in an upright position, with the transducer just lateral to the vertebral column and angled toward the thoracic aorta.
63. An aneurysm is any abnormal bulging of the otherwise normal vessel.
64. b
65. c
66. c
67. d
68. b
69. b
70. a. 75%
    b. 50%
    c. 25%
    d. 75%
71. The dissection occurs along the aortic media, with formation of a separate blood-filled false channel.
72. a
73. b
74. true
75. b
76. a
77. b
78. c
79. true
80. d

Answers to Clinical Studies

1. It would be helpful to know if the patient was an alcoholic, if there had been any trauma to the abdominal area, or if he had experienced this type of pain previously. The sonographer should look especially for pancreatic disease.

2. The differential diagnosis for a pulsatile abdominal mass in a young male would be retroperitoneal tumor, lymphoma, or AIDS. It would be unlikely that the aorta would be dilated at this age, unless the patient had cystic medial necrosis.

3. The sonographer would carefully examine the right upper quadrant, especially the liver, gallbladder, and pancreas. Enlargement of the liver and spleen should be noted. Look for the presence of ascites. Evaluate the liver texture for signs of cirrhosis. Evaluate the thickness of the gallbladder wall and look for enlargement or calcifications within the pancreas.

4. Patients with Marfan's syndrome have cystic medial necrosis of their vascular walls, which causes the walls to become weak and aneurysmal, with dissection as a

complication. You would particularly want to investigate the entire aorta, from the root through the arch, down the thoracic aorta, and into the abdominal aorta.

Other arterial vessels should also be examined.

5. Abe may initially have severe back pain if a dissection were to occur.

Answers to Case Reviews

1. (Figure 3-12)
   a. aorta
   b. inferior vena cava
   c. superior mesenteric artery
   d. superior mesenteric vein
   e. left renal vein
   f. right renal artery
   g. right renal vein
   h. gastroduodenal artery
   i. splenic vein
   j. main portal vein
   k. right portal vein
   l. left portal vein
   m. right hepatic vein
   n. middle hepatic vein
   o. left hepatic vein

2. (Figure 3-13) The patient usually presents with hepatosplenomegaly on ultrasound examination. The parenchymal pattern of the liver may be normal or may show diffuse echogenic infiltrative changes. Look for additional masses in the spleen, retroperitoneum, and/or scrotum. Lymphoma masses usually present as hypoechoic.

   The enlarged nodes along the aorta and inferior vena cava may "simulate" an abdominal aortic aneurysm with transmitted pulsations. The nodes may be posterior, elevating the great vessels in an anterior direction, or completely surrounding the aorta and inferior vena cava, causing compression of these vessels. Color Doppler may be useful to help delineate the vascular channel when the vessel is compressed by the enlarged nodes.

3. (Figure 3-14) Thrombosis of the aorta usually occurs at the site of atherosclerotic narrowing of the vessel. In addition, an aneurysm is present, with progressive weakening of the aortic lumen.

   On the ultrasound, careful examination of the abdominal aorta should be made. If an aneurysm is present, analysis of the aortic wall should be noted to look for calcification and narrowing of the lumen. As the aneurysm increases, the normal lumen remains the same; therefore the blood "pools" along the pathway of low flow to cause accumulation of thrombus. The thrombus may appear as very low level echoes to hyperechoic echoes (over a period of time).

   Color Doppler is very helpful to delineate the normal lumen diameter and is useful to measure changes in the diameter over a period of time.

   The patient will have pain with the reduction in the size

of the aortic lumen (secondary to thrombus). This occurs as the resistance to blood flow increases.

4. (Figure 3-15) This is a coronal oblique view. The patient is rolled into a left lateral decubitus position. The transducer is longitudinal along the right midaxillary line. The plane of sector should bisect the right lobe of the liver, the inferior vena cava, and the aorta. Usually the renal arteries and veins are well seen in this view.
   a. aorta
   b. inferior vena cava
   c. right renal artery
   d. left renal artery

   This view is used to record accurate Doppler measurements for the renal artery and veins. It is useful to delineate the renal vessels when searching for thrombus or tumor formation.

5. (Figure 3-16) A fusiform aneurysm is the most common type of aneurysm found. It usually is located at the level of the umbilicus, at the site of the bifurcation of the aorta, well below the renal arteries. The sonographer should be careful to examine the walls of the aortic lumen to look for thickening and calcification. The presence of thrombus should also be evaluated. Analysis of both iliac arteries should be made to look for extension of the aneurysm.

6. (Figure 3-17) This ultrasound shows a large abdominal aortic aneurysm, measuring 6.0 cm in the widest dimension. It is important to evaluate this aneurysm in both A-P and longitudinal dimensions and to note its relationship to the renal arteries. If an aneurysm extends beyond the renal arteries, the occurrence of thrombosis of the renal vessels is increased (with resulting hypertension). The low back pain could be significant in detecting an early, slow leak in the aneurysm. Generally, the aneurysm should be symmetrical in shape, without a "double" lumen surrounding the aortic wall.

7. (Figure 3-18) Your first thought would be to rule out a dissecting aortic aneurysm. Bleeding occurs between the aortic intima and the media. This condition is commonly associated with atherosclerosis. On the ultrasound, first measure the maximum size of the aorta to see if there has been an increase in size. Look for irregularities around the wall of the aorta (irregular walls, double lumen, false channel, or flap of the actual dissection). Use color Doppler to outline the lumen of the vessel and to see if flow reversal occurs in the false lumen channel.

CHAPTER
4
The Liver

OBJECTIVES

At the completion of this chapter, students will show orally, in writing, or by demonstration that they will be able to:

1. Describe the location and size of the liver.
2. Describe the position, size, and boundaries of the lobes of the liver.
3. Describe the location, shape, and function of the four fossae of the liver.
4. Describe the formation and tracts of the vascular and biliary structures in the liver.
5. Illustrate the surface anatomy and internal anatomy of the liver and adjacent structures in cross-section and sagittal planes.
6. Explain the appearance, frequency, and significance of congenital anomalies (e.g., Reidel's lobe)
7. Explain the functions of the liver.
8. Select the pertinent laboratory tests and other diagnostic tests for liver evaluation.
9. Explain the function of laboratory and other diagnostic tests for liver evaluation.
10. Differentiate between sonographic appearances of the following diseases by explaining the clinical significance of masses that affect the liver:

   a. Focal anomalies
   b. Cystic lesions
   c. Congenital
   d. Infection and inflammatory lesions
   e. Benign neoplasms of the liver
   f. Malignant tumors of the liver
   g. Traumatic lesions of the liver
   h. Diffuse hepatic disease
11. Differentiate between the sonographic appearances of intrahepatic and extrahepatic biliary obstruction.
12. Describe the sonographic appearance by explaining the clinical significance of the liver secondary to congestive heart failure.
13. Create high-quality diagnostic scans that demonstrate the appropriate anatomy in all planes pertinent to the liver.
14. Select the correct equipment settings appropriate to individual body habitus.
15. Distinguish between the normal and abnormal appearance of the liver.

To further enhance learning, students should use marking pens to color the anatomic illustrations that follow.

LIVER

FIGURE 4-1
Anterior View of the Liver

Lobes of the Liver

The liver occupies almost all of the right hypochondrium, the greater part of the epigastrium, and usually the left hypochondrium to the mammillary line. It is divided into three regions: the right lobe, left lobe, and caudate lobe.

Right Lobe (FIGURE 4-1)
The largest of the three lobes, the right lobe is six times larger than the left lobe. It occupies the right hypochondrium and is bordered on its upper surface by the falciform ligament, on its posterior surface by the left sagittal fossa, and on its anterior by the umbilical notch. The inferior and posterior surfaces are marked by the fossae of three structures: the porta hepatis, the gallbladder, and the inferior vena cava.

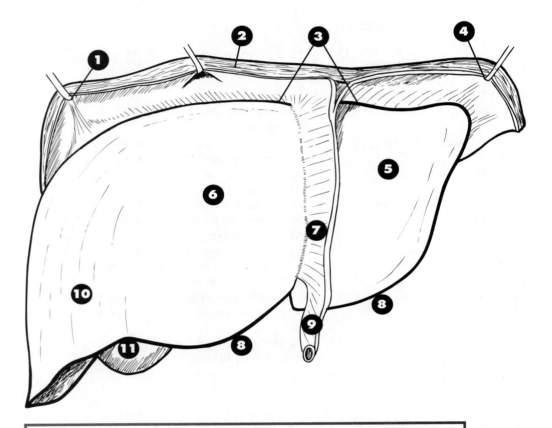

1	right triangular ligament	7	falciform ligament
2	diaphragm (pulled up)	8	inferior margin
3	coronary ligament	9	ligamentum teres
4	left triangular ligament	10	costal impression
5	left lobe	11	gallbladder
6	right lobe		

FIGURE 4-2
Superior View of the Liver

Left Lobe (FIGURE 4-2)
The left lobe lies in the epigastric and left hypochondriac regions. Its upper surface is molded onto the diaphragm. Its under-surface includes the gastric impression and the omental tuberosity.

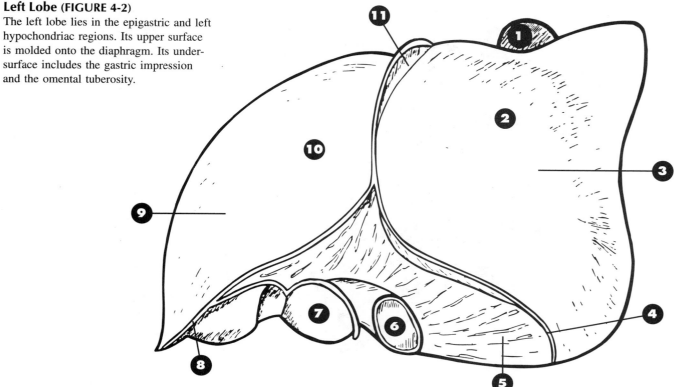

1	fundus of the gallbladder
2	right lobe
3	diaphragmatic surface
4	coronary ligament
5	bare area
6	inferior vena cava
7	caudate lobe
8	left triangular ligament
9	diaphragmatic surface
10	left lobe
11	falciform ligament

FIGURE 4-3
Posterior View of the Diaphragmatic Surface of the Liver

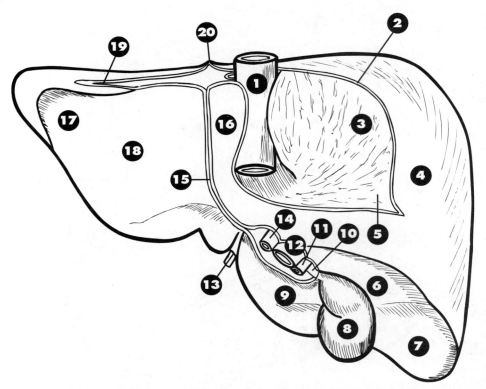

Caudate Lobe (FIGURE 4-3)

The small caudate lobe is located on the posterosuperior surface of the right lobe, opposite the tenth and eleventh thoracic vertebrae. It is bounded on the bottom by the porta hepatis, on the right by the fossa of the inferior vena cava, and on the left by the fossa of the venous duct.

1	inferior vena cava	12	portal vein
2	coronary ligaments	13	ligamentum teres
3	bare area	14	hepatic artery
4	right lobe	15	attachment of the lesser omentum
5	right triangular ligament	16	caudate lobe
6	renal impression	17	gastric impression
7	colic impression	18	left lobe
8	gallbladder	19	left triangular ligament
9	quadrate lobe	20	falciform ligament
10	cystic duct		
11	hepatic duct		

FIGURE 4-4
Vascular System of the Liver

Portal and Hepatic Venous Anatomy (FIGURE 4-4)

The portal veins carry blood from the bowel to the liver; the hepatic veins drain the blood from the liver into the inferior vena cava. The hepatic arteries carry oxygenated blood from the aorta to the liver. The bile ducts transport bile, manufactured in the liver, to the duodenum.

Main Portal Vein

The main portal vein approaches the porta hepatis in a rightward, cephalad, and slightly posterior direction within the hepatoduodenal ligament. It comes into contact with the anterior surface of the inferior vena cava near the porta hepatis

and serves to locate the liver hilum, where it divides into right and left portal veins.

Right Portal Vein

The right portal vein is the larger branch and requires a more posterior and caudal approach. The anterior division closely parallels the anterior abdominal wall.

Left Portal Vein

The left portal vein is more anterior and cranial than is the right portal vein. The main portal vein elongates at the origin of the left portal vein.

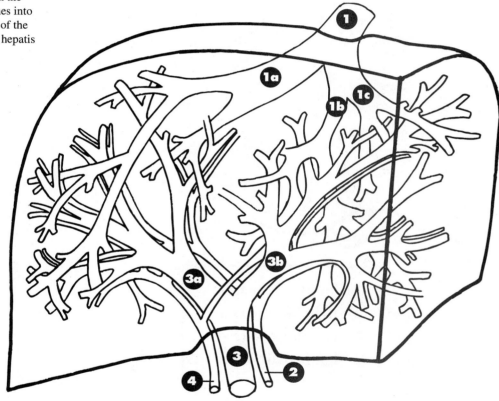

1	**hepatic veins**		**3**	**portal vein**
1a	**right hepatic vein**		**3a**	**right portal**
1b	**middle hepatic vein**		**3b**	**left portal**
1c	**left hepatic vein**		**4**	**bile duct**
2	**hepatic artery**			

FIGURE 4-5
Hepatic Veins

Hepatic Veins (FIGURE 77)

The hepatic veins are divided into three components: right, middle, and left. The right hepatic vein is the largest and enters the right lateral aspect of the inferior vena cava. The middle hepatic vein enters the anterior or right anterior surface of the inferior vena cava. The left hepatic vein enters the left anterior surface of the inferior vena cava.

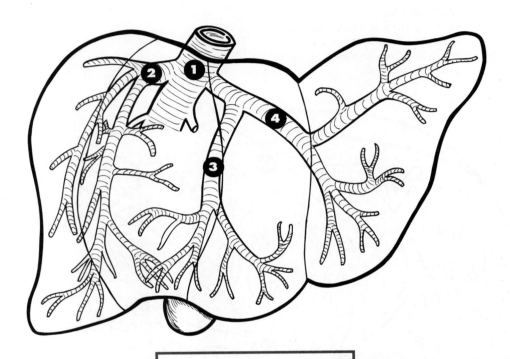

1	inferior vena cava
2	right hepatic vein
3	middle hepatic vein
4	left hepatic vein

FIGURE 4-6
Divisions of the Liver

Segmental Liver Anatomy

The liver is divided into two lobes, right and left, each of which has two segments (Figure 4-6). The right lobe is divided into anterior and posterior segments, the left lobe into medial and lateral segments. The caudate lobe is the posterior portion of the liver lying between the fossa of the inferior vena cava and the fissure of the ligamentum venosum. The caudate lobe receives portal venous and hepatic arterial blood from both the right and left systems.

Functional Division of the Liver

The purpose of a functional division is to separate the liver into component parts according to blood supply and biliary drainage so that one component can be removed in the event of tumor invasion or trauma.

The right functional lobe includes everything to the right of a plane through the gallbladder fossa and inferior vena cava. The left functional lobe includes everything to the left of this plane.

Ligaments and Fissures

There are several important ligaments and fissures in the liver. The falciform ligament extends from the umbilicus to the diaphragm in a parasagittal plane. Within this ligament is a round fibrous cord, the ligamentum teres, which is a remnant of the old umbilical vein. In the anteroposterior axis the falciform ligament extends from the right rectus muscle to the bare area of the liver.

The bare area of the liver is where the peritoneal reflections from the liver onto the diaphragm leave an irregular triangle of liver without peritoneal covering. The peritoneal reflection around the bare area is called the coronary ligament. The caudal part of the coronary ligament is reflected onto the diaphragm and the right kidney and is called the hepatorenal ligament. Below this is a potential peritoneal space, the hepatorenal pouch, (Morison's pouch), which is bounded by the liver, kidney, colon, and duodenum.

Both the falciform ligament and the ligamentum teres divide the medial segments of the left lobe. The fissure for the ligamentum venosum separates the left lobe from the caudate lobe.

Relational Anatomy

The fundus of the stomach lies posterior and lateral to the left lobe of the liver. The duodenum lies adjacent to the right and medial aspects of the left lobes of the liver. The pancreas is usually just inferior to the liver. The posterior border impinges on the right kidney, inferior vena cava, and aorta. The diaphragm covers the superior border of the liver.

Subphrenic Spaces

The right and left anterior subphrenic spaces lie between the diaphragm and the liver on each side of the falciform ligament. The right posterior subphrenic space lies amid the right lobe of the liver, the right kidney, and the right colic flexure. The right extraperitoneal space lies between the layers of the coronary ligament between the liver and diaphragm.

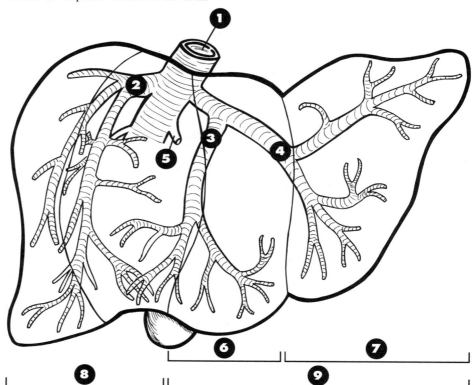

1	inferior vena cava	6	medial segment
2	right hepatic vein	7	lateral segment
3	middle hepatic vein	8	right lobe
4	left hepatic vein	9	left lobe
5	caudate lobe		

Liver Review Notes

GENERAL ANATOMY

- The liver is a segmental organ with well-defined vascular cleavage planes.
- The liver lies inferior to the diaphragm and is the largest and one of the most complex organs in the body.
- A single liver cell can carry on more than 500 separate metabolic activities.
- The right lobe of the liver is larger than the left.
- Each liver lobe is divided into thousands of microscopic **lobules,** which are the functional units of the liver.
- A lobule consists of several plates of liver cells.
- Oxygenated blood is brought to the liver by the **hepatic arteries.**
- The liver also receives blood from the **portal vein,** which delivers nutrients just absorbed from the intestine.
- Small branches of the hepatic arteries and the hepatic portal vein deliver blood to the tiny **hepatic sinusoids,** thereby allowing blood from the hepatic arteries and hepatic portal vein to mix.
- The liver sinusoids are partially lined with phagocytic Kupffer's cells, which remove bacteria, foreign matter, and weakened blood cells.
- Blood from the liver sinusoids is eventually delivered to the hepatic veins, which conduct blood toward the heart.

FUNCTIONS OF THE LIVER

The numerous functions of the liver include the following:

1. The liver secretes bile, which is important in the digestion of fats. **Bilirubin,** a pigment released when red blood cells are broken down, is excreted in the bile.
2. The liver removes nutrients from the blood.
3. The liver converts glucose to glycogen and stores it. When glucose is needed, the liver breaks down the glycogen and releases glucose into the blood.
4. The liver stores iron and certain vitamins.
5. The liver converts excess amino acids to fatty acids and urea.
6. The liver performs many important functions in the metabolism of proteins, fats, and carbohydrates.
7. The liver manufactures many of the plasma proteins found in the blood.
8. The liver detoxifies many drugs and poisons that enter the body.
9. The liver phagocytizes bacteria and weakened red blood cells.

LIVER SIZE AND SHAPE

- Dependent on the size of the lateral segment of the left lobe liver (LLL) and the length of the right lobe liver (RLL)

Left Lobe Liver

- The LLL is always smaller than the RLL.
- The LLL varies considerably in size and shape.
- The LLL may be congenitally small or atrophic, which may be a result of interference with the left portal venous supply when the ductus venosus closes at birth.
- The degree to which the LLL (especially the lateral segment) extends toward the left and the craniocaudal dimension are key features in ultrasonic visualization of the pancreatic region.
- The body habitus of the small LLL affects remaining abdominal structures (aorta, IVC, prevertebral vessels, and gallbladder) to be overlaid by the bowel.

Right Lobe Liver

- The length of the RLL determines the clarity of the right kidney in the supine position.
- The longer the RLL, the less likely the interference of bowel gas by the hepatic flexure.

Reidel's Lobe

- More commonly found in women
- Tonguelike projection of the RLL that may extend to the iliac crest
- Usually positioned anteriorly

PORTAL VEINS

Main Portal Vein

- The main portal vein (MPV) enters the porta hepatis in a rightward, cephalic, and slightly posterior direction within the hepatoduodenal ligament.
- The main portal vein comes into contact with the IVC.
- This point of contact of the portal vein with the IVC serves as a general indicator of the location of the liver hilus.
- The MPV appears elongated at the origin of the left portal vein (LPV).
- The major divisions of the right portal vein (RPV) and LPV course centrally within the segments (intrasegmental) and do not cross intersegmental divisions.
- This intrasegmental coursing is seen only at the bifurcation of the PV and represents a precise indicator of the porta hepatis location. The IVC is seen posteriorly. The elongation occurs in an anterior and cranial direction.

Left Portal Vein

- The LPV is smaller, more anterior, and more cranial.
- The LPV branches into medial and lateral segments.
- After branching from the MPV, the LPV moves cranially along the anterior surface of the caudate lobe and then abruptly turns anteriorly.

- The LPV extends branches to the caudate lobe and then divides into medial and lateral segments.
- The LPV travels within a canal that contains large amounts of connective tissue; this thick, echogenic linear band can be seen coursing horizontally through the lateral segment of the LLL.
- The LPV is in contact with the fissure of the ligamentum venosum.

Right Portal Vein

- The RPV is larger, more posterior, and more caudal.
- The RPV branches into anterior and posterior divisions.
- The course of the anterior division of the RPV is parallel with the anterior abdominal wall.

HEPATIC VEINS

Note: The major hepatic veins course between the lobes and segments (interlobar and intersegmental).

Right Hepatic Vein

- Largest hepatic vein
- Entrance to IVC at right lateral aspect
- Division of anterior and posterior segments of RLL

Middle Hepatic Vein

- Entrance at anterior or right anterior surface of IVC

Left Hepatic Vein

- Smallest hepatic vein
- Entrance at left anterior surface of IVC or directly into right atrium

Differences Between Portal and Hepatic Veins
- HVs—course between hepatic lobes and segments
- PVs—course within lobar segments
- HVs—drain toward right atrium
- PVs—emanate from porta hepatis
- HVs—increase in caliber toward diaphragm
- PVs—increase in caliber at level of porta hepatis
- PVs—have high amplitude reflections
- HVs—do not have high amplitude reflections
- PVs—course centrally within the segments
- HVs—course between lobes and segments

SEGMENTAL LIVER ANATOMY

RLL: anterior and posterior segments
LLL: medial and lateral segments

Fissures

Main lobar fissure
- The fissure divides the liver into true anatomic right and left lobes.
- The fissure is found in a line joining the gallbladder fossa with the IVC.

- The MHV courses within the main lobar fissure.
- This vein divides the RLL and LLL or the anterior segment of the RLL from the medial segment of the LLL.

Right Segmental Fissure
- This fissure divides the anterior and posterior segments of the RLL.
- The anterior and posterior divisions of the RPV course centrally through these segments.
- The RHV (transverse and sagittal) courses within the right segmental fissure and bisects the anteroposterior right portal dimensions.

Left Segmental Fissure
- The fissure divides the LLL into medial and lateral segments.
- The portion of the falciform ligament that contains the ligamentum teres hepatis courses in the caudal aspect of the left intersegmental fissure.

Left Intersegmental Fissure
- The fissure is divided into cranial, middle, and caudal segments.
- The LHV courses within the cranial aspect of the left intersegmental fissure and divides the cephalic portions of the medial and lateral segments of the left hepatic lobe.
- The falciform ligament (remnant of the fetal portion of the ventral mesentery) extends between the LPV and anterior abdominal wall.
  - Divides the caudal portions of the medial and lateral left hepatic segments.

Ligamentum Teres (obliterated umbilical vein)
- Runs in the inferior or free edge of the falciform ligament
- Seen transversely as a rounded structure generating high amplitude echoes and an acoustic shadow

Middle Third of Left Intersegmental Fissure
- The observed course of the LPV is as follows: Initially, it courses over the anterior surface of the caudate lobe and generally toward the patient's left side.
- Before the branches to the lateral and medial segments arise, the LPV makes an abrupt anterior turn; this occurs in the left intersegmental fissure and can be used as an indicator of the middle third of the fissure that divides the medial and lateral segments of the left lobe.

Caudate Lobe

- The caudate lobe is the posterior portion of the liver lying between the fossa of the IVC and the fissure of the ligamentum venosum.
- The proximal LPV courses over the anterior margin of the inferior caudate lobe, separating it from the more anterior left hepatic lobe.

Caudate Process

- The hepatic tissue extends obliquely and rightward from the inferior portion of the caudate lobe to the right lobe.
- This tonguelike process lies between the IVC and MPV and medial portion of the RLL.
- The caudate process may pass between the MPV and IVC.
- The fissure along which the ligamentum venosum courses is the most important of those structures useful in defining the caudate lobe.
- The left anterior margin of the caudate lobe is separated from the lateral segment of the left hepatic lobe by the intervening fissure of the ligamentum venosum.

Gastrohepatic Ligament

- This ligament inserts into the fissure of the ligamentum venosum.
- The caudate lobe is situated immediately posterior to where the gastrohepatic ligament inserts into the fissure of the ligamentum venosum.
- The left margin of the caudate lobe forms the hepatic boundary of the superior recess of the lesser sac.
- The caudate lobe lies cephalic to the bifurcation of the MPV.
- The posterior surface of the proximal LPV serves as an accurate anatomic boundary of the anterior caudate lobe margin.

Vascular Supply to the Caudate Lobe

- The right and left portal triads give off portal venous and hepatic arterial branches to the caudate lobe and receive bile duct tributaries.
- As the caudate lobe enlarges, the initial LPV segment shows increasing deflection from the course of the MPV.
- As the initial LPV segment courses over the anterior portion of the inferior caudate lobe, it divides into several caudate lobe branches before reaching the intersegmental fissure.
- The caudate lobe is drained by a series of short venous channels that extend directly from the posterior aspect of the caudate lobe into the IVC adjoining the posterior margin of the caudate lobe.

LIVER PHYSIOLOGY

The Liver and Bile in Digestion

Liver Structure in Relation to Bile Formation

- The liver is the largest gland in the body.
- The formation of bile is a major exocrine function.
- Each liver lobule is part of a hexagon in which the lobules are connected peripherally to incoming blood and centrally to a vein that drains the blood.

- The liver receives blood from two sources: the hepatic artery and the portal vein.
- The blood leaves the liver via the hepatic vein.
- The liver cells (**hepatocytes**) are packed in walls of cells that are separated by blood sinusoids.
- The incoming arterial blood and portal blood are mixed as they flow into sinusoids.
- Hepatocytes take oxygen and nutrients from this blood and then flow into the hepatic vein.
- Hepatocytes form bile and secrete it into small **canaliculi,** which coalesce to form first the smaller and then the larger **bile ducts.**
- In these ducts, bile flows in the opposite direction of blood to prevent mixing.
- The bile ducts coalesce to form the **hepatic duct,** which emerges from the liver.
- The hepatic duct bifurcates to form the **cystic duct,** which leads to the gallbladder and the **common bile duct;** together with the **pancreatic duct,** they empty into the duodenum.
- The **sphincter of Oddi** regulates bile outflow from the common bile duct into the duodenum. (When this sphincter is closed, the bile accumulates in the common bile duct, flowing back into the cystic duct and the gallbladder, where it is stored temporarily. After meals, the gallbladder contracts, releasing bile into the duodenum.)

Bile Composition

- The bile is composed of 97% water, bile salts and pigments, and inorganic salts (sodium chloride and sodium bicarbonate). All of the elements are produced by liver cells.
- Bile salts (or acids) are formed from cholesterol within the hepatocytes.
- To form bile pigments, bilirubin, which is the metabolite of heme formed during red blood cell destruction, is taken up from blood and conjugated to glucuronic acids to form the yellow bilirubin glucuronide.
- Most bile salts are reabsorbed by the intestines and delivered back to the liver; bile pigments are excreted with the feces.

Bile Function

- Only the salts play an important role. (Pigments are excretory products.)
- Typical bile salts are fat-solubilizing agents; they can mix with fat and water, thus increasing fat solubility.
- In the presence of bile salts, large fat droplets in the chyme become dispersed, forming smaller fat particles, a process called *emulsification.*
- Fats can be digested by the water-soluble enzyme **lipase,** which comes from the pancreas.

Metabolism of Proteins

Role of the Liver

- The amino acids within the liver cells form a pool that can be used to make the various proteins of the liver and blood in addition to glucose, fats, and energy (ATP).
- Amino acids can be exchanged with a second similar pool in the blood, which in turn exchanges amino acids with a third pool within the tissue cells.
- The liver is a major center for the synthesis and degradation of amino acids and proteins.
- The liver forms and secretes most of the blood proteins.
  - Albumin transports hormones and fatty acids and is responsible for plasma osmotic pressure.
  - Globulins are enzymes that transport hormones.
  - Fibrinogen is used in blood clotting.
- The amino acids in the liver can be used as fuel to obtain ATP; however, only during starvation are the amino acids catabolized as fuels.
- Ammonia is formed during the deamination of amino acids.

    Ammonia can be toxic to the liver or other tissues. The liver detoxifies ammonia by converting it into urea, which is a water-soluble substance.

Metabolism of Fat

Fat Metabolism in Liver

- The liver is capable of forming, degrading, and storing fats.
- The liver has the ability to achieve metabolic interconversion among fats, carbohydrates, and proteins.
- The liver (through fat metabolism) can make cholesterol and form ketone bodies.

Metabolic Physiology of Carbohydrates

Glucose and Liver

- Simple sugars freely enter the liver cells, where they are converted to glucose.
- The glucose pool in the liver can be easily exchanged with that in the blood. (Only the liver can actually release glucose; when the blood glucose level is low, the liver releases glucose into the blood; when the glucose level is high, the liver cells take up and store glucose.)
- Glucose in liver cells can be produced from other sources:
  - Proteins are broken down to form amino acids.
  - Deamination of amino acids leads to pyruvic acid, which can be converted to glucose by reverse glycolysis, a process called *gluconeogenesis.*
- Glycerol is liberated by lipolysis, which is a breakdown of triglycerides in the liver and fat cells.
- Lactic acid is usually formed in the muscles and delivered to the liver via the blood. In the liver, lactate is converted first to pyruvate and then to glucose through reverse steps of glycolysis.

Formation and Source of Blood

- The bulk of plasma proteins are manufactured by the liver; various sources in the body contribute other dissolved plasma constituents.
- Blood cells are formed mainly in the bone marrow.

Hormonal Regulation of Blood Sugar

- The liver is the major organ regulating the balance of blood sugar and carbohydrate metabolism.
- The liver has enzymes that convert glycogen to glucose, glycerol to glucose, and vice versa, and amino acids to glucose and the reverse.
- The liver cannot synthesize glucose from fatty acids.
- Through the portal vein, the liver has direct access to the carbohydrates absorbed from the intestine, which makes it the center for the synthesis, delivery, storage, and production of glucose.
- The liver has a special enzyme to free glucose and is the only organ that can secrete glucose into the blood when its level of this substance exceeds the blood level. This gives the liver the unique roles of glucose exchanger and glucostat.

LABORATORY DATA

Liver Function Tests

The term *liver function tests* refers to a group of various laboratory tests established to provide the clinician with an analysis of how the liver is performing under normal and diseased conditions.

In patients with known liver disease, a number of laboratory tests are used to help in the diagnosis. In addition to the clinical findings and abnormal blood tests, elevated urine bilirubin and urobilinogen levels may serve as clues to the presence of liver disease. A combination of serum tests is listed as follows:

1. Aspartate aminotransferase (AST or SGOT)
2. Alanine aminotransferase (ALT or SGPT)
3. Lactic acid dehydrogenase (LDH)
4. Alkaline phosphatase (Alk Phos)
5. Bilirubin (indirect, direct, and total)
6. Prothrombin time
7. Albumin and globulins

Aspartate Aminotransferase (AST or SGOT). AST is an enzyme present in tissues that have a high rate of metabolic activity, one of which is the liver. As a result of death or injury to the producing cells, AST is released into the bloodstream in abnormally high levels. Any disease that causes injury to the cells causes an elevation in AST levels. This enzyme is also produced in other tissues with high metabolic rates, and thus an elevation does not always mean liver disease is present. Significant elevations are characteristic of acute hepatitis and cirrhosis. AST is also elevated in patients with hepatic necrosis, acute hepatitis, and infectious mononucleosis.

Alanine Aminotransferase (ALT or SGPT). ALT is more specific than AST for evaluating liver function. Its level is slightly elevated in acute cirrhosis, hepatic metastasis, and pancreatitis. There is a mild to moderate increase in obstructive jaundice. Hepatocellular disease and infectious or toxic hepatitis show moderate to increased levels. (In alcoholic hepatitis, the AST level is higher).

Lactic Acid Dehydrogenase (LDH). LDH is found in the tissues of several systems, including the kidneys, heart, skeletal muscle, brain, liver, and lungs. Cellular injury and death cause LDH to increase. The test for LDH shows a moderate increase in infectious mononucleosis and mild elevation in hepatitis, cirrhosis, and obstructive jaundice. Its primary use is in the detection of myocardial or pulmonary infarction.

Alkaline Phosphatase (Alk Phos). Alkaline phosphatase is produced by the liver, bones, intestines, and placenta. It may be a good indicator of intrahepatic or extrahepatic obstruction, hepatic carcinoma, abscess, or cirrhosis. In hepatitis and cirrhosis the enzyme's level is moderately elevated.

Bilirubin. Bilirubin is a product of the breakdown of hemoglobin in tired red blood cells. The liver converts these byproducts into bile pigments, which, along with other factors, are secreted as bile by the liver cells into the bile ducts. Following are three ways this cycle can be disturbed:

1. An excessive amount of red blood cell destruction
2. Malfunction of liver cells
3. Blockage of ducts leading from cells

These disturbances cause a rise in serum bilirubin levels, which flows into the tissues and gives the skin a jaundiced, or yellow, color.

Indirect Bilirubin. Also known as *unconjugated bilirubin,* indirect bilirubin has elevated levels with increased red blood cell destruction, such as occurs with anemias, trauma from a hematoma, and hemorrhagic pulmonary infarct.

Direct Bilirubin. Also known as *conjugated bilirubin,* this product circulates in the blood and is excreted into the bile after it reaches the liver and is conjugated with glucuronide. Elevation of the direct bilirubin level is usually related to obstructive jaundice caused by stones or neoplasm.

Total Bilirubin. Specific liver diseases may cause an elevation of both direct and indirect (total) bilirubin levels, but the increase in the direct level is more marked. The diseases that cause elevation in total bilirubin levels are hepatic metastasis, hepatitis, lymphoma, cholestasis secondary to drugs, and cirrhosis.

Prothrombin Time. Prothrombin is a liver enzyme that is part of the blood-clotting mechanism. The production of prothrombin depends on an adequate intake and use of vitamin K. It is increased in the presence of liver disease with cellular damage, such as with cirrhosis and metastatic disease.

Albumin and Globulins. Depressed synthesis of proteins, especially serum albumin and the plasma coagulation factors, is a sensitive test for metabolic derangement of the liver. In patients with hepatocellular damage, a low serum albumin level suggests decreased protein synthesis. A prolonged prothrombin time indicates a poor prognosis. Chronic liver diseases commonly show an elevation of the level of gamma globulins.

Serum Tests Summary

The best method for diagnosing liver disease is a liver biopsy examination. Serum tests provide indirect information about hepatic pathophysiology. Significant elevations of AST and ALT may indicate marked damage to liver cells and suggest acute hepatitis, although increases in these enzymes may also occur in chronic liver disease. Prominent elevations of alkaline phosphatase and bilirubin (especially conjugated bilirubin) levels suggest biliary obstruction. Significant depression of serum albumin levels and prolongation of plasma prothrombin time suggest serious metabolic derangement of the liver. Elevation of serum gamma globulin levels raises the possibility of chronic hepatitis, cirrhosis, or both.

LIVER PATHOLOGY
Benign Neoplasms of the Liver
Mesenchyma Hamartoma

- Mesenchyma hamartoma are rare.
- These neoplasms occur in children under 2 years of age.
- They may enlarge to produce an abdominal mass.
- They are composed of well-differentiated ductal structures surrounded by loose mesenchymal connective tissue (probably lymphangiomatous in origin).
- Flow patterns seen on ultrasound examination are well-defined and predominantly anechoic with some trabeculation or transonic with a reticular, lacelike configuration.

Cavernous Hemangioma

- Cavernous hemangioma is the most common benign tumor of the liver.
- The incidence is 0.4% to 7.3%.

- Cavernous hemangioma is composed of a large network of vascular endothelium-lined spaces filled with red blood cells.
- Cavernous hemangioma is more frequently seen in women.
- A cavernous hemangioma may enlarge slowly.
- The liver is marked by degeneration, fibrosis, and calcification.
- Flow patterns seen on ultrasound examination are homogenous, echodense, and sharply marginated.
- Echogenicity is caused by multiple interfaces between the walls of the cavernous sinuses and blood within them.
- Some lesions are complex or anechoic with acoustic enhancement.
- Posterior enhancement is correlated with hypervascularity on angiogram.
- Approximately 73% of lesions occur in the right lobe of the liver.
- Cavernous hemangioma is located in a subcapsular position.
- Cavernous hemangioma is small (2 to 3 cm).
- Cavernous hemangioma has round, oval, or lobulated borders.
- The differential diagnosis includes hepatocellular CA, liver cell adenoma, focal nodular hyperplasia, and solitary metastasis.

Infantile Hemangioendothelioma

- The tumor is the most common symptomatic vascular liver tumor in children.
- Approximately 85% occur before 6 months of age.
- The tumor is more commonly seen in females by a 2:1 ratio.
- The tumor grows rapidly and then regresses gradually.
- Complications include thrombocytopenia, angiopathic anemia, gastrointestinal bleeding, and intraabdominal rupture with hemorrhage.
- The mass is round, smooth, multilobular or irregular, and well demarcated.
- Central areas are seen in large lesions of infarction, hemorrhage, fibrosis and foci of dysmorphic calcification.
- Flow patterns seen on ultrasound examination are hyperechoic, hypoechoic, and diffuse.
- Multiple lucent lesions vary from 1 to 3 cm, with few low-level and hyperechoic margins.
- Large veins that drain and dilated proximal abdominal aorta may be seen with arteriovenous shunting.

Focal Nodular Hyperplasia

- This rare, benign tumor is usually discovered by imaging.
- This tumor is more commonly seen in females under 40 years of age.

- There is an increased incidence with use of oral contraceptives.
- Patients usually show no symptoms.
- The tumor is located near the free edge of the liver (subcapsular).
- The tumor is solitary, well circumscribed, nonencapsulated, and multinodular.
- The tumor is composed of normal hepatocytes, Kupffer's cells, bile duct elements, and fibrous connective tissue.
- Multiple nodules are separated by bands of fibrous tissue, often radiating from a large central scar.
- Flow patterns seen on ultrasound examination are slightly less echogenic than the liver, hyperechoic, or may appear as a mass isosonic to the normal liver.
- Characteristics are similar to the surrounding liver.
- Dense, nonshadowing linear or stellate group of echoes in a solitary hepatic mass may be seen.

Liver Cell Adenoma

- Liver cell adenoma represents normal or slightly atypical hepatocytes that frequently contain areas of bile stasis and focal hemorrhage or necrosis but do not contain bile ducts or Kupffer's cells.
- The mass is solitary, marginated, and encapsulated.
- The mass is more commonly seen in females.
- There is an increased incidence with use of oral contraceptives.
- Patients exhibit symptoms.
- Palpable mass or severe RUQ pain is caused by rupture with bleeding into tumor.
- If bleeding occurs, the mass may be lucent or of a greater density than the liver.
- The mass often looks similar to focal nodular hyperplasia.
- This lesion has been reported in Type I glycogen storage disease (GSD); in GSD there is an 8% incidence of adenoma; in Type I GSD, there is a 40% incidence.
  - On ultrasound examination, the mass appears solitary or as a multiple hyperechoic solid lesion.
  - The mass increases in size and becomes heterogeneous with hypoechoic foci secondary to necrosis or hemorrhage.
  - Acoustic enhancement is increased.

Lipoma

- This rare, benign primary solid tumor is derived from mesenchymal elements.
- The tumor is nonencapsulated.
- The tumor is in continuity with normal liver.
- Flow patterns seen on ultrasound examination are hyperechoic (multiple fat and nonfat interfaces).
- A posterior shadow is seen as a result of diminished penetration of the sound beam.

Malignant Tumors

Hepatoblastoma

- Hepatoblastoma is a rare malignant tumor.
- Hepatoblastoma is seen in infancy and early childhood.
- The patient has abdominal enlargement with hepatomegaly.
- Calcification of the liver may be present.
- The alpha-fetoprotein (AFP) level is increased.
- Two types of hepatoblastoma are the following:
  1. Epithelial—sheets of cells resembling fetal liver cells or undifferentiated embryonal cells
  2. Mixed—epithelial, mesenchymal connective tissue and other elements, particularly osteoid tissue.
- Flow patterns seen on ultrasound examination are echogenic or cystic with internal septations.

Hepatocellular Carcinoma

- The pathogenesis of hepatocellular carcinoma (HCC) is related to hepatocarcinogens in foods, cirrhosis, and chronic hepatitis B viral infection.
- Approximately 80% of HCC occurs in livers with pre-existing cirrhosis, most frequently in those with post-necrotic or macronodular cirrhosis (13% to 23%) and alcoholic cirrhosis (3.2%).
- The overall incidence of HCC with cirrhosis in the United States is 5%.
- There are several morphologic patterns, including solitary massive tumor, multiple nodules throughout the liver, and diffuse infiltrative types. All of these cause liver enlargement.
- HCC tends to invade hepatic veins, producing Budd-Chiari syndrome.
- Thrombosis or tumor invasion of portal system is seen in 30% to 68% of patients with HCC; in 13% the tumor invades the hepatic veins and can invade the biliary tree.
- HCC sometimes destroys the portal venous radicle wall and invades the vessel lumen.
- The tumor grows within the vessel, with its blood supply coming from the capillary bed, surrounding vein, and/or adjacent bile duct.
- Patients have palpable mass in the liver, liver enlargement, unexplained mild fever, and signs of cirrhosis; HCC is suspected in a patient with cirrhosis who suddenly worsens or has a sudden, progressive enlargement of the liver with bloody ascites.
- Liver function tests show surprisingly little abnormality other than for cirrhosis.
- Approximately 70% of patients with HCC have elevated AFP levels.
- Flow patterns seen on ultrasound examination are discrete echogenic, discrete echofree, mixed, isoechoic, and diffusely infiltrative.

Metastases

- Metastases is the most common form of neoplastic involvement of the liver.
- Primary sites of metastases include the gastrointestinal tract (colon), breast, and lung.
- Dissemination of the tumor to the liver occurs via the portal vein, lymphatics, hepatic artery, and less frequently, by direct extension.
- There is usually enlargement of the liver.
- Typically there are multiple nodes throughout both lobes of the liver.
- Flow patterns seen on ultrasound examination are discrete hypoechoic, discrete echogenic, anechoic, and diffuse inhomogeneity.
- The majority of metastases are from a primary colon lesion (54%) and hepatomas (25%).
- There is a high correlation between hyperechoic metastases and colon CA.
- On follow-up after chemotherapy, assessments are made of any changes, progression or decrease in size or extent, and pattern changes.
- As metastatic nodules increase rapidly in size and outgrow their blood supply, central necrosis and hemorrhage are possible. Metastases may be distinguished from uncomplicated hepatic cysts by observing wall thickness, mural nodules, septations, and fluid to fluid levels.
- Metastatic sarcomas tend to undergo degenerative changes more frequently than metastatic CA.
- Calcification of metastasis corresponds to partial involution; it is always associated with polymetastatic hepatic condition and does not affect prognosis. This condition has an acoustic shadow on ultrasound examination. Carcinoma of the colon is most frequently associated with calcification.
  1. On ultrasound examination, most cases of hypervascular lesions correspond to hyperechoic patterns. The most common hypervascular masses include renal cell carcinoma, carcinoid tumors, choriocarcinoma, transitional cell carcinoma, islet cell carcinoma, papillary cell carcinoma of the pancreas, and HCC.
  2. Hypovascular lesions furnish hypoechoic lesions. These lesions also have necrosis and ischemic areas resulting from neoplastic thrombosis.
- Hepatic lymphomas have hypoechoic wave patterns on ultrasound examination.
- With both Hodgkin's and non-Hodgkin's lymphomas, wave patterns are hypoechoic and diffuse. (There is no correlation between the type of Hodgkin's lymphoma and ultrasound appearances.)
- With non-Hodgkin's lymphoma, there are target and echogenic wave patterns.
- With Burkitt's lymphoma, intrahepatic lucent is seen.

- With leukemia, wave patterns show multiple discrete hepatic masses; e.g., they are solid with no acoustic enhancements. Many may have a "bulls-eye" appearance, with a dense center resulting from necrosis.
- In children, the most common forms of metastases are neuroblastoma, Wilms' tumor, and leukemia.
  - On ultrasound examination, neuroblastoma shows a densely reflective pattern with liver involvement similar to hepatoma, hepatoblastoma, and Wilms' tumor. (In Wilms' tumor, the lungs are involved.)
  - Wilms' tumor shows a densely reflective pattern, often with lucencies resulting from necrosis or hypoechoic lesions.
  - Metastatic adenocarcinoma is unusual in children.

Diffuse Disease

- Hepatocellular disease affects the hepatocytes and interferes with liver function enzymes.
- Diffuse hepatocellular disease affects the hepatocytes and interferes with liver function.
- The hepatocyte is a parenchymal liver cell that performs all the functions ascribed to the liver.
- A measurement of this abnormality is done through the series of liver function tests.
- The hepatic enzyme levels are elevated with cell necrosis.
- With cholestasis (interruption in the flow of bile through any part of the biliary system, from the liver to the duodenum), the alkaline phosphatase and direct bilirubin levels increase.
- Likewise, when there are defects in protein synthesis, there may be elevated serum bilirubin levels and decreased serum albumin and clotting factor levels.
- Fatty infiltration implies increased lipid accumulation in the hepatocytes and is the result of significant injury to the liver or a systemic disorder leading to impaired or excessive metabolism of fat.
- Fatty infiltration is a benign process and may be reversible.
- Common causes of fatty liver include the following: alcoholic liver disease, diabetes mellitus, obesity, severe hepatitis, chronic illness, and steroids.
- Moderate to severe fatty infiltration shows increased echogenicity on ultrasound examination.
- Enlargement of the lobe affected by the fatty infiltration is evident.
- Visualization of the portal vein structures may be difficult because of the increased attenuation of the ultrasound.
- Thus it becomes more difficult to see the outline of the portal vein and hepatic vein borders.
- Following are the three grades of liver texture that have been defined in sonography for classification of fatty infiltration:

- Grade 1: There is a slight diffuse increase in fine echoes in the hepatic parenchyma, with normal visualization of the diaphragm and intrahepatic vessel borders.
- Grade 2: There is a moderate diffuse increase in fine echoes with slightly impaired visualization of the intrahepatic vessels and diaphragm.
- Grade 3: There is a marked increase in fine echoes with poor or no visualization of the intrahepatic vessel borders, diaphragm, and posterior portion of the right lobe of the liver.
- Fatty infiltration is not always uniform throughout the liver parenchyma.
- It is not uncommon to see a patchy distribution of fat, especially in the right lobe of the liver.
- The fat does not displace normal vascular architecture.
- The other characteristic of fatty infiltration is focal sparing.
- This condition should be suspected in patients who have masslike hypoechoic areas in typical locations in a liver that is otherwise increased in echogenicity.
- The most common areas of focal sparing are anterior to the gallbladder or the portal vein, and the posterior portion of the left lobe of the liver.
- Patients with hepatitis may initially present with flu and gastrointestinal symptoms, including loss of appetite, nausea, vomiting, and fatigue.
- Jaundice may occur in severe cases of hepatitis.
- Lab values show abnormal liver function tests, with an increase in the ASP, AST, and bilirubin.

Acute Hepatitis

- In acute hepatitis, damage to the liver may range from a mild disease to massive necrosis and liver failure.
- Hepatosplenomegaly is present, and the gallbladder wall is thickened.

Chronic Hepatitis

- Chronic hepatitis exists when there is clinical or biochemical evidence of hepatic inflammation for at least 3 to 6 months.
- Chronic persistent hepatitis is a benign, self-limiting process.
- Chronic active hepatitis usually progresses to cirrhosis and liver failure.
- On ultrasound examination, the liver parenchyma is coarse, with decreased brightness of the portal triads; however, the degree of attenuation is not as great as seen in fatty infiltration.
- The liver does not increase in size with chronic hepatitis.
- Fibrosis may be evident, which may produce soft shadowing posteriorly.

Cirrhosis
- The essential features of cirrhosis are simultaneous parenchymal necrosis, regeneration, and diffuse fibrosis, resulting in disorganization of lobular architecture.
- The disease process is chronic and progressive, with liver cell failure and portal hypertension as the end stage.
- Cirrhosis is most commonly the result of chronic alcohol abuse but can be the result of nutritional deprivation, hepatitis, or other infection.
- The diagnosis of cirrhosis by ultrasound examination may be difficult.
- Specific findings may show coarsening of the liver parenchyma secondary to fibrosis and nodularity.
- Increased attenuation may be present, with decreased vascular markings.
- Hepatosplenomegaly may be present, with ascites surrounding the liver.
- Chronic cirrhosis may show nodularity of the liver edge, especially if ascites is present.
- The hepatic fissures may be accentuated.
- The isoechoic regenerating nodules may be seen throughout the liver parenchyma.
- Portal hypertension may be present with or without abnormal Doppler flow patterns.
- Patients who have cirrhosis have an increased incidence of developing hepatoma tumors within the liver parenchyma.

Biliary Obstruction Proximal to the Cystic Duct
- Biliary obstruction proximal to the cystic duct can be caused by carcinoma of the common bile duct, or of metastatic tumor invasion of the porta hepatis.
- Clinically the patient may be jaundiced, and may experience pruritus (itching).
- The liver function tests would show an elevation in the direct bilirubin and alkaline phosphatase levels.
- On a sonogram, carcinoma of the common bile duct would appear as a tubular branching with dilated intrahepatic ducts that are best seen in the periphery of the liver.
- It may be difficult to image a discrete mass lesion.
- The gallbladder is of normal size, even after a fatty meal is administered.

Biliary Obstruction Distal to the Cystic Duct
- A biliary obstruction distal to the cystic duct may be caused by stones in the common duct, an extrahepatic mass in the porta hepatis, or stricture of the common duct.
- Clinically, common duct stones cause right upper quadrant pain, jaundice, pruritus, and an increase in direct bilirubin and alkaline phosphatase.
- On ultrasound examination, the dilated intrahepatic ducts are seen in the periphery of the liver.

- The size of the gallbladder is variable, but it is usually small.
- Gallstones are often present and appear as hyperechoic lesions along the posterior floor of the gallbladder, with a sharp posterior acoustic shadow.
- Careful evaluation of the common duct may show shadowy stones within the dilated duct.

Extrahepatic Mass
- An extrahepatic mass in the area of the porta hepatis would cause the same clinical signs as biliary obstruction.
- On ultrasound examination, an irregular, ill defined, hypoechoic, and inhomogeneous lesion may be seen in the area of the porta hepatis.
- There is intrahepatic ductal dilation with a hydropic gallbladder.
- The lesion may arise from the lymph nodes or from pancreatitis, pseudocyst, or carcinoma in the head of the pancreas.

Amebic Abscess
- An amebic abscess is a collection of pus formed by disintegrated tissue in a cavity, usually in the liver, caused by the protozoan parasite *Entamoeba histolytica*.
- The infection is primarily a disease of the colon but can spread to the liver, lungs, and brain.
- Amebiasis is contracted by ingesting the cysts through contaminated water and food.
- The amebic parasites reach the liver parenchyma via the portal vein.
- The amebae usually affect the colon and cecum, and the parasitic organism remains within the gastrointestinal tract.
- If the organism invades the colon mucosa, it may travel to the liver via the portal venous system.
- Patients may not show symptoms or may have gastrointestinal symptoms such as abdominal pain, diarrhea, leukocytosis, and low fever.
- The ultrasound appearance of amebic abscess is variable and nonspecific.
- The abscess may be round or oval and may have a lack of significantly defined wall echoes.
- The lesion is hypoechoic compared with normal liver parenchyma and may show low-level echoes at higher sensitivity.
- There may be some internal echoes along the posterior margin secondary to debris.
- Distal enhancement may be seen beyond the lesion.
- Some organisms may rupture through the diaphragm into the hepatic capsule.

Echinococcal Cyst of the Liver
- Hepatic echinococcosis is an infectious cystic disease that is common in sheepherding areas of the world but is seldom encountered within the United States.

- On ultrasound examination, several patterns may occur, from a simple cyst to a complex mass with acoustic enhancement.
- The shape of the cyst may be oval or spherical, and may have regularity of the walls. Calcifications may occur.
- Septations are very frequent; e.g., there is a honeycomb appearance with fluid collections; water lily sign, which shows a detachment and collapse of the germinal layer; or cyst within a cyst.

- Sometimes the liver may contain multiple parent cysts in both lobes of the liver; the cyst with the thick walls occupies a different part of the liver.
- The tissue between the cysts indicates that each cyst is a separate parent cyst and not a daughter cyst.
- If a daughter cyst is found, it is specific for echinococcal disease.

Review Exercise A • Liver Physiology

1. What is the largest gland in the body? _____

   _____

   _____

2. The formation of bile is a major _____ function. _____

3. Name the two sources that supply blood to the liver. _____

   _____

   _____

4. How does the blood leave the liver? _____

   _____

5. What is the name of the liver cells? _____

   _____

   _____

6. Describe the pathway of the blood as it flows into the liver. _____

   _____

   _____

7. Trace the path of bile after the hepatocytes form bile in the liver. _____

   _____

   _____

8. What is the function of the sphincter of Oddi? _____

   _____

   _____

   _____

9. What is the composition of bile? _____

   _____

   _____

   _____

   _____

10. Describe the role of the liver in the metabolism of proteins. _____

    _____

    _____

    _____

11. Discuss the role of fat metabolism in the liver. _____

    _____

    _____

    _____

12. What is the metabolic physiology of carbohydrates in the liver? _____

_____

_____

_____

13. What is the role of the liver in the formation and source of blood? _____

_____

_____

_____

_____

14. What role does the liver play in the hormonal regulation of blood sugar? _____

_____

_____

_____

_____

Review Exercise B • Laboratory Tests for the Liver

Questions 1 to 5: define the terms and their functions in detecting liver disease.

1. AST (SGOT): _____

_____

_____

2. ASP (SGPT): _____

_____

_____

3. LDH: _____

_____

_____

4. Alkaline phosphatase: _____

_____

_____

5. Bilirubin (indirect and direct): _____

_____

_____

_____

6. What diseases cause an elevation of both direct and indirect bilirubin? _____

_____

_____

Review Exercise C • Pathology of the Liver

1. What does an ultrasound evaluation of the liver parenchyma include? _____

_____

_____

_____

_____

2. What happens to the hepatic parenchyma pattern with disease? _____

_____

_____

_____

3. How does diffuse hepatocellular disease affect the hepatocytes in the liver? _____

_____

_____

_____

_____

4. What is the effect of fatty infiltration on the liver? _____

_____

_____

_____

_____

_____

_____

5. Name the common causes of fatty liver. _____

_____

_____

6. Describe the ultrasound appearance of fatty infiltration of the liver. _____

_____

_____

_____

7. Name the three grades of liver texture defined in sonography for classifying fatty infiltration. _____

_____

_____

8. Describe the clinical findings in a patient with hepatitis. _____

_____

_____

_____

9. Describe the difference between acute and chronic hepatitis. _____

_____

_____

_____

10. What is the ultrasound appearance of hepatitis? _____

_____

_____

_____

11. Describe the complications of cirrhosis of the liver. _____

_____

_____

_____

12. Discuss the ultrasound findings of a cirrhotic liver. _____

_____

_____

_____

13. What is the significance of biliary obstruction proximal to the cystic duct? _____

_____

_____

_____

14. What is the significance of biliary obstruction distal to the cystic duct? _____

_____

_____

_____

_____

15. What would an extrahepatic mass show on ultrasound examination? _____

_____

_____

16. Discuss the cause, ultrasound findings, and symptoms of a patient with a hepatic cyst. _____

_____

_____

_____

17. Name the three basic types of abscess formation in the liver. _____

_____

_____

18. Describe the clinical symptoms and ultrasound appearance of a pyogenic hepatic abscess. _____

_____

_____

_____

19. Describe the characteristic findings of an amebic abscess. _____

_____

_____

_____

20. Describe the ultrasound appearance of an echinococcal cyst of the liver. _____

_____

_____

_____

_____

21. What is the definition of a neoplasm? _____

_____

22. Describe the findings of a cavernous hemangioma. _____

_____

_____

_____

23. What are the clinical symptoms and ultrasound findings of a liver adenoma? _____

_____

_____

_____

24. Describe the ultrasound findings and incidence of focal nodular hyperplasia. _____

_____

_____

_____

25. Discuss the three patterns of hepatocellular carcinoma. _____

_____

_____

_____

_____

26. Name the primary sites that cause metastatic disease to spread to the liver. _____

_____

_____

_____

27. What are the clinical and ultrasound findings of metastatic liver disease? _____

_____

_____

_____

28. Describe the appearance of lymphoma of the liver. _____

_____

_____

_____

29. Discuss the incidence and findings of liver trauma. _____

_____

_____

_____

30. What is the role of ultrasound in liver transplantation? _____

_____

_____

_____

31. What complications may arise after liver transplant? _____

_____

_____

_____

32. Discuss the development of portal venous hypertension and its effects on the hepatic system. _____

_____

_____

_____

33. Discuss the development of collateral circulation. _____

_____

_____

34. What are the clinical findings in a patient with portal hypertension? _____

_____

_____

_____

_____

35. What is a recannalized umbilical vein? _____

_____

_____

_____

36. Discuss the various portal caval shunts available and what considerations the sonographer should have before the examination. _____

_____

_____

_____

Review Exercise D • Liver Terminology

For 1 to 20, match the following terms with the definitions listed on p 137.

1. _____ Caudate lobe

2. _____ Ligamentum teres (Use for 2 answers)

3. _____ Quadrate lobe

4. _____ Falciform ligament

5. _____ Fissure for the ligamentum venosum

6. _____ Neck of the gallbladder

7. _____ Right lobe of liver

8. _____ Left lobe of liver

9. _____ Reidel's lobe of liver

10. _____ Functional right lobe

11. _____ Functional left lobe

12. _____ Portal triad

13. _____ Porta hepatis

14. _____ Bare area

15. _____ Lesser sac

16. _____ Portal veins

17. _____ Hepatic veins

18. _____ Hepatic arteries

19. _____ Bile ducts

20. _____ "Mickey Mouse sign"

21. Name the three fossa important to liver anatomy: _____

_____

22. The fundus of the stomach lies anterior and medial to the left lobe of the liver (true or false).

23. The duodenum lies inferior to the caudate lobe and adjacent to the right lobe of the liver (true or false).

24. The pancreas is usually posterior and inferior to the right and left lobes of the liver (true or false).

25. If the far right lateral border of the liver is scanned, the following structures would be identified: _____

_____

26. Which vascular structure passes through the right lobe of the liver to pierce the diaphragm and empty into the right atrium?

27. The liver is suspended from the diaphragm and anterior abdominal wall by the:

    a. ligamentum teres

    b. round ligament

    c. falciform ligament

    d. square ligament

28. What is the name of the space between the liver and the diaphragm that is a common site for abscess formation?

29. What is the significance of Morison's pouch? Where is it located?

30. Define these terms and give an example of each:

    a. homogeneous:

    b. anechoic:

    c. echogenic:

    d. acoustic enhancement:

    e. shadow effect:

DEFINITIONS: LIVER TERMINOLOGY

  a. Echogenic focus in the left lobe of the liver; remnant of the fetal ductus venosus

  b. Obsolete term for the medial segment of the left lobe of the liver

  c. Referred to as a "sling" that separates the left lobe from the rest of the liver

  d. Rounded termination of the falciform ligament, remnant of the umbilical vein

  e. Arises from the celiac axis

  f. Portal vein, hepatic artery, common bile duct

  g. Lobe of the liver that lies posterior to the left lobe, anterior to the IVC

  h. Separates the left lobe from the caudate lobe

  i. Lies between the right and quadrate lobes of the liver

  j. Tonguelike projection of the right lobe of the liver

  k. Run longitudinally within the liver parenchyma

  l. Run transversely within the liver parenchyma

  m. Area of no peritoneal covering of the liver

  n. This lobe is supplied by the left portal vein and left hepatic artery

  o. Everything to the right of a plane through the gallbladder fossa and IVC

  p. The "door" of the liver

  q. Largest lobe of the liver

  r. Everything to the left of the plane through the gallbladder fossa and IVC

  s. Of the tubular structures within the liver, these have more acoustic enhancement

  t. Enclosed portion of the peritoneal space behind the liver and stomach

  u. Transverse section through the CBD, portal vein, and hepatic artery

Review Exercise E • Liver Segments

Match the following terms with their definitions.

Structure:

a. RHV

b. MHV

c. LHV

d. RPV (anterior)

e. RPV (posterior)

f. LPV (initial)

g. LPV (ascending)

h. IVC fossa

i. GB fossa

j. Ligamentum teres

k. Fissure of the ligamentum venosum

1. _____ (Use three answers) These structures separate the right and left lobes of the liver.

2. _____ This separates the caudate lobe from the lateral segment of the left lobe of the liver.

3. _____ This courses centrally in the anterior segment of the RLL.

4. _____ This separates the caudate lobe posteriorly from the medial segment of the LL anteriorly.

5. _____ This divides the medial and lateral segments of the LL.

6. _____ This divides cephalic aspects of the medial and lateral segments of the LL.

7. _____ This divides the caudal aspect of the LL into medial and lateral segments.

8. _____ This divides the cephalic aspect of the anterior and posterior segments of the RLL.

9. _____ This courses centrally in the posterior segment of the RLL.

Self-Test A • The Liver

1. The liver is suspended from the diaphragm and anterior abdominal wall by the:

   a. ligamentum teres

   b. round ligament

   c. falciform ligament

   d. square ligament

2. Fatty infiltration may be seen in all patients except those with:

   a. diabetes mellitus

   b. chronic alcoholism

   c. hepatoportal fistula

   d. hepatitis

3. The brightly reflective echo patterns in the liver may be caused by an increase in hepatic fat content (true or false).

4. Fatty infiltration of the liver is always uniform (true or false).

5. Sonographic findings of acute hepatitis include:

   a. accentuated brightness, more extensive demonstration of portal vein radicles, and overall decreased echogenicity of liver

   b. decreased brightness and echogenicity of liver

   c. increased brightness and echogenicity of liver; no demonstration of portal vein radicles

   d. ascites, decreased brightness, and echogenicity

6. The primary cause of portal hypertension is:

   a. hepatitis

   b. cirrhosis

   c. FNH

   d. glycogen storage disease

7. Portal hypertension is followed by several clinical signs. Which of the following is not correct?

   a. ascites

   b. collateral vessels

   c. splenomegaly

   d. hepatitis

8. The normal flow in the portal system is:

   a. hepatofugal

   b. hepatopedal

   c. hepatoflugal

   d. hepatopetal

9. Budd-Chiari syndrome is a rare disorder caused by obstruction of:

   a. portal veins

   b. hepatic veins

   c. the superior mesenteric vein

   d. the splenic vein

10. In Budd-Chiari syndrome the liver becomes:

    a. shrunken and echogenic

    b. enlarged and tender with ascites

    c. enlarged without ascites

    d. isoechoic

11. All of the following are true regarding the features most often observed in an intrahepatic mass except:

    a. anterior displacement of the right kidney

    b. displacement of the hepatic vascular radicles

    c. external bulging of the liver capsule

    d. focal inhomogeneity within the liver capsule

12. What percent of patients with polycystic kidney disease have cysts in the liver?

    a. 10%

    b. 25% to 50%

    c. 70%

    d. 85%

13. Echinococcal cysts have the highest incidence in countries where:

    a. fishing is common

    b. rock climbing is prevalent

    c. poultry is abundant

    d. sheep grazing is common

14. Clinical signs of liver infection include:

    a. elevated liver function

    b. anemia

    c. fever, pain

    d. normal liver function

15. The most common ultrasound findings in a patient with candidiasis are:

    a. wheels in wheels

    b. bull's eye or target

    c. spokes in spokes

    d. a and b

    e. b and c

16. The most common benign tumor of the liver is:

    a. cavernous hemangioma

    b. mesenchyma hamartoma

    c. infantile hemangioendothelioma

    d. adenoma

17. What benign liver tumor has been found in patients with Type I glycogen storage disease?

    a. lipoma

    b. adenoma

    c. focal nodular hyperplasia

    d. hamartoma

18. What liver tumor is a rare, benign, primary solid tumor comprised of fatty tissue?

    a. cavernous lipangioma

    b. lipoma

    c. hamartoma

    d. hyperplastic lipotoma

19. Patients who have hepatocellular carcinoma are likely to have had:

    a. cirrhosis

    b. hemochromatosis

    c. adenosis

    d. carcinosis

20. Hepatocellular carcinoma tends to present itself:

    a. as an incidental finding

    b. with normal AFP tests

    c. with a shrunken liver

    d. with Budd-Chiari syndrome

21. The most common form of neoplastic involvement of the liver is:

    a. hepatocellular carcinoma

    b. metastases

    c. hepatoma

    d. hamartoma

22. On ultrasound examination, Burkitt's lymphoma may show:

    a. diffuse liver disease

    b. starry night echo pattern

    c. isoechoic focal mass

    d. hyperechoic focal mass

23. The left portal vein lies more posterior and cranial than the right portal vein (true or false).

24. (Choose 2 answers) The right lobe of the liver is divided into the:

    a. anterior segment

    b. posterior segment

    c. medial segment

    d. lateral segment

25. (Choose 2 answers) The left lobe of the liver is divided into the:

   a. anterior segment

   b. medial segment

   c. posterior segment

   d. lateral segment

26. The quadrate lobe is a portion of the:

   a. anterior segment

   b. medial segment

   c. posterior segment

   d. lateral segment

27. The ligamentum teres is located in which fissure?

   a. right intersegmental

   b. left intersegmental

   c. lateral lobar

   d. main lobar

28. The fissure of the ligamentum venosum is located between which lobes of the liver?

   a. right and left

   b. left and caudate

   c. caudate and right

29. The fossae of the RPV and gallbladder are found in the:

   a. main lobar fissure

   b. left intersegmental fissure

   c. right intersegmental fissure

   d. left lobar fissure

30. The falciform ligament extends from the umbilicus to the diaphragm in a parasagittal plane containing the:

   a. ligamentum venosum

   b. ligamentum teres

   c. quadratus ligamentum

   d. ligamentum falciformis

31. The lesser sac is an enclosed portion of the peritoneal space located:

   a. posterior to the liver and stomach

   b. anterior to the liver and stomach

   c. medial to the liver and stomach

   d. lateral to the liver and stomach

32. The portal veins carry _____ blood from the _____.

    a. unoxygenated; spleen to the liver   c. unoxygenated; bowel to liver

    b. oxygenated; bowel to the liver   d. oxygenated; aorta to liver

33. In patients with biliary obstruction, the elevation of SGPT and SGOT is:

    a. high

    b. moderately high

    c. moderate

    d. mild

34. In severe hepatocellular destruction, the SGOT and SGPT are:

    a. high

    b. moderately high

    c. moderate

    d. mild

35. Elevation of alkaline phosphatase is associated with:

    a. biliary obstruction

    b. tumor lesion in the liver

    c. hepatocellular disease

    d. cystic disease of the liver

36. Elevation of serum bilirubin results in:

    a. hepatocellular disease

    b. ascites

    c. jaundice

    d. hemolysis

37. When restriction to flow is advanced, increased venous pressure occurs and blood is forced to bypass the liver via collateral channels. This condition is called:

    a. varices

    b. cirrhosis

    c. portal hypertension

    d. obstructive vascular liver disease

38. (Choose 3 answers) Fatty infiltration of the liver may be characterized in its early stage by:

    a. hepatomegaly

    b. small, shrunken liver

    c. ascites

    d. decreased echogenicity

    e. increased echogenicity

    f. increased vascularity

    g. decreased vascularity

39. Focal nodular hyperplasia (FNH) of the liver may be distinguished from cirrhosis by:

    a. discrete nodular lesions throughout the liver

    b. discrete nodular lesions in one portion of the liver

    c. diffuse inhomogeneity of the liver parenchyma

    d. diffuse homogeneity of the liver parenchyma

40. In a patient with portal hypertension, a Doppler flow study would show:

    a. hepatopedal flow in the portal system

    b. hepatofugal flow in the portal system

    c. distended portal structures with turbulent flow

    d. small portal structures with decreased flow

41. Diminished vascular structures within the liver parenchyma most likely represents:

    a. cirrhosis

    b. obstructive portal disease

    c. Budd-Chiari syndrome

    d. acute viral hepatitis

Self-Test B • The Liver

1. The _____ of the normal liver is used to evaluate other organs and glands in the body.

    a. size

    b. parenchyma

    c. border

    d. caudate lobe

2. In relationship to question #1, the following can be said (use the terms *more, less,* or *same*):

    a. The kidneys are _____ echogenic than the liver.

    b. The spleen is _____ echogenic than the liver.

    c. The pancreas is _____ echogenic than the liver.

3. The liver occupies which three abdominal regions?

4. Downward displacement of the liver may be caused by:

5. Upward displacement of the liver may be caused by:

6. Use the terms *RL* [right lobe], *LL* [left lobe], and *CL* [caudate lobe] to identify which lobe of the liver is being described in each of the following descriptions:

    _____ a. Lies in the left hypochondriac region

    _____ b. Situated on the posterosuperior surface of the right lobe

    _____ c. Undersurface includes the gastric impression

_____ d. Largest lobe of liver

_____ e. Bounded below by the porta hepatis

_____ f. Bordered on upper surface by the falciform ligament

_____ g. Bordered anteriorly by umbilical notch

_____ h. Inferior and posterior surfaces marked by three fossae

_____ i. Riedel's lobe can sometimes be seen as an anterior projection

7. Which vessel approaches the porta hepatis in a rightward, cephalic, and slightly posterior direction within the hepatoduodenal ligament?

a. right portal vein

b. left portal vein

c. main portal vein

d. hepatic vein

8. The right portal vein is the larger of the two and requires a more posterior and more caudal approach (true or false).

9. The left portal vein lies more posterior and cranial than the right portal vein (true or false).

10. The hepatic veins lie within a canal containing large amounts of connective tissue, which results in the visualization of an echogenic linear band coursing through the central portion of the lateral segment of the left lobe (true or false).

11. Label which hepatic vein courses into the inferior vena cava (use the terms _right, middle,_ and _left_).

_____ enters the anterior of right anterior surface of the IVC

_____ largest, enters the right lateral aspect of the IVC

_____ smallest, enters the left anterior surface of the IVC

12. The best way to distinguish hepatic from portal vessels is to trace their points of origin. Complete these sentences:

_____ course between the hepatic lobes and segments; the major branches course

within the lobar segments.

_____ drain toward the right atrium; the _____ emanate from

the porta hepatis.

13. (Choose 2 answers) The right lobe of the liver is divided into the:

a. anterior segment

b. posterior segment

c. medial segment

d. lateral segment

14. (Choose 2 answers) The left lobe of the liver is divided into the:

a. anterior segment

b. medial segment

c. posterior segment

d. lateral segment

15. Identify these fissures found within the liver:

    a. right intersegmental fissure

    b. main lobar fissure

    c. left intersegmental fissure

      _____ separates right and left lobes

      _____ divides cephalic aspect of anterior and posterior segments of right hepatic lobe and courses between anterior and posterior branches of RPV

      _____ divides cephalic aspects of medial and lateral segments of left lobe

16. The ligamentum teres is located in which fissure?

    a. right intersegmental

    b. left intersegmental

    c. main lobar

17. The fissure of the ligamentum venosum is located between which lobes of the liver?

    a. Right, medial lobe of left

    b. Left lateral lobe, and right

    c. Caudate, lateral lobe of left

18. The fossae of the IVC and gallbladder are found in the:

    a. main lobar fissure

    b. left intersegmental fissure

    c. right intersegmental fissure

    d. left lobar fissure

19. The falciform ligament extends from the umbilicus to the diaphragm in a parasagittal plane containing the:

    a. ligamentum venosum

    b. ligamentum teres

    c. quadratus ligamentum

    d. ligamentum falciformis

20. The fissure of the ligamentum venosum separates the:

    a. right lobe from the caudate lobe

    b. caudate lobe from the quadrate lobe

    c. left lobe from the right lobe

    d. left lobe from the caudate lobe

21. The lesser sac is an enclosed portion of the peritoneal space located:

    a. posterior to the liver and stomach

    b. anterior to the liver and stomach

    c. medial to the liver and stomach

    d. lateral to the liver and stomach

22. The portal veins carry _____ blood from the:

    a. unoxygenated; spleen to the liver

    b. oxygenated; bowel to the liver

    c. unoxygenated; bowel to liver

    d. oxygenated; aorta to liver

23. The liver is the major center of (fill in answers):

    a.

    b.

    c.

24. Diseases affecting the liver may be classified as:

    a. cystic

    b. hepatocellular

    c. obstructive

    d. b and c

25. Viral hepatitis is an example of obstructive liver disease (true or false).

26. Hepatocellular disease is generally treated surgically, while obstructive disease is treated medically (true or false).

27. The liver functions as a major site for conversion of dietary sugars into glucose (true or false).

28. In severe liver disease the body may become:

    a. hyperglycemic

    b. hypoglycemic

    c. glucose dependent

    d. glucose comatose

29. The liver is a principal site for metabolism of fats. Fats are transported to the body or stored in the liver. The failure of the liver to convert fat to glucose may contribute to:

    a. hypoglycemia

    b. fatty liver

    c. hepatosis

    d. a and b

30. The liver produces many proteins, especially albumin. This protein functions to maintain oncotic pressure within the vascular system. When the liver is diseased with abnormal albumin levels, what develops?

    a. cirrhosis

    b. edema

    c. hypoalbuminemia

    d. hepatitis

31. _____ are protein catalysts used throughout the body in all metabolic processes.

32. The presence of increased quantities of _____ in the blood is a very sensitive indicator of hepatocellular disorder.

33. In patients with biliary obstruction, the elevation of ALT and AST is:

    a. high

    b. moderately high

    c. normal

    d. mild to moderate

34. In severe hepatocellular destruction, the ALT and AST are:

    a. high

    b. moderately high

    c. normal

    d. mild to moderate

35. Elevation of alkaline phosphatase is associated with all except:

    a. echinococcal disease

    b. tumor lesion in liver

    c. metastatic liver disease

    d. cholangiocarcinoma

36. (Choose 2 answers) Detoxification of the waste products in the liver includes:

    a. ammonium converted to urea

    b. bilirubin

    c. albumin

    d. alkaline phosphatase

37. In hematologic diseases associated with abrupt breakdown of large numbers of RBC, the liver may receive more bilirubin from the renal system than it can detoxify (true or false).

38. The level of indirect bilirubin will be decreased in hematologic diseases (true or false).

39. In biliary obstruction, the hepatocytes pick up bilirubin but cannot dispose of it (true or false).

40. Therefore, in biliary obstruction, the indirect bilirubin predominates (true or false).

41. In hepatocellular disease the bilirubin is excreted into the blood when the hepatocytes are damaged (true or false).

42. Elevation of serum bilirubin results in:

    a. hepatocellular disease

    b. ascites

    c. jaundice

    d. hemolysis

43. _____ is the excretory product of the liver.

    a. Bile

    b. Nitrogen

    c. Ammonia

    d. Alkaline phosphatase

44. The primary functions of bile are:

   a. removal of waste products excreted by the liver

   b. hemolysis of blood products

   c. emulsification of intestinal fat

   d. a and c

45. When restriction to flow is advanced, increased venous pressure occurs and blood is forced to bypass the liver via collateral channels. These collateral channels are called:

   a. varices

   b. cirrhosis

   c. portal hypertension

   d. obstructive vascular liver disease

46. Normal sonographic demonstration of the sagittal view of the liver shows the liver dimension to measure under:

   a. 10 cm

   b. 20 cm

   c. 12 cm

   d. 15 cm

47. To image the near field of the liver, the following should be done:

   a. change the transducer from 5.0 to 7.5 MHz

   b. change from a linear to a sector transducer

   c. change from a sector to a curved array transducer

   d. increase the near gain

48. The evaluation of the liver parenchyma includes the assessment of

_____ ; _____ ; and _____ .

49. In acute viral hepatitis, the sonographer would identify these findings in the liver:

   a. small, shrunken liver

   b. splenomegaly

   c. tenderness over liver

   d. portal hypertension

50. (Choose 2 answers) Fatty infiltration of the liver may be characterized in its early stages by:

   a. hepatomegaly

   b. small, shrunken liver

   c. ascites

   d. decreased echogenicity

   e. increased echogenicity

   f. increased vascularity

   g. decreased vascularity

   h. increased attenuation

51. (Choose 4 answers) Cirrhosis of the liver may be characterized by:

    a. hepatomegaly

    b. small, shrunken liver

    c. increased vascular structures

    d. decreased vascular structures

    e. diffuse homogeneity

    f. inhomogeneity

    g. ascites

52. Focal nodular hyperplasia of the liver may be distinguished from cirrhosis by:

    a. discrete nodular lesions throughout the liver

    b. discrete nodular lesions in one portion of the liver

    c. diffuse inhomogeneity of the liver parenchyma

    d. diffuse homogeneity of the liver parenchyma

53. Cystic disease within the liver is always congenital (true or false).

54. Cysts may be defined from nodular lesions in the liver by all except:

    a. dense, reflective borders

    b. anechoic characteristics

    c. well-defined borders

    d. posterior enhancement

55. In patients with polycystic renal disease, at least what percent will have associated polycystic liver disease?

    a. 30% to 50%

    b. 45% to 60%

    c. 30% to 40%

    d. 20% to 30%

56. In patients with polycystic liver disease, what percent will have associated polycystic renal disease?

    a. 50%

    b. 60%

    c. 40%

    d. 30%

57. A well-defined lesion that is sonolucent and good through transmission may be undoubtedly reported as a simple cyst (true or false).

58. The three basic locations for liver abscess pockets to form are:

    a. subhepatic, subphrenic, intrahepatic

    b. subhepatic, subdiaphragmatic, subphrenic

    c. subhepatic, parapancreatic, extrahepatic

    d. intrahepatic, extrahepatic, infrahepatic

59. Typical symptoms a patient may have with an abscess formation are all of the following except:

   a. decreased white blood count

   b. fever

   c. pain

   d. increased white blood count

60. How can one distinguish an abscess collection from a simple liver cyst?

61. A collection inferior to the liver and anterior to the right kidney is called:

   a. a subdiaphragmatic abscess

   b. a pararenal abscess

   c. an infrahepatic abscess

   d. a subcapsular abscess

62. How can one distinguish a subphrenic abscess from a pleural effusion?

63. Jim MacDonald, a sheep farmer, arrives at the hospital with right upper quadrant pain, fever, and elevated white blood cell count. He states that 3 months ago he was kicked in the ribs. An irregular mass showing low-level echoes is found on the sonogram. What is your differential diagnosis?

   a. amebic abscess

   b. hematoma

   c. echinococcal cyst

   d. hepatic abscess

64. Larry Jones was admitted to the ER after a fight with complaints of severe RUQ pain. Blood tests showed RBC was decreased liver function tests (LFTS) were normal, and ALP were almost normal. An emergency ultrasound scan was ordered to help with the diagnosis. What would you expect to find?

   a. cholecystitis

   b. cirrhosis

   c. hematoma

   d. viral hepatitis

65. Benign liver tumors generally associated with oral contraceptives are

   a. estroma

   b. adenoma

   c. hemangioma

   d. Addison's angioma

66. The vascular tumor composed of blood vessel cells with nonspecific sonographic findings is

   a. adenoma

   b. hemangioma

   c. Ewing's angioma

   d. hamartoma

67. In adults the primary hepatic tumor that is malignant is the

    a. hepatoblastoma

    b. hamartoma

    c. hepatoma

    d. cystic hemangioma

68. The most common intrahepatic neoplasm is

    a. hepatoblastoma

    b. hamartoma

    c. hepatoma

    d. metastatic liver disease

69. Patients with lymphoma have hepatic involvement that shows sonographically as hepatomegaly with a normal liver pattern or a diffuse alteration of echo architecture (true or false).

70. Biliary obstruction proximal to the cystic duct can be carcinoma of the CBD or hepatic metastases in the porta hepatis (true or false).

71. A patient with hepatic metastasis in the porta hepatis would present with abnormal hepatocellular function (true or false).

72. Dilated intrahepatic bile ducts may be seen with all of the following except:

    a. intrahepatic mass in the area of the porta hepatis

    b. gallstones in the fundus of the gallbladder

    c. obstructive stone in the cystic duct

    d. lymphadenopathy in the porta hepatis

Self-Test C • Liver: Diffuse Disease

1. Hepatocellular disease can be defined as a process that affects the:

    a. spherocytes and interferes with liver function

    b. phagocytes and doesn't interfere with liver function

    c. phagocytes and interferes with liver function

    d. hepatocytes and interferes with liver function

2. In fatty infiltration, fat in the liver cells implies significant injury to the liver (true or false).

3. In patients with chronic hepatitis, the sonographic findings are:

    a. increased brightness of liver, increased echogenicity

    b. decreased brightness of liver, decreased number of portal vein radicles, increased liver echogenicity, coarse echo pattern

    c. decreased brightness of liver, increased number of portal vein radicles

    d. increased brightness of liver, decreased echogenicity, decreased portal vein radicles

4. Describe the sonographic progression of cirrhosis.

    a.

    b.

    c.

5. What happens to the liver as fibrosis evolves?

   a. increased liver size, increased portal radicles

   b. decreased liver size, nodularity

   c. increased liver size, increased attenuation

   d. no change in liver size, increased attenuation

6. Increased attenuation means that there is increased visualization through transmission (true or false).

7. In glycogen storage disease, Type I is the most common. This is also known as:

   a. von Gierke's disease

   b. von Gussel's disease

   c. von Gerpe's disease

   d. von Slurpie's disease

8. In Type I glycogen storage disease, the following is noted:

   a. echogenic small liver

   b. echogenic large liver, hepatic adenomas

   c. normal texture, increased liver, adenoma

   d. normal texture, decreased liver, FNH

9. Normal measurement of the portal vein is:

   a. 0.1 cm

   b. 1.3 cm

   c. 1.7 cm

   d. 2.2 cm

10. In a patient with cirrhosis, there is a marked increase in extrahepatic resistance leading to less variation as a result of respiration on the portal vein (true or false).

11. In a patient with portal hypertension and chronic liver disease, if a shunt is present, the portal vein may:

   a. increase in caliber

   b. decrease in caliber

   c. collapse

   d. rupture

12. The most common portosystemic venous collaterals in portal hypertension are _____ ; _____ ; _____ ; _____ ; and _____ .

13. A patent umbilical vein must measure at least _____ to be significant.

   a. 1 mm

   b. 5 mm

   c. 3 mm

   d. 7 mm

14. Extrahepatic obstruction is most often related to thrombosis or direct invasion of the portal vein by cancer involving adjacent organs (true or false).

15. Other structures that should be evaluated for tumor extension from the liver are

_____ ; _____ ; and _____ .

16. In a patient with portal vein thrombosis, the liver is not enlarged or tender (true or false).

17. In a patient with Budd-Chiari syndrome, the caudate lobe specifically enlarges and appears hypoechoic (true or false).

18. All of the following are true regarding the features most often observed in an extrahepatic mass except:

    a. internal invagination of the liver capsule

    b. posterior shift of the IVC

    c. discontinuity of the liver capsule

    d. anteromedial shift of the IVC

19. All of the following are true regarding the features most often observed in an intrahepatic mass except:

    a. anterior displacement of the right kidney

    b. displacement of the hepatic vascular radicles

    c. external bulging of the liver capsule

    d. focal inhomogeneity within the liver capsule

20. Congenital cysts arise from developmental defects in the formation of the bile ducts (true or false).

21. Congenital cysts have all but one of the following features:

    a. vary in diameter

    b. do not cause hepatomegaly

    c. are usually palpable

    d. are lined with epithelium

22. Hepatic cysts are always found because the patient has with right upper quadrant pain and distress (true or false).

23. The most common site for the Echniococcal virus to grow is the:

    a. lungs

    b. liver

    c. bones

    d. brain

24. Complete cyst wall calcification in the Echniococcal cyst indicates an inactive lesion (true or false).

25. The routes for bacteria to gain access to the liver include the _____ ;

_____ ; _____ ; _____ ; and

_____ .

26. Clinical signs of infection include:

    a. elevated liver function

    b. anemia

    c. fever, pain

    d. normal liver function

27. The amebic abscess may reach the liver through:

    a. hepatic artery

    b. gastroduodenal artery

    c. hepatorectal artery

    d. portal vein

28. What benign liver tumor is located near the free edge of the liver, is solitary, well-circumscribed, and is a nonencapsulated multi-nodular mass?

    a. cavernous hemangioma

    b. adenoma

    c. focal nodular hyperplasia

    d. lipoma

29. The rare hepatic malignant tumor seen in infancy and childhood is:

    a. adenoma

    b. Wilms'

    c. adenolipoma

    d. hepatoblastoma

30. The primary sites of tumor invasion of the liver are from: _____ ; _____ ; and _____ .

31. Cancer of the colon is the cancer most frequently associated with calcification (true or false).

32. The most common ultrasound finding in a patient with lymphoma is a _____ mass.

33. In patients with leukemia, there may be multiple discrete hepatic masses. These lesions have been observed to be anechoic (true or false).

Case Reviews

1. A 54-year-old female arrives at the hospital with nonspecific abdominal pain that has been continuing for the past 6 months. The patient states that the discomfort does not change when she has a six-pack of beer. Describe the ultrasound findings (Figure 4-7).

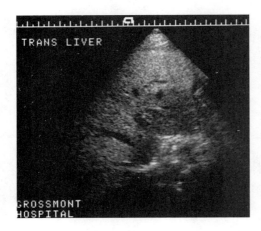

2. A 32-year-old male with AIDS has right upper quadrant pain. Significant symptoms include loss of appetite, nausea, fatigue, and abnormal liver function tests. Describe the ultrasound findings (Figure 4-8).

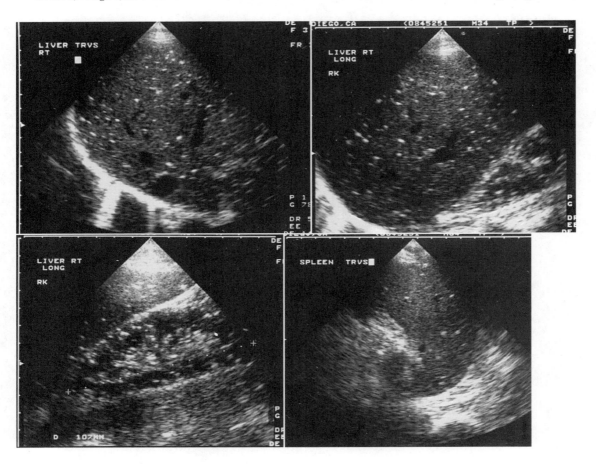

3. A 37-year-old alcoholic arrives at the hospital with increasing abdominal girth, anorexia, nausea, and vomiting. Describe the ultrasound findings (Figure 4-9).

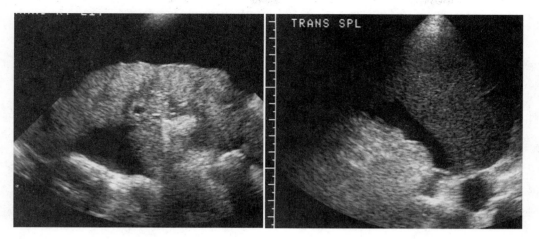

4. A 56-year-old male with palpable abdominal mass has a history of alcoholism, abdominal pain, hepatospleno-megaly, and weight loss. Describe the ultrasound findings (Figure 4-10).

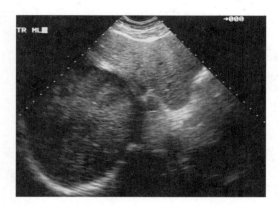

5. A 16-year-old female returns from Mexico with right upper quadrant pain, fever, and nausea. Describe the ultrasound findings (Figure 4-11).

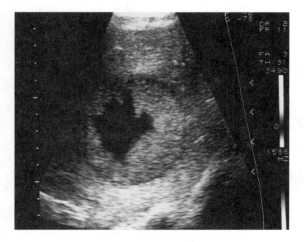

6. A 58-year-old female from the Middle East arrives at the hospital with right upper quadrant pain and hepatomegaly. Describe the ultrasound findings (Figure 4-12).

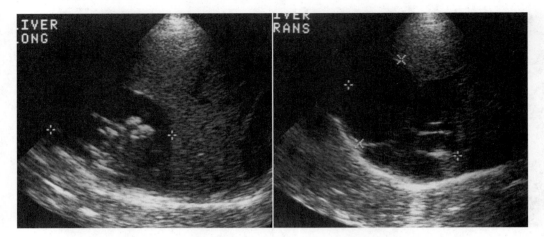

7. A 32-year-old female who has been taking birth control pills for the past 10 years has right upper quadrant pain. Lab results for liver function were within normal limits. Describe the ultrasound findings (Figure 4-13).

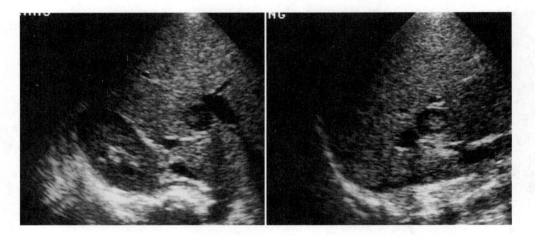

8. A 34-year-old patient with adenocarcinoma of the colon has had hepatomegaly and weight loss over the past 2 months. Describe the ultrasound findings (Figure 4-14).

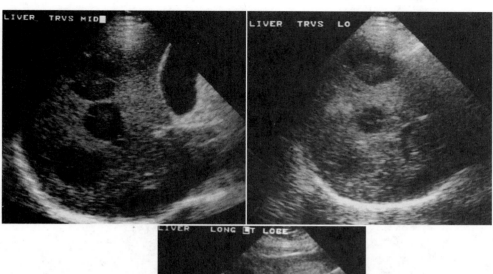

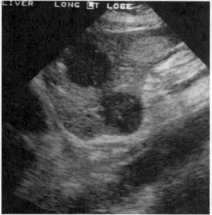

9. A 54-year-old male with lymphoma arrives at the hospital with hepatomegaly. His liver function test results are abnormal. Describe the ultrasound findings (Figure 4-15).

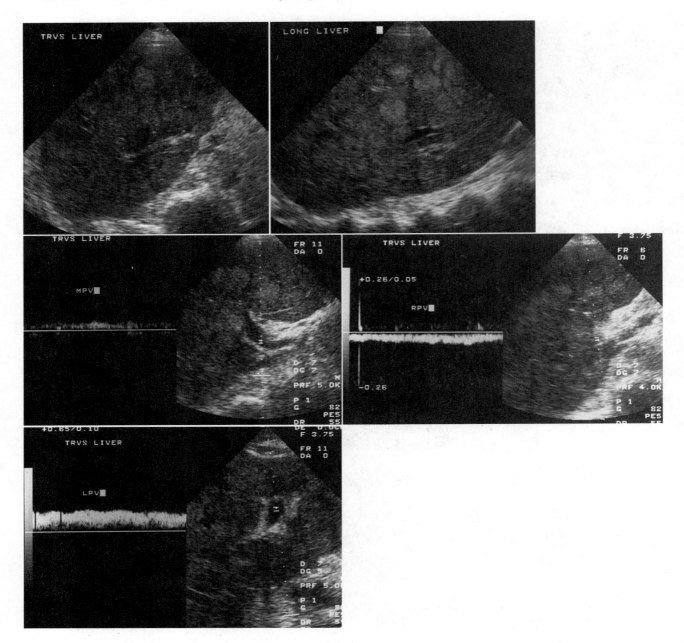

10. A 40-year-old male with portal hypertension is sent to have an ultrasound examination for further evaluation of portal venous flow. Describe the ultrasound findings (Figure 4-16).

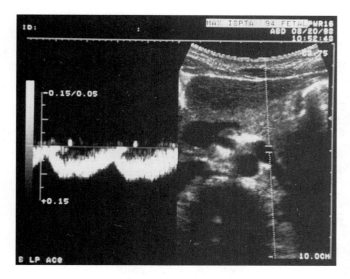

11. A 47-year-old alcoholic has abdominal pain, nausea, and vomiting. Describe the ultrasound findings (Figure 4-17).

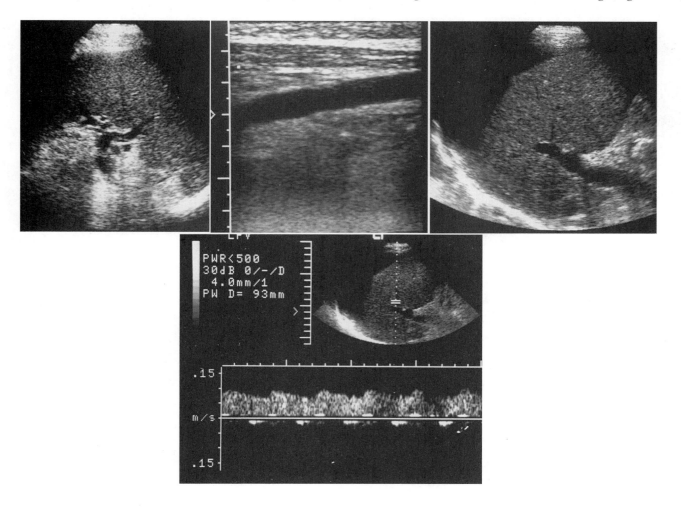

12. A 54-year-old male has a postportocaval shunt. Describe the ultrasound findings (Figure 4-18).

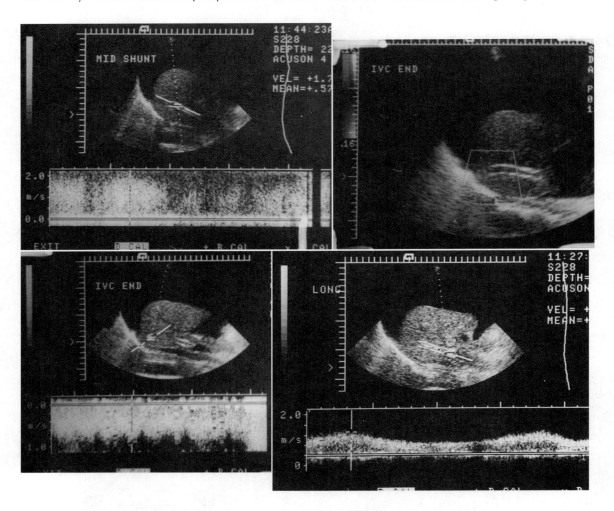

Answers to Review Exercise A

1. The liver is the largest gland in the body.
2. The formation of bile is a major exocrine function.
3. The liver receives blood from two sources: The hepatic artery and the portal vein.
4. The blood leaves the liver via the hepatic vein.
5. The liver cells are called *hepatocytes* and are packed in the walls of cells that are separated by blood sinusoids.
6. The incoming arterial blood and portal blood are mixed as they flow into the liver sinusoids. The hepatocytes take oxygen and nutrients from this blood, and then the blood flows into the hepatic veins.
7. The hepatocytes form bile and secrete it into small canaliculi, which coalesce to form first the smaller and then the larger bile ducts. In these ducts, bile flows in the opposite direction of blood to prevent mixing.

    The bile ducts coalesce to form the hepatic duct, which emerges from the liver. The hepatic duct bifurcates to form the cystic duct, which leads to the gallbladder and the common bile duct; together with the pancreatic duct they empty into the duodenum.
8. The sphincter of oddi regulates bile flow from the common bile duct into the duodenum. (When this sphincter is closed, the bile accumulates in the common bile duct, flowing back into the cystic duct and the gallbladder, where it is stored temporarily. After meals, the gallbladder contracts, releasing bile into the duodenum).
9. Bile is composed of 97% water, bile salts and pigments, and inorganic salts (sodium chloride and sodium bicarbonate). All of these elements are produced by liver cells.

    Bile salts (or acids) are formed from cholesterol within the hepatocytes. To form bile pigments, bilirubin, which is the metabolite of heme formed during red blood cell destruction, is taken up from the blood and conjugated to glucuronic acids to form the yellow bilirubin glucuronide.

    Most bile salts are reabsorbed by the intestines and delivered back to the liver; bile pigments are excreted with the feces.
10. The amino acids within the liver cells form a pool that can be used to make the various proteins of the liver and blood as well as glucose, fats, and energy (ATP). The amino acids can be exchanged with a second similar pool in the blood, which in turn exchanges amino acids with a third pool within the tissue cells. The liver is a major center for the synthesis and degradation of amino acids and proteins. The liver forms and secretes most of the blood proteins.

    Albumin transports hormones and fatty acids and is responsible for plasma osmotic pressure. Globulins are enzymes that transport hormones. Fibrinogen is used in blood clotting.

    The amino acids in the liver can be used as fuel to obtain ATP; however, only during starvation are the amino acids catabolized as fuels.

    Ammonia is formed during the deamination of amino acids. Ammonia can be toxic to the liver or other tissues. The liver detoxifies ammonia by converting it into urea, which is a water-soluble substance.
11. The liver is capable of forming, degrading, and storing fats. It has the ability to achieve to achieve metabolic interconversion among fats, carbohydrates, and proteins. The liver (through fat metabolism) can make cholesterol and form ketone bodies.
12. Simple sugars freely enter the liver cells, where they are converted to glucose. The glucose pool in the liver can be easily exchanged with that in the blood. (Only the liver can actually release glucose; when the blood glucose is low, the liver releases glucose into the blood; when the glucose level is high, the liver cells take up and store glucose.)

    Glucose in liver cells can be produced from other sources:
    - Proteins are broken down to form amino acids.
    - Deamination of amino acids leads to pyruvic acid, which can be converted to glucose by reverse glycolysis.
    - Glycerol is liberated by lipolysis, which is the breakdown of triglycerides in the liver and fat cells.
    - Lactic acid is usually formed in the muscles and delivered to the liver via the blood. In the liver, lactate is converted first to pyruvate and then to glucose through reverse steps of glycolysis.
13. The bulk of plasma proteins are manufactured by the liver; various sources in the body contribute other dissolved plasma constituents. Blood cells are formed mainly in the bone marrow.
14. The liver is the major organ regulating the balance of blood sugar and carbohydrate metabolism. The liver has enzymes that convert glycogen to glucose, glycerol to glucose, and vice versa, and amino acids to glucose and the reverse. The liver cannot synthesize glucose from fatty acids.

    Through the portal vein, the liver has direct access to the carbohydrates absorbed from the intestine, which makes it the center for the synthesis, delivery, storage, and production of glucose.

    The liver has a special enzyme to free glucose and is the only organ that can secrete glucose into the blood when the level of this substance exceeds the blood level. This gives the liver the unique roles of glucose exchanger and glucostat.

Answers to Review Exercise B

1. AST/SGOT (serum glutamic oxalacetic transaminase) is an enzyme present in tissues that have a high rate of metabolic activity. It is released into the bloodstream in abnormally high levels as a result of death or injury to the producing cells. AST is produced in many types of tissues, including the liver. It is elevated in cirrhosis of the liver (10 to 100 times the normal level) and in hepatic necrosis, acute hepatitis, and infectious mononucleosis.

2. ASP/SGPT (serum glutamic pyruvic transaminase) is more specific for evaluating liver function. Its level is mildly increased in acute cirrhosis, hepatic metastasis, and pancreatitis. There is a mild to moderate increase in obstructive jaundice and a moderate to marked increase in hepatocellular disease and in infectious or toxic hepatitis.

3. LDH (lactic acid dehydrogenase) is an enzyme found in many tissues. An increase in normal level indicates cellular injury and death. It is not specific for hepatic function. LDH is moderately increased in infectious mononucleosis and mildly elevated in hepatitis, cirrhosis, and obstructive jaundice.

4. Alkaline phosphatase is an enzyme produced by the liver, bones, and placenta. It is markedly increased in obstructive jaundice, hepatic carcinoma, abscess, and cirrhosis and is moderately elevated in hepatitis and less active cases of cirrhosis

5. Bilirubin is a product that results from the breakdown of hemoglobin in tired red blood cells. Liver cells convert these byproducts into bile pigments, which, along with bile salts, are secreted as bile by the liver cells into the bile ducts. The production cycle can be disrupted in three ways: an excessive amount of red blood cell destruction; a malfunction of liver cells; and a blockage of ducts leading from cells. Disruptions cause an increase in serum bilirubin, which eventually leaks into tissues and gives the skin a jaundiced, or yellow, color.

   Indirect bilirubin is unconjugated bilirubin. Elevated levels are seen with increased red blood cell destruction such as occurs with anemia, trauma from a hematoma, and hemorrhage.

   Direct bilirubin is conjugated bilirubin, which circulates freely in the blood, reaches the liver, is conjugated with gluronide, and is excreted into bile. Elevated levels are caused by obstructive jaundice, an obstruction of the biliary system caused by stones or neoplasm.

6. Total bilirubin is the elevation of both direct (more marked) and indirect levels in hepatic metastasis, hepatitis, lymphoma, cholestasis secondary to drugs, and cirrhosis.

Answers to Review Exercise C

1. The evaluation of the liver parenchyma includes the assessment of its size, configuration, homogeneity, and contour. The determination of liver volume can be made from serial scans in an effort to detect subtle increases in size or hepatomegaly.

2. As in other organ systems, the hepatic parenchyma pattern changes with disease processes. Hepatocellular disease affects the hepatocytes and interferes with liver function enzymes. The detection of cirrhosis, ascites, or fatty liver patterns may be seen with the ultrasound examination. Intrahepatic, extrahepatic, subhepatic, and subdiaphragmatic masses may be outlined, and their internal compositions recognized as specific echo patterns in efforts to provide a differential diagnosis for the clinician.

3. Diffuse hepatocellular disease affects the hepatocytes and interferes with liver function. The hepatocyte is a parenchymal liver cell that performs all the functions ascribed to the liver.

   A measurement of this abnormality is done through the series of liver function tests. The hepatic enzyme levels are elevated with cell necrosis. With cholestasis (interruption in the flow of bile through any part of the biliary system, from the liver to the duodenum), the alkaline phosphatase and direct bilirubin levels increase. Likewise, when there are defects in protein synthesis, there may be elevated serum bilirubin levels and decreased serum albumin and clotting factor levels.

4. Fatty infiltration implies increased lipid accumulation in the hepatocytes and is the result of significant injury to the liver or a systemic disorder leading to impaired or excessive metabolism of fat. Fatty infiltration is a benign process and may be reversible.

5. Common causes of fatty liver include the following: alcoholic liver disease, diabetes mellitus, obesity, severe hepatitis, chronic illness, and steroids.

6. Moderate to severe fatty infiltration shows increased echogenicity on ultrasound examination. Enlargement of the lobe affected by the fatty infiltration is evident. Visualization of the portal vein structures may be difficult because of the increased attenuation of the ultrasound. Thus it becomes more difficult to see the outline of the portal vein and hepatic vein borders.

7. Following are the three grades of liver texture that have been defined in sonography for classification of fatty infiltration:

Grade 1: There is a slight diffuse increase in fine echoes in the hepatic parenchyma, with normal visualization of the diaphragm and intrahepatic vessel borders.

Grade 2: There is a moderate diffuse increase in fine echoes with slightly impaired visualization of the intrahepatic vessels and diaphragm.

Grade 3: There is a marked increase in fine echoes with poor or no visualization of the intrahepatic vessel borders, diaphragm, and posterior portion of the right lobe of the liver.

Fatty infiltration is not always uniform throughout the liver parenchyma. It is not uncommon to see a patchy distribution of fat, especially in the right lobe of the liver. The fat does not displace normal vascular architecture.

The other characteristic of fatty infiltration is focal sparing. This condition should be suspected in patients who have masslike hypoechoic areas in typical locations in a liver that is otherwise increased in echogenicity. The most common areas of focal sparing are anterior to the gallbladder or the portal vein, and the posterior portion of the left lobe of the liver.

8. Patients with hepatitis may initially present with flu and gastrointestinal symptoms, including loss of appetite, nausea, vomiting, and fatigue. Jaundice may occur in severe cases. Lab values show abnormal liver function tests, with increases in the ASP, AST, and bilirubin.

9. In acute hepatitis, damage to the liver may range from a mild disease to massive necrosis and liver failure. Hepatosplenomegaly is present, and the gallbladder wall is thickened.

Chronic hepatitis exists when there is clinical or biochemical evidence of hepatic inflammation for at least 3 to 6 months. Chronic persistent hepatitis is a benign, self-limiting process. Chronic active hepatitis usually progresses to cirrhosis and liver failure.

10. On ultrasound examination, the liver parenchyma is coarse, with decreased brightness of the portal triads; however, the degree of attenuation is not as great as seen in fatty infiltration. The liver does not increase in size with chronic hepatitis. Fibrosis may be evident, which may produce soft shadowing posteriorly.

11. The essential features of cirrhosis are simultaneous parenchymal necrosis, regeneration, and diffuse fibrosis, resulting in disorganization of lobular architecture. The disease process is chronic and progressive, with liver cell failure and portal hypertension as the end stage. Cirrhosis is most commonly the result of chronic alcohol abuse but can be the result of nutritional deprivation, hepatitis, or other infection.

12. The diagnosis of cirrhosis by ultrasound examination may be difficult. Specific findings may show coarsening of the liver parenchyma secondary to fibrosis and nodularity. Increased attenuation may be present, with decreased vascular markings. Hepatosplenomegaly may be present, with ascites surrounding the liver. Chronic cirrhosis may show nodularity of the liver edge, especially if ascites is present. The hepatic fissures may be accentuated. The isoechoic regenerating nodules may be seen throughout the liver parenchyma. Portal hypertension may be present with or without abnormal Doppler flow patterns. Patients who have cirrhosis have an increased incidence of developing hepatoma tumors within the liver parenchyma.

13. Biliary obstruction proximal to the cystic duct can be caused by carcinoma of the common bile duct, or of metastatic tumor invasion of the porta hepatis. Clinically the patient may be jaundiced, and may experience pruritus (itching).

The liver function tests would show an elevation in the direct bilirubin and alkaline phosphatase levels.

On a Sonogram, carcinoma of the common bile duct would appear as a tubular branching with dilated intrahepatic ducts that are best seen in the periphery of the liver. It may be difficult to image a discrete mass lesion. The gallbladder is of normal size, even after a fatty meal is administered.

14. A biliary obstruction distal to the cystic duct may be caused by stones in the common duct, an extrahepatic mass in the porta hepatis, or stricture of the common duct. Clinically, common duct stones cause right upper quadrant pain, jaundice, pruritus, and an increase in direct bilirubin and alkaline phosphatase.

On ultrasound examination, the dilated intrahepatic ducts are seen in the periphery of the liver. The size of the gallbladder is variable, but it is usually small. Gallstones are often present and appear as hyperechoic lesions along the posterior floor of the gallbladder, with a sharp posterior acoustic shadow. Careful evaluation of the common duct may show shadowy stones within the dilated duct.

15. An extrahepatic mass in the area of the porta hepatis would cause the same clinical signs as biliary obstruction. On ultrasound examination, an irregular, ill-defined, hypoechoic, and inhomogeneous lesion may be seen in the area of the porta hepatis. There is intrahepatic ductal dilation with a hydropic gallbladder. The lesion may arise from the lymph nodes or from pancreatitis, pseudocyst, or carcinoma in the head of the pancreas.

16. Hepatic cysts may be congenital or acquired, solitary or multiple. Patients are often asymptomatic, except those who have large cysts that may compress the hepatic vasculature or ductal system.

Types of cystic lesions within the liver may include simple or congenital hepatic cysts; traumatic, parasitic, or inflammatory cysts; or they may be polycystic or a pseudocyst.

Simple hepatic cysts. The ultrasound finding of a simple hepatic cyst is usually an incidental discovery because most patients are asymptomatic. As the cyst grows, it may cause pain or a mass effect to suggest a more serious condition such as infection, abscess, or necrotic lesion. Hepatic cysts occur more often in females than in males. On ultrasound examination, the cyst walls are thin with well-defined borders, and the flow patterns are anechoic with distal posterior enhancement. Infrequently, cysts will contain fine linear internal septae. Complications such as hemorrhage may occur and cause pain. Calcification may be seen within the cyst wall, which may cause shadowing.

Congenital hepatic cysts. A solitary congenital cyst of the liver is rare and usually is an incidental lesion. This abnormality arises from developmental defects in the formation of bile ducts. The mass is usually solitary and may vary in size from tiny to as large as 20 cm. The cyst is usually found on the anterior undersurface of the liver. It usually does not cause liver enlargement and is found in the right lobe of the liver more often than in the left lobe.

Polycystic liver disease. Polycystic liver disease is autosomal dominant and affects 1 out of 500 people. At least 25% to 50% of patients with polycystic renal disease have one to several hepatic cysts. In patients with polycystic liver disease, 60% will have associated polycystic renal disease. The cysts are small, under 2 to 3 cm, and multiple throughout the hepatic parenchyma. Cysts within the porta hepatis may enlarge and cause biliary obstruction. Histologically they appear similar to simple hepatic cysts. It may be very difficult to assess an abscess formation or neoplastic lesion in a patient with polycystic liver disease.

On ultrasound examination, the cysts generally appear as anechoic, with well-defined borders with acoustic enhancement. The differential diagnosis for a cystic lesion would include necrotic metastasis, echinococcal cyst, hematoma, hepatic cystadenocarcinoma, or abscess.

17. There are three basic types of abscess formation in the liver: intrahepatic, subhepatic, and subphrenic.

18. The search for an abscess must be made to locate solitary or multiple lesions within the liver, or to search for abnormal fluid collections in Morison's pouch, in the subdiaphragmatic or subphrenic space.

Clinically the patient has fever, pain, pleuritis, nausea, vomiting, and diarrhea. Elevated liver function tests, leukocytosis, and anemia are present.

The ultrasound appearance of pyogenic abscess may be variable, depending on the internal consistency of the mass. The size varies from 1 cm to very large. The right central lobe of the liver is the most common location for abscess development. The abscess may be hypoechoic with round or ovoid margins and acoustic enhancement, or it may be complex with irregular walls and some debris along the posterior margin. It may have a fluid level, or if gas is present, it may be hyperechoic with dirty shadowing.

19. An amebic abscess is a collection of pus formed by disintegrated tissue in a cavity, usually in the liver, caused by the protozoan parasite *Entamoeba histolytica*. The infection is primarily a disease of the colon but it can also spread to the liver, lungs, and brain. Amebiasis is contracted by ingesting the cysts through contaminated water and food. The amebic parasites reach the liver parenchyma via the portal vein. The amebae usually affect the colon and cecum, and the parasitic organism remains within the gastrointestinal tract. If the organism invades the colon mucosa, it may travel to the liver via the portal venous system.

Patients may not show symptoms or may have gastrointestinal symptoms such as abdominal pain, diarrhea, leukocytosis, and low fever.

The ultrasound appearance of amebic abscess is variable and nonspecific. The abscess may be round or oval and may have a lack of significantly defined wall echoes. The lesion is hypoechoic compared with normal liver parenchyma and may show low-level echoes at higher sensitivity. There may be some internal echoes along the posterior margin secondary to debris. Distal enhancement may be seen beyond the lesion. Some organisms may rupture through the diaphragm into the hepatic capsule.

20. Hepatic echinococcosis is an infectious cystic disease that is common in sheepherding areas of the world but is seldom encountered within the United States.

On ultrasound examination, several patterns may occur, from a simple cyst to a complex mass with acoustic enhancement. The shape of the cyst may be oval or spherical, and may have regularity of the walls. Calcifications may occur. Septations are very frequent, e.g., honeycomb appearance with fluid collections; water lily sign, which shows a detachment and collapse of the germinal layer; or cyst within a cyst. Sometimes the liver may contain multiple parent cysts in both lobes of the liver; the cyst with the thick walls occupies a different part of the liver. The tissue between the cysts indicates that each cyst is a separate parent cyst and not a daughter cyst. If a daughter cyst is found, it is specific for echinococcal disease.

21. A neoplasm is any new growth of new tissue, either benign or malignant. If the neoplasm is benign, growth

occurs locally, but does not spread or invade surrounding structures. It may push surrounding structures aside or adhere to them. A malignant mass is uncontrolled and is prone to metastasize to nearby or distant structures via the blood stream and lymph nodes.

22. A hemangioma is a benign, congenital tumor consisting of large, blood-filled cystic spaces. Cavernous hemangioma is the most common benign tumor of the liver. The tumor is found more frequently in females. Patients are usually asymptomatic, although a small percent of the tumors may bleed, causing right upper quadrant pain. Hemangiomas enlarge slowly and undergo degeneration, fibrosis, and calcification. They are found in the subcapsular hepatic parenchyma or in the posterior right lobe more often than in the left lobe of the liver.

    The ultrasound appearance of hemangioma is typical in that most are hyperechoic with acoustic enhancement. They are either round, oval, or lobulated, with well-defined borders. The larger hemangiomas may have a mixed pattern as a result of necrosis. The hemangioma may become more heterogeneous as it undergoes degeneration and fibrous replacement. It may also project with calcifications, which appear as complex or anechoic echo pattern.

23. A liver adenoma, or lesion, is found more commonly in women and has been related to oral contraceptive useage. Patients may have right upper quadrant pain secondary to rupture, with bleeding into the tumor. There is increased incidence in patients with Type I glycogon storage disease or von Gierke's disease. On ultrasound examination, the mass may look similar to focal nodular hyperplasia. It is hyperechoic with a central hypoechoic area caused by hemorrhage. The lesion may be solitary or multiple. If the lesion ruptures, fluid should be found in the peritoneal cavity.

24. This lesion is found in women under 40 years of age. There is an increased incidence among women who use oral contraceptives, and there is increased bleeding within the tumor in these patients. In these cases, the patient is without symptoms. Lesions occur in the right lobe of the liver. There may be more than one mass; many are located along the subcapsular area of the liver; some are pendunculated; and many have a central scar.

    On ultrasound examination, the lesions appear well-defined and show hyperechoic to isoechoic patterns as compared with the liver. The internal linear echoes may be seen within the lesions if multiple nodules are together.

25. The carcinoma may appear in one of three patterns: as a solitary massive tumor, multiple nodules throughout the liver, or as diffuse infiltrative masses in the liver. All of the patterns cause hepatomegaly.

    The carcinoma can be very invasive and is seen to invade the hepatic veins to produce Budd-Chiari syndrome. The portal venous system may also be invaded with tumor or thrombosis. The hepatocellular carcinoma has a tendency to destroy the portal venous radicle walls with invasion into the lumen of the vessel.

26. The primary sites of metastatic disease are found in the colon, breast, and lung. The majority of metastases arise from a primary colon or from a hepatoma.

27. In metastatic liver disease, clinically the patient has hepatomegaly, abnormal liver function tests, weight loss, and decreased appetite. It is typical for this disease to occur in multiple nodes throughout both lobes of the liver.

    The ultrasound patterns of metastatic tumor involvement in the liver vary. Three specific patterns have been described: 1) well-defined hypoechoic mass; 2) well-defined echogenic mass; and 3) diffuse distortion of normal homogeneous parenchymal pattern without focal mass. The hypovascular lesions produce hypoechoic patterns in the liver as a result of necrosis and ischemic areas from neoplastic thrombosis. Most cases of hypervascular lesions correspond to hyperechoic patterns.

    The common primary masses include renal cell carcinoma, carcinoid, choriocarcinoma, transitional cell carcinoma, islet cell carcinoma, and hepatocellular carcinoma. The echogenic lesions are common with colon primary tumors and may present with calcification. Target-type metastases or bulls-eye patterns are the result of edema around the tumor or necrosis or hemorrhage within the tumor. As the nodules increase rapidly in size and outgrow their blood supply, central necrosis and hemorrhage may result.

    Various combinations of these patterns can be seen simultaneously in a patient with metastatic liver disease. The first abnormality is hepatomegaly or alterations in contour, especially on the lateral segment of the left lobe. The lesions may be solitary or multiple, variable in size and shape, and may have sharp or ill-defined margins. Metastases may be extensive or localized to produce an inhomogeneous parenchymal pattern.

28. Patients with lymphoma of the liver have hepatomegaly, with a normal or diffuse alteration of parenchymal echoes. A focal hypoechoic mass may sometimes be seen. The presence of splenomegaly or retroperitoneal nodes may help confirm the diagnosis of lymphadenopathy.

    Hodgkin's lymphoma appears with hypoechoic and diffuse ultrasound patterns in the liver.

    Non-Hodgkin's lymphoma may appear with target

and echogenic mass lesions. Burkitt's lymphoma may appear intrahepatic and lucent.

29. The liver is the third most common organ injured in the abdomen after the spleen and kidney. Laceration of the liver occurs in 3% of trauma patients and is frequently associated with other injured organs. The need for surgery is determined by the size of the laceration, the amount of hemoperitoneum, and the patient's clinical status. The right lobe is more often affected than the left. The degree of trauma is variable and may include small lacerations, large lacerations with hematomas, subcapsular hematomas, or capsular disruptions.

    Ultrasound examination is not used as commonly as other imaging modalities to localize the extent of a laceration because of the difficulty in detecting small lacerations in the dome of the right lobe of the liver. Intraperitoneal fluid should be assessed along the flanks and into the pelvis.

    Intrahepatic hematomas are hyperechoic in the first 24 hours and are hypoechoic and sonolucent thereafter as a result of the resolution of the blood within the area. Septations and internal echoes develop 1 to 4 weeks after the trauma. A subcapsular hematoma may appear as anechoic, hypoechoic, septated lenticular, or curvilinear. It may be differentiated from ascitic fluid in that it occurs unilateral, along the area of laceration. The degree of homogenicity depends on the age of the laceration.

30. Ultrasound examination can play a significant role in the preoperative and postoperative evaluation of hepatic transplantation. The primary function of the ultrasound examination is the evaluation of the portal venous system, the hepatic artery, the inferior vena cava, and the liver parenchymal pattern. The vascular structures should be assessed for their size and patency in the preoperative evaluation. The examination of the liver parenchyma should be made to rule out the presence of hepatic architecture disruption. The sonographer should also evaluate the biliary system to look for dilation and to evaluate the portosystemic collateral vessels.

31. Hepatic artery thrombosis is the most serious complication of liver transplantation. Postoperatively, evaluation of the hepatic artery is made with Doppler and color-flow ultrasound in the area of the porta hepatis. The normal hepatic artery flow is a low-resistance arterial signal. Thrombosis may be detected when there is absence of this signal. In the adult patient, the development of collateral vessels in the region of the hepatic artery is absent. However, in children, collateral formation of hepatic artery circulation may be present. Thus the scans should be made within 24 and 48 hours postoperatively and weekly thereafter to assess for change in velocity flow pattern.

The development of anastomotic stenoses is another problem that may occur in the transplant patient. The flow pattern of this complication shows a turbulent, high velocity signal indicative of hepatic artery stenosis. Portal vein thrombosis may also occur in the postoperative period. Air in the portal vein may be seen as brightly, echogenic moving targets within the portal venous system.

Compromise of the inferior vena cava is another complication of transplantation. A fatal complication is hepatic necrosis associated with thrombosis of the hepatic artery or portal vein. Massive necrosis takes the forms of gangrene of the liver and air in the hepatic parenchyma.

32. The development of increased pressure in the portal splenic venous system is the cause of portal hypertension. The hypertension develops when hepatopedal flow (toward the liver) is impeded by thrombus or tumor invasion. The blood becomes obstructed as it passes through the liver to the hepatic veins and is diverted to collateral pathways in the upper abdomen.

    There are two ways portal hypertension may develop. One is through increased resistance to flow, and the other is in increased portal blood flow. The most common mechanism for increased resistance to flow occurs in patients with cirrhosis.

    Patients that have increased portal blood flow may have an arteriovenous fistula or splenomegaly secondary to a hematologic disorder.

33. The development of collateral circulation occurs when the normal venous channels become obstructed. This diverted blood flow causes embryologic channels to reopen; blood flows hepatofugally (away from the liver) and is diverted into collateral vessels.

    The collateral channels may be the gastric veins (coronary veins), esophageal veins, recanalized umbilical vein, and splenorenal, gastrorenal, retroperitoneal, hemorrhoidal and intestinal veins.

    The most common collateral pathways are through the coronary and esophageal veins, which is the case in 80% to 90% of patients with portal hypertension. Varices, tortuous dilations of veins, may develop because of increased pressure in the portal vein, usually secondary to cirrhosis. Bleeding from the varices occurs with increased pressure.

34. In hypertension, clinically the patient would present with ascites, hepatosplenomegaly, gastrointestinal bleeding, elevated liver enzymes, jaundice, and hematemesis.

35. The umbilical vein may become recanalized secondary to portal hypertension. This vessel is best seen on the longitudinal plane near the midline, as a tubular structure coursing posterior to the medial surface of the left lobe of the liver. On transverse scans, a bulls-

eye pattern is seen within the ligamentum teres as the enlarged umbilical vein.

36. There are basically three types of shunts: the portocaval, mesocaval, and splenorenal. It is the responsibility of the sonographer to know specifically which type of shunt the patient has in place to image the flow patterns correctly.

The portocaval shunt attaches the main portal vein at the superior mesenteric vein–splenic vein confluence to the anterior aspect of the inferior vena cava.

The mesocaval shunt attaches the middistal superior mesenteric vein to the inferior vena cava. This shunt may be difficult to image if overlying bowel gas is present.

The splenorenal shunt attaches the splenic vein to the left renal vein. The shunt and connecting vessel should be documented with real-time, pulsed Doppler and color Doppler to determine flow patterns and patency.

Answers to Review Exercise D

1. g
2. a, d
3. b
4. c
5. h
6. i
7. q
8. n
9. j
10. o
11. r
12. f
13. p
14. m
15. t

16. l
17. k
18. e
19. s
20. u
21. IVC; right kidney; gallbladder
22. false
23. true
24. true
25. liver; right kidney; diaphragm
26. IVC
27. c
28. subdiaphragmatic space
29. Morison's pouch collects abscess

or free fluid. It is located anterior to the right kidney and posterior to the right lobe of the liver.
30. a. uniform texture pattern; example: liver
b. without echoes; example: cyst, bladder
c. echo-producing; example: solid mass
d. increased posterior through transmission; example: cyst
e. calcification that prohibits sound from passing through; example: gallstones, air pockets.

Answers to Review Exercise E

1. b, h, i
2. k
3. d

4. f
5. g
6. c

7. j
8. a
9. e

Answers to Self-Test A

1. c
2. c
3. false
4. false
5. a
6. b
7. d
8. d
9. b
10. b
11. a
12. b
13. d
14. c

15. b
16. a
17. b
18. b
19. a
20. d
21. b
22. b
23. false
24. a, b
25. b, d
26. b
27. b
28. b

29. a
30. b
31. a
32. b
33. d
34. a
35. a
36. c
37. a
38. a, e, g
39. b
40. b
41. a

Answers to Self-Test B

1. b
2. a less; b same; c same to more
3. right hypochondrium; epigastrium; left hypochondrium
4. tumor infiltration; cirrhosis; ascites; subphrenic abscess
5. ascites; dilation of the colon; abdominal tumors
6. a. LL
   b. CL
   c. LL
   d. RL
   e. CL
   f. RL
   g. LL
   h. RL
   i. RL
7. c
8. true
9. false
10. false
11. middle; right; left
12. hepatic veins; portal; hepatic veins; portal veins
13. a, b
14. b, d
15. b; a; c
16. b
17. c
18. a
19. b
20. d
21. a
22. b
23. metabolism; detoxification; storage
24. d
25. false
26. false
27. true
28. b
29. d
30. b
31. amino acids
32. bilirubin
33. d
34. a

35. a
36. a, b
37. true
38. false
39. true
40. false
41. true
42. c
43. a
44. d
45. a
46. d
47. c
48. size; configuration; contour
49. c
50. a, e
51. b, d, f, g
52. b
53. false
54. a
55. a
56. b
57. false
58. a
59. a
60. A simple liver cyst has smooth, well-defined borders with no internal echoes and with good through transmission. An abscess may have smooth or irregular borders, with low-level internal echoes or debris along the posterior wall.
61. a
62. A pleural effusion is above the diaphragm; a subphrenic abscess is below the diaphragm.
63. c
64. c
65. b
66. b
67. c
68. d
69. true
70. true
71. true
72. b

Answers to Self-Test C

1. d
2. true
3. b
4. a. normal to hepatomegaly, increased density and attenuation
   b. coarse, dense liver parenchyma. Liver begins to shrink; ascites may develop
   c. shrunken, coarse, nodular, and echogenic liver, decreased portal radicles, massive ascites

5. d

6. false

7. a

8. b

9. b

10. false

11. b

12. esophageal; gastric; splenic; umbilical; rectal;

13. c

14. true

15. inferior vena cava; hepatic veins; portal veins

16. true

17. true

18. b

19. a

20. true

21. c

22. false

23. b

24. true

25. portal vein; lymphatics; biliary system; laceration; trauma

26. d

27. d

28. c

29. d

30. colon; breast; lung

31. true

32. hypoechoic to isoechoic

33. false

Answers to Case Reviews

1. (Figure 4-7) The transverse image of the liver shows a nonuniform pattern within the liver parenchyma, with specific focal sparing of the caudate lobe. Fat infiltration does not always affect the entire liver uniformly; there may be localized areas of fat distribution throughout the liver, predominantly in the right and caudate lobes.

2. (Figure 4-8) Acute hepatitis appears as an inflammation of the liver, with accentuated brightness, echogenic walls of the portal veins, and decreased echogenicity of the liver. Thickening of the gallbladder wall may also be noted. Hepatosplenomegaly is usually present.

  The scans also show signs of pneumocystic disease, with multiple areas of calcification throughout the liver, kidney, and spleen.

  A, Liver, transverse with multiple calcifications.

  B, Liver, longitudinal.

  C, Right kidney, longitudinal with multiple calcifications.

  D, Spleen, transverse with few calcifications.

3. (Figure 4-9) Chronic cirrhosis shows ascites surrounding the liver with nodularity of the anterior liver edge. The liver texture is very coarse and echogenic secondary to fibrosis and distorted intrahepatic vascular structures. The size of the liver is shrunken.

4. (Figure 4-10) This patient is well known to the gastroenterology staff for having chronic bouts of cirrhosis and hepatitis. A large hyperechoic mass is found in the right lobe of the liver. The patient is diagnosed with a liver hepatoma and chronic cirrhosis. It has been reported that 80% of hepatocellular carcinomas occur in livers with preexisting cirrhosis.

5. (Figure 4-11) A large, complex mass is seen in the right lobe of the liver consistent with an amebic

abscess. The amebic parasites reach the liver through the entrance of the portal system.

6. (Figure 4-12) A large, complex mass consistent with an echinococcal cyst is shown in the right lobe of the liver. The ultrasound pattern is hypoechoic, with oval walls and multiple echogenic foci within. The low-level echoes represent hydatid sand within the mass.

7. (Figure 4-13) A well-circumscribed solid mass consistent with a small hepatic adenoma is seen in the right lobe of the liver. The adenoma generally appears hyperechoic but may present with complex characteristics if hemorrhage has occurred. The size may vary from small to over 14 cm.

8. (Figure 4-14) The liver is enlarged, with diffuse abnormalities throughout the liver parenchyma. These masses represent metastatic disease as well-defined hypoechoic lesions throughout the right lobe of the liver. The target lesion appears as a hypoechoic ring with an echogenic center, which is also known as the "bull's eye" sign.

9. (Figure 4-15) Ultrasound findings show Metastatic disease; specifically, hepatomegaly with diffuse iso-echoic lesions throughout the liver parenchyma. Decreased flow is noted in the main portal vein secondary to compression of the portal system from the multiple lesions.

10. (Figure 4-16) The splenic vein shows flow reversal in this patient, with portal hypertension and thrombosis of the main portal vein.

11. (Figure 4-17) A patient with cirrhosis and hepatosplenomegaly shows a recannalized umbilical vein with normal flow in the left portal vein.

  A, Spleen, transverse view of the prominent splenic vein.

  B, Recannalized umbilical vein, longitudinal view.

  C, Liver, longitudinal view of the dilated portal

vein, shrunken liver, with coarse parenchymal echo pattern and surrounding ascites.

D, Duplex of the portal vein with hepatopedal flow.

12. (Figure 4-18) The shunt should be evaluated at its proximal, mid, and distal ends to make sure turbulent flow is present. The bright, echogenic tubular structure *(B)* represents the gortex shunt material.

A, Liver, longitudinal view of the portal shunt with the Doppler curser within the flow pattern. A high velocity shunt flow pattern was seen.

B, Liver, longitudinal view of the bright gortex shunt at the entrance into the inferior vena cava.

C, Liver, longitudinal view of the shunt as it flows into the inferior vena cava.

D, Liver, longitudinal view of the normal portal flow into the liver.

CHAPTER
5
The Biliary System

OBJECTIVES

At the completion of this chapter, students will show orally, in writing, or by demonstration that they will be able to:

1. Describe the internal, surface, and relational anatomies of the gallbladder.
2. Know the size and position of the biliary system by recognizing the normal sonographic pattern of each of the following:
   a. gallbladder
   b. cystic duct
   c. hepatic ducts
   d. common bile duct
   e. vaterian system
   f. related arterial, venous, and lymphatic systems
3. Illustrate the cross-sectional anatomy of the hepatobiliary system and adjacent structures.
4. Describe congenital anomalies that affect the gallbladder, hepatic, cystic, and common bile ducts.
5. Explain the production, composition, and function of bile.
6. Select the pertinent laboratory tests and diagnostic procedures.
7. Explain the use of laboratory tests in evaluating the function of the biliary system.
8. Differentiate among the sonographic appearances of the following diseases by explaining the effect of the pathologic process on the gallbladder:
   a. jaundice
   b. cholelithiasis
   c. cholecystitis
   d. cholesterosis

e. diverticulosis
f. benign tumors
g. carcinoma
h. abscess, gangrenous cholecystitis
i. pericholecystic fluid
j. wall changes
k. sludge
l. polyps
m. porcelain gallbladder
n. emphysematous cholecystitis
o. sclerosing cholangitis

9. Differentiate among the sonographic appearances of the following abnormalities of the hepatobiliary tree by explaining the clinical significance of each:
   a. choledocholithiasis
   b. cholangitis
   c. choledocal cyst
   d. benign tumors
   e. carcinoma
   f. biliary cirrhosis
   g. cholangiocarcinoma (Klatzkin's tumor)
10. Create high quality diagnostic scans demonstrating the appropriate anatomy in all planes pertinent to the biliary system.
11. Select the correct equipment settings appropriate to individual body habitus.
12. Distinguish between normal and abnormal appearances of the biliary system.

To further enhance learning, students should use marking pens to color the anatomic illustrations that follow.

GALLBLADDER AND BILIARY SYSTEM

FIGURE 5-1
Anterior View of the Biliary System

The extrahepatic biliary apparatus consists of the right and left hepatic ducts, the common hepatic duct, the common bile duct, the gallbladder, and the cystic duct (Figure 5-1).

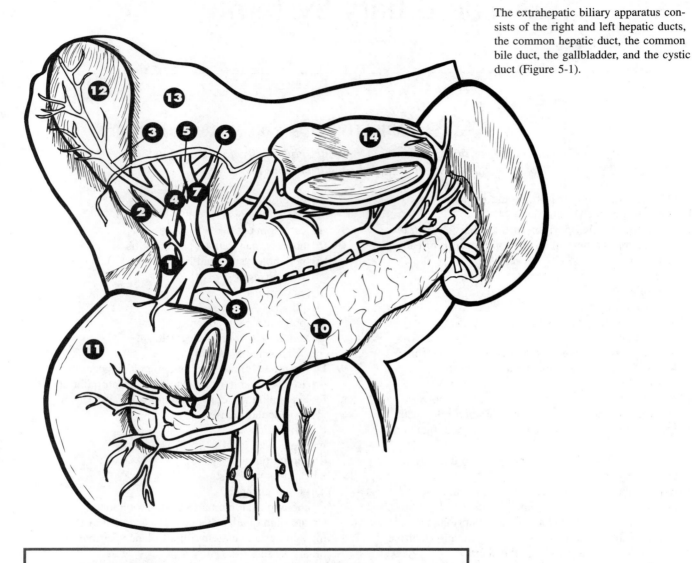

1	common bile duct	8	portal vein
2	cystic duct	9	common hepatic artery
3	cystic artery	10	pancreas
4	common hepatic duct	11	duodenum
5	middle hepatic artery	12	gallbladder
6	left hepatic artery	13	liver
7	proper hepatic artery	14	stomach

FIGURE 5-2
Gallbladder and Bile Ducts

Hepatic Ducts (FIGURE 5-2)

The right and left hepatic ducts emerge from the right lobe of the liver in the porta hepatis to form the common hepatic duct. The hepatic duct passes caudally and medially and runs parallel to the portal vein.

The common hepatic duct is approximately 4 mm in diameter and descends into the edge of the lesser omentum. It is joined by the cystic duct to form the common bile duct.

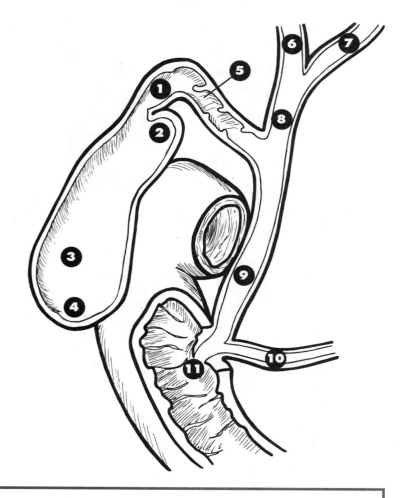

1	neck of gallbladder	7	left hepatic duct
2	Hartmann's pouch	8	common hepatic duct
3	body of the gallbladder	9	common bile duct
4	fundus of the gallbladder	10	pancreatic duct
5	cystic duct	11	Vater's ampulla
6	right hepatic duct		

FIGURE 5-3
Gallbladder and Bile Ducts

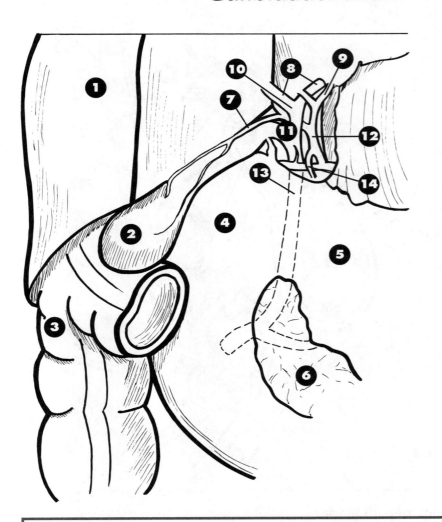

Common Bile Duct
(FIGURE 5-3)

The common bile duct has a diameter of less than 6 mm. In the first part of its course it lies in the right free edge of the lesser omentum. In the second part it is situated posterior to the first part of the duodenum. In the third part it lies in a groove on the posterior surface of the head of the pancreas. It ends by piercing the medial wall of the second part of the duodenum. There, it is joined by the main pancreatic duct, and together they open through the small ampulla of Vater into the duodenal wall. The ends of both ducts and the ampulla are surrounded by circular muscle fibers known as the sphincter of Oddi.

The proximal portion of the common bile duct is lateral to the hepatic artery and anterior to the portal vein. The duct becomes more posterior after it descends behind the duodenal bulb and enters the pancreas. The distal duct lies parallel to the anterior wall of the vena cava.

Within the liver parenchyma, the bile ducts follow the same course as the portal venous and hepatic arterial branches. All of the structures are encased in a common collagenous sheath forming the portal triad.

1	liver	8	right and left hepatic ducts
2	gallbladder	9	right and left hepatic arteries
3	colon	10	common hepatic duct
4	duodenum	11	cystic duct
5	stomach	12	proper hepatic artery
6	pancreas	13	common bile duct
7	cystic artery	14	right gastric artery

FIGURE 5-4
Posterior View of the Diaphragmatic
Surface of the Gallbladder

Gallbladder

The gallbladder is a pear-shaped sac in the anterior aspect of the right upper quadrant, closely related to the visceral surface of the liver (Fig. 5-4)). It is divided into the fundus, body, and neck. The fundus usually projects below the inferior margin of the liver, where it comes into contact with the anterior abdominal wall at the level of the ninth right costal cartilage. The body generally lies in contact with the visceral surface of the liver and is directed upward, backward, and to the left. The neck becomes continuous with the cystic duct, which turns into the lesser omentum to join the right side of the common hepatic duct to form the common bile duct.

The neck of the gallbladder is oriented posteromedially toward the porta hepatis; the fundus is lateral, caudal, and anterior to the neck.

The arterial supply of the gallbladder is from the cystic artery, a branch of the right hepatic artery. The cystic vein drains directly into the portal vein. A number of smaller arteries and veins run between the liver and the gallbladder.

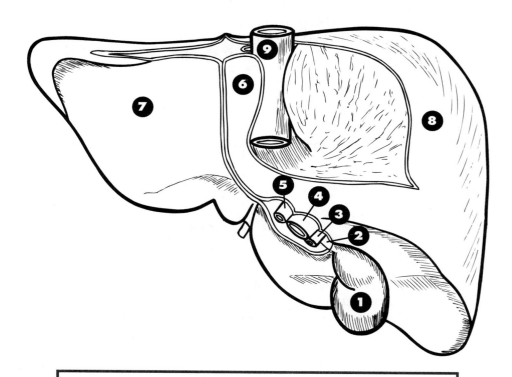

1	gallbladder	6	caudate lobe of the liver
2	cystic duct	7	left lobe of the liver
3	hepatic duct	8	right lobe of the liver
4	portal vein	9	inferior vena cava
5	hepatic artery		

Gallbladder Review Notes

GALLBLADDER PHYSIOLOGY

The primary functions of the extrahepatic biliary tract are the transportation of bile from the liver to the intestine and the regulation of its flow. Since the liver secretes approximately 1 to 2 liters of bile per day, this is an important function.

When the gallbladder and bile ducts are functioning normally, they respond in a fairly uniform manner during the various phases of digestion. Concentration of bile in the gallbladder occurs during a state of fasting. It is forced into the gallbladder by an increased pressure within the common bile duct that is produced by the action of the sphincter of Oddi at the distal end of the gallbladder.

During the fasting state, very little bile flows into the duodenum. Stimulation produced by the influence of food causes the gallbladder to contract, resulting in an outpouring of bile into the duodenum. When the stomach is emptied, duodenal peristalsis diminishes, the gallbladder relaxes, the tonus of the sphincter of Oddi increases slightly, and thus very little bile passes into the duodenum. Small amounts of bile secreted by the liver are retained in the common duct and forced into the gallbladder.

Removal of the Gallbladder

When the gallbladder is removed, there is loss of tonus of the sphincter of Oddi, and pressure within the common bile duct drops to that of intraabdominal pressure. Bile is no longer retained in the bile ducts but is free to flow into the duodenum during fasting and digestive phases.

Dilation of the extrahepatic bile ducts, which is usually less than 1 centimeter, occurs after cholecystectomy.

Secretion is largely caused by a bile salt–dependent mechanism, and ductal flow is controlled by secretion. Bile salts form micelles, and solubilize triglyceride fat and assist in its absorption together with calcium, cholesterol, and fat-soluble vitamins from the intestine.

Bile is the principle means of excretion of bilirubin and cholesterol. The products of steroid hormones are also excreted in the bile. It is also the way drugs and poisons such as salts of heavy metals are excreted. The bile salts from the intestine stimulate the liver to make more bile. Bile salts activate intestinal and pancreatic enzymes.

Clinical Symptoms of Gallbladder Disease

Some of the clinical signs and symptoms of gallbladder disease are:

- Fat intolerance
- Midepigastric pain
- Jaundice
- Abdominal pain
- Chills and fever

Gallbladder Terminology

adenomyomatosis small polypoid masses arising from gallbladder wall; causes RUQ pain

biliary atresia a condition in which the bile ducts become narrowed; affects infants a few months old

bilirubin yellowish pigment in the bile formed by red cell breakdown. Causes jaundice if present in increased amounts and is elevated in all types of jaundice. Can be measured in the urine and serum. Direct elevation of the bilirubin level is usually caused by obstructive jaundice

cholangitis inflammation of a bile duct

cholecystitis inflammation of the gallbladder

choledochal cyst fusiform dilation of the common duct that causes obstruction

choledochojejunostomy a surgical procedure in which the bile duct is anastomosed to the jejunum; food and air may reflex into the bile ducts

choledocholithiasis gallstone in the bile duct

cholelithiasis gallstones in the gallbladder or the biliary tree

cholesterosis a variant of adenomyomatosis, in which cholesterol polyps arise from the gallbladder wall

cirrhosis diffuse disease of the liver with fibrosis; causes portal hypertension

collaterals dilated veins that appear when portal hypertension is present; seen in the region of the porta hepatis and pancreas

Courvoisier's sign an RUQ mass with painless jaundice implies that there is a carcinomatous mass in the head of the pancreas causing biliary duct obstruction. (A palpable mass indicates a hydroptic gallbladder)

fatty infiltration diffuse involvement of the liver with fat; associated with ETOH, obesity, diabetes mellitus, steroid overadministration, jejunoileal bypass, and malnutrition

Glisson's capsule layer of fibrous tissue that surrounds the bile ducts, hepatic arteries, and portal veins within the liver as they travel together; also surrounds the liver

Hartmann's pouch portion of the gallbladder that lies nearest the cystic duct where stones often collect

hepatitis inflammation of the liver as a result of viral infections transmitted by fecal-oral (type A) route or hematogenous (type B) route; disease may be acute or may become chronic after an acute episode

jaundice yellow pigmentation of the skin caused by excessive bilirubin accumulation; the severity of disease is best judged by the appearance of the sclerae

phrygian cap variant gallbladder shape in which the fundus of the gallbladder is tilted and has a partial septum

portal hypertension increased portal venous pressure usually caused by liver disease; leads to dilation of the portal vein with splenic and superior mesenteric vein enlargement, splenomegaly, and formation of collaterals; may be caused by portal vein thrombosis

pruritus itching, which may be caused by an excessive amount of bilirubin; is found in patients with obstructive jaundice

serum enzymes SGOT, SGPT, LDH, alkaline phosphatase are liver enzymes released from damaged hepatic cells. They are elevated with both obstructive and intrinsic liver disease. The alkaline phosphatase is higher in obstruction, whereas the others are higher in intrinsic liver disease

sphincter of Oddi opening of the common bile duct (CBD) and pancreatic duct into the duodenum

Pathology and Congenital Anomalies

Biliary Dyspepsia

Biliary dyspepsia consists of a feeling of fullness, indigestion, and belching that occurs soon after the ingestion of food. Dyspepsia may occur whether or not the gallbladder is infected. It may be caused by an insufficient amount of bile present in the duodenum at the beginning of a meal to produce proper fat digestion. Removal of the diseased gallbladder is accompanied by a loss of tonus of the sphincter of Oddi, and the unimpaired flow of bile into the duodenum both in the fasting state and during feeding provides an adequate amount of bile in the duodenum to permit proper digestion. This seems to be a logical explanation for relief of dyspepsia. Mild forms of dyspepsia can be relieved by the ingestion of bile salts.

Biliary Dyskinesia

Biliary dyskinesia is a functional disorder of the biliary tract, especially spasm of the sphincter of Oddi. Biliary colic without jaundice or fever results from the contraction of the gallbladder. Treatment is by ingestion of antispasmodics.

Choledocholithiasis

The majority of stones in the CBD have migrated from the gallbladder. Common duct stones are usually associated with calculous cholecystitis. Stones tend to affect Vater's ampulla and may project into the duodenum. This explains the importance for surgeons to check the CBD when removing the gallbladder.

Cholangitis

Bile may become infected as a result of the intestines turning dark brown and opaque. The CBD is thickened and dilated, especially in Vater's ampulla. Cholangitis abscesses are seen in severe or prolonged infection. Malaise and fever followed by sweating and shivering develop during cholangitis. In severe cases, the patient suffers from lethargy, prostration, and shock. Because of increasing pressure in the biliary tree, pus accumulates. Decompression of the CBD is necessary.

Biliary Fistula

After a cholecystostomy or T-tube choledochotomy, a biliary fistula may occur. Only under certain circumstances does a fistula occur after gallstones, carcinoma of the gallbladder, or trauma. If possible, the bile lost should be returned to the patient. Hemorrhage into the biliary tree may follow trauma, aneurysms of the hepatic artery or one of its branches, biopsy of the liver, tumors of the tract, gallstones, or inflammation of the liver.

Strictures

A stricture may occur if biliary pressure is raised, perhaps by a residual common duct stone. Usually after biliary tract surgery, benign strictures of the CBD appear. Prolonged T-tube drainage of the CBD, cholecystostomy, rough probing of the bile duct for calculi, and attempts at operative cholangiography, especially with a normal size duct, have resulted in infected bile.

Choledochal Cysts

Description

Choledochal cysts are possibly the result of pancreatic juices refluxing into the bile duct because of the anomalous junction of the pancreatic duct into the distal common bile duct, thereby causing duct wall abnormality, weakness, and outpouching of ductal walls.

Laboratory Values

- Laboratory values indicate that these cysts are rare and occur more commonly in females than in males, with a ratio of 4:1.
- There is an increased incidence in infants, although the cysts may occur in adults.
- The cysts may be associated with gallstones, pancreatitis, or cirrhosis.

- The patient may have an abdominal mass, pain, fever, or jaundice.
- Diagnosis may be confirmed with an HIDA scan.

Pathology

- The majority of cases are thought to be congenital and caused by bile reflux.
- The pathologic process may involve cystic dilation of the biliary system.

Sonographic Appearance

- On ultrasound examination, a choledochal cyst may appear as a true cyst.
- The cyst will be located in the RUQ.
- There may or may not be apparent communication with the biliary system.

Cysts Are Classified by Anatomy

- I—Localized cystic dilation of CBD
- II—Diverticulum from CBD
- III—Invagination of CBD into duodenum
- IV—Dilation of CBD and common hepatic duct (CHD)

NEOPLASMS OF THE GALLBLADDER

Benign Tumors

- True benign tumors of the gallbladder are very rare
- An **adenoma** is the most common type of benign tumor.
- It appears as a flat elevation located in the body of the gallbladder.
- Adenomas almost always occur in or near the fundus and must be distinguished pathologically from adenomyomatosis.
- **Adenomyomatosis** is a hyperplastic change in the gallbladder wall.
- **Papillomas** may occur singly or in groups and may be scattered over a large part of the mucosal surface of the gallbladder.
  - These are not precursors to cancer.
  - On OCG, the tumor is better seen after partial contraction of the gallbladder.
  - Compression and various patient positions show that the lesion is not freely moveable within the gallbladder.

Pseudotumors of the Gallbladder

- A cholesterol polyp is the most common pseudotumor.
- Other masses that may occur include mucosal hyperplasia, inflammatory polyps, mucous cysts, and granulomata caused by parasitic infections.

Ultrasound Findings

- On ultrasound examination, benign tumors appear as small elevations in the gallbladder lumen.

- These elevations maintain their initial location during position changes, and there is no acoustic shadow behind a papillomatous elevation.
- Intraparietal diverticula would suggest an adenomyomatosis.

Carcinoma

Malignant tumors are encountered in three clinical situations:

- Rarely, carcinoma may appear during a screening examination of the abdomen as an intravesicular mass. Later, a pathologic examination of the mass may find it to be malignant. (Small intravesicular tumors appear either as polypoid masses without acoustic shadowing, or as areas of localized wall thickening.)
- More frequently, carcinoma is found after palpation of a right upper quadrant mass.
- In most cases, malignant tumors are found during the evaluation of a jaundiced patient.

Characteristics of Malignant Gallbladder Masses

- On ultrasound examination, the global shape of the malignant mass is similar to the shape of the gallbladder.
- The echotexture of the mass is heterogeneous, solid, or semisolid.
- A malignant tumor is free of shadows.
- The gallbladder wall is markedly thickened.
- Adjacent liver tissue in the hilar area is often heterogeneous because of direct spread of the tumor.
- A dilated biliary duct will appear as a "shotgun" sign.
- Carcinoma of the gallbladder is almost never detected at a resectable stage.
- Obstruction of the cystic duct by the tumor or lymph nodes occurs early in the course of the disease and causes the gallbladder to be nonvisual on OCG.
- One documented case of noninvasive papillary adenocarcinoma showed that the tumor was evident as a solitary, fixed defect in a well-opacified gallbladder.

Causes of Fixed Filling Defects in an Opacified Gallbladder

- Cholesterosis: a condition resulting from a disturbance in the metabolism of lipids, and is characterized by deposits of cholesterol in tissue
- Adenomyomatosis
- Adherent gallstone
- Adenoma
- Papilloma: a benign papillary tumor
- Carcinoid
- Carcinoma
- Metastases
- Mucosal hyperplasia

- Inflammatory polyp
- Epithelial cyst
- Mucous retention cyst
- Spurious, or false, defect of the infundibulum
- Heterotopic pancreatic or gastric tissue
- Parasitic granuloma
- Metachromatic sulfatides
- Varices
- Arterial tortuosity and aneurysm

Malignant Tumors

- Primary carcinoma of the gallbladder is nearly always a rapidly progressive disease, with a mortality rate approaching 100%.
- It is associated with cholelithiasis in about 80% to 90% of cases, although as yet there is no direct proof that gallstones are the carcinogenic agents.
- Patients with a porcelain gallbladder have an increased incidence of carcinoma.
- This is two times as common as carcinoma of the bile ducts and occurs most frequently in women 60 years of age and older.
- Carcinoma arises in the body and rarely in the cystic duct.
- The tumor infiltrates the gallbladder locally or diffusely.
- The tumor causes thickening and rigidity of the gallbladder wall.
- The adjacent part of the liver is often invaded by direct spread of the tumor, extending through tissue spaces, the ducts of Luschka, and/or the lymph channels.
- Obstruction of the cystic duct is caused by direct extension of the tumor or extrinsic compression by involved lymph nodes that occurs early.
- The tumor is columnar cell adenocarcinoma, sometimes mucinous in type.
- Squamous cell carcinoma occurs but is unusual.
- Metastatic cancer of the gallbladder is usually a result of melanoma.
  - It is usually accompanied by liver metastases.
  - Most patients have no symptoms that relate to the gallbladder unless there is complicating acute cholecystitis.

Tumors Arising from Extrahepatic Bile Ducts

- Tumors arising from the CBD and ampullar cancer have the same ultrasound features as pancreatic tumors.
- A specific pattern exists when the ampulloma bulges inside a dilated common bile duct.

- Cancer of the biliary convergence or of the hepatic duct usually infiltrates the ductal wall without bulging outside.
- It is difficult to image these tumors; diagnosis is indirect, with biliary dilation above the tumor.

Tumors Arising from Intrahepatic Bile Ducts

- These tumors have the same features as primary tumors of the liver.
- There is associated dilation of intrahepatic ducts.
- There is a pattern of rare cystic cholangiocarcinoma.

GALLBLADDER PERILS
Gallbladder Wall Thickness

- Common causes for more than 2 mm of thickening of the gallbladder wall include the following:
  - hypoalbumin
  - AIDS
  - CHF
  - cholecystitis
  - cholecystitis/adenocarcinoma
  - nonfasting
  - hepatitis
  - tumor
  - ascites
  - drugs
  - hydration (rapid)
  - TPN
- Common causes for a false positive result of a gallstone examination include the following:
  - polyp
  - adenomyosis
  - sludge ball
  - duodenal gas
  - clips
  - biliary air
  - porcelain gallbladder
  - gallbladder agenesis
- Common causes for a false negative result of a gallstone examination include the following:
  - contracted gallbladder
  - duct/neck
  - very small
  - geographic location/technique
  - sludge ball
  - gallstone in fundal cap

Review Exercise A • Gallbladder Physiology

1. What are the primary functions of the extrahepatic biliary tract? _____

_____

_____

_____

2. What is the function of the sphincter of ODDI? _____

_____

_____

_____

3. What is the role of the duodenum in the release of bile? _____

_____

_____

_____

_____

4. What occurs when the gallbladder is removed? _____

_____

_____

_____

5. What are the functions of bile? _____

_____

_____

6. What are the clinical symptoms of gallbladder disease? _____

_____

_____

_____

Review Exercise B • Gallbladder Definitions

Define the following terms:

1. Adenomyomatosis: _____

2. Biliary atresia: _____

3. Bilirubin: _____

4. Choledochal cyst: _____

5. Cholangitis: _____

6. Cholecystitis: _____

7. Choledochojejunostomy: _____

8. Choledocholithiasis: _____

9. Cholelithiasis: _____

10. Cholesterosis: _____

11. Cirrhosis: _____

12. Collaterals: _____

13. Courvoisier's sign: _____

14. Fatty infiltration: _____

15. Glisson's capsule: _____

16. Hartmann's pouch: _____

17. Hepatitis: _____

18. Jaundice: _____

19. Phrygian cap: _____

20. Portal hypertension: _____

21. Pruritus: _____

22. Serum enzymes: _____

23. Sphincter of Oddi: _____

Review Exercise C • Jaundice

Fill in the blanks using the terms from the list below.

adenomyomatosis   choledocholithiasis   Hartmann's Pouch
biliary atresia   cholelithiasis   hepatitis
bilirubin   cholesterosis   jaundice phrygian cap
choledochal cyst   cirrhosis collaterals   portal hypertension
cholangitis   Courvoisier's Sign   pruritus
cholecystitis   fatty infiltration
choledochogejunostomy   Glisson's Capsule

1. _____ yellowish pigment in bile formed by red cell breakdown.

2. _____ condition causing RUQ pain in which small polypoid masses arise from
the gallbladder wall.

3. _____ increased portal venous pressure usually caused by liver disease.

4. _____ inflammation of the gallbladder.

5. _____ a right upper quadrant mass with painless jaundice implies that there is a carcinomatous mass in the head of the pancreas that is causing biliary duct obstruction.

6. _____ variant gallbladder shape in which the fundus of the gallbladder is tilted and
has a partial septum.

7. _____ surgical procedure in which the bile duct is anastomosed to jejunum; food and air
may relux into the bile ducts.

8. _____ gallstone in a bile duct.

9. _____ gallstones in the gallbladder or biliary tree.

10. _____ variant of adenomyomatosis in which cholesterol polyps arise from the gallbladder wall.

11. _____ portion of the gallbladder that lies nearest the cystic duct where stones often collect.

12. _____ condition in which the bile ducts become narrowed.

13. _____ diffuse involvement of the liver with fat.

14. _____ inflammation of the liver caused by a viral infection transmitted by fecal-oral (type A) or hematogenous (type B) route.

15. _____ itching.

16. _____ yellow pigmentation of the skin as a result of excessive bilirubin accumulation.

17. _____ a fusiform dilation of the common duct that causes obstruction.

18. _____ layer of fibrous tissue that surrounds the bile ducts, hepatic arteries, and portal veins within the liver as they travel together.

19. _____ dilated veins that appear when portal hypertension is present.

20. _____ diffuse disease of the liver with fibrosis.

21. The portal vein can be distinguished from the common duct because the portal vein has echogenic walls and branches toward the diaphragm (true or false).

22. The hepatic veins are easily distinguishable from portal veins because they empty into the IVC (true or false).

23. The left hepatic artery crosses between the common duct and the portal vein (true or false).

24. One can easily detect diffuse liver disease with sonography (true or false).

25. In patients with hemolytic anemia, the liver appears shrunken in size (true or false).

26. Which of the following describe biliary ducts?

   a. Run anterior to portal veins

   b. Run inferior to portal veins

   c. Have regular walls, branch into right and left

   d. Have irregular walls, branch repeatedly

   e. Show acoustic enhancement

   f. Show no acoustic enhancement

   g. Will dilate with valsalva maneuver

   h. Will not dilate with valsalva maneuver

   i. If dilated, will show the "double barrel shotgun" sign.

Review Exercise D • Neoplasms of the Gallbladder • Benign Tumors

1. What is the most common benign tumor of the gallbladder? _____

2. What are adenomyomatosis and papillomas of the gallbladder? _____

_____

_____

3. What should the sonographer look for to distinguish between a benign tumor and a gallstone? _____

_____

_____

_____

4. What are the frequency and findings in carcinoma of the gallbladder? _____

_____

_____

_____

_____

5. Name the causes of fixed filling defects in an opacified gallbladder. _____

_____

_____

_____

6. What is a porcelain gallbladder? _____

_____

_____

_____

7. Describe the ultrasound appearance of carcinoma of the gallbladder. _____

_____

_____

_____

8. Metastatic cancer of the gallbladder is usually caused by what condition? _____

_____

_____

_____

9. Discuss the ultrasound appearance of tumors arising from extrahepatic bile ducts. _____

_____

_____

_____

10. Discuss the ultrasound appearance of tumors arising from intrahepatic bile ducts. _____

_____

_____

_____

_____

Self-Test • Gallbladder and Biliary System

1. The extrahepatic biliary system consists of the:

   a. hepatic ducts, common bile duct

   b. common bile duct, gallbladder, cystic duct

   c. common hepatic duct, common bile duct, gallbladder, cystic duct

   d. hepatic duct, cystic duct, common bile duct, pancreatic duct

2. Name the structures in Figure 5-1.

1. _____	6. _____	11. _____
2. _____	7. _____	12. _____
3. _____	8. _____	13. _____
4. _____	9. _____	14. _____
5. _____	10. _____	

FIGURE 5-1

Anterior View of the Biliary System

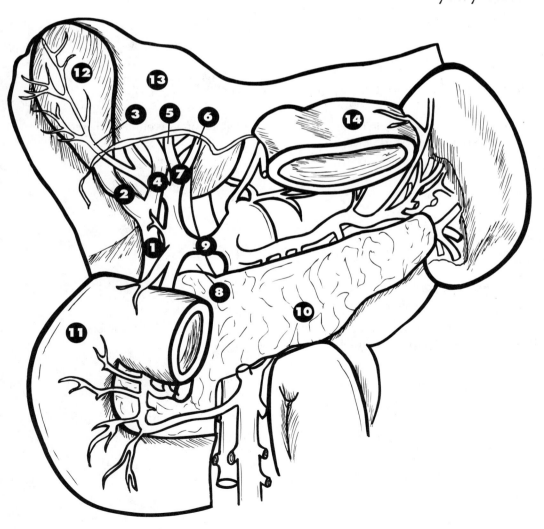

3. What is Hartmann's pouch?

4. In normal patients, the common hepatic duct is larger than the common bile duct (true or false).

5. Within the liver parenchyma, the bile ducts follow the same course as the portal venous and hepatic arterial branches (true or false).

6. The arterial supply of the gallbladder is from the _____ .

7. List at least seven causes of gallbladder wall thickening.

   a.

   b.

   c.

   d.

   e.

   f.

   g.

8. What does it mean when a patient has jaundice?

9. What is pneumobilia? When would the sonographer see this?

10. What is CCK and what does CCK do?

11. What type of food causes the greatest CCK reaction?

12. What is a porcelain gallbladder?

13. What is acute cholecystitis?

14. What characteristics might be found by a sonographer when scanning a patient with acute cholecystitis?

15. If a patient has choledocholithiasis and the stone is located in the CBD, which areas would be dilated if the stone was there for a prolonged period of time?

    a. the pancreatic duct

    b. the distal CBD

    c. the proximal CBD

    d. the common hepatic duct

    e. the right hepatic duct

    f. the left hepatic duct

16. If a patient has a Klatzkin's tumor, which areas of the biliary tree may be dilated?

17. If there is an obstructive stone in the CBD and you ask the patient to eat a fatty meal and come back in 45 minutes, the diameter of the CBD (proximal to the stone) would:

    a. decrease in size

    b. stay the same

    c. increase in size

18. The right and left hepatic ducts emerge from the right lobe of the liver in the porta hepatis and unite to form the:

    a. cystic duct

    b. common hepatic duct

    c. common bile duct

    d. common pancreatic duct

19. This duct passes caudally and medially and runs _____ with the portal vein.

    a. perpendicular

    b. parallel

    c. horizontal

    d. lateral

20. The diameter of the common hepatic duct is:

    a. 2 mm

    b. 3 mm

    c. 4 mm

    d. 5 mm

21. The hepatic duct is joined by the _____ to form the _____ .

    a. pancreatic duct; cystic duct

    b. common bile duct; cystic duct

    c. cystic duct; common bile duct

    d. right hepatic duct; common bile duct

22. In a 60-year-old adult, the normal common bile duct should not measure more than:

    a. 5 mm

    b. 6 mm

    c. 8 mm

    d. 10 mm

23. The distal portion of the common bile duct is lateral to the hepatic artery and anterior to the portal vein (true or false).

24. The distal duct lies _____ with the anterior wall of the IVC.

    a. perpendicular

    b. lateral

    c. parallel

    d. horizontal

25. The cystic duct connects the _____ of the gallbladder with the common hepatic duct

to form the _____ .

    a. fundus; CHD

    b. fundus; CBD

    c. neck; CBD

    d. body; CHD

26. The walls of the gallbladder generally measure less than _____ .

    a. 1 to 2 mm

    b. 2 to 3 mm

    c. 3 to 4 mm

    d. 4 to 5 mm

27. A phrygian cap of the gallbladder is:

    a. calcification of the gallbladder wall

    b. septations within the organ

    c. folding of the fundus

    d. partial septation

28. Hartmann's pouch is formed:

    a. when septations divide the neck from the cystic duct

    b. when the gallbladder folds back on itself at the neck

    c. when the gallbladder is partially septated

    d. when the fundus is folded

29. The function of the gallbladder is:

    a. storage for enzymes

    b. storage for extra cholesterol

    c. reservoir for bile

    d. reservoir for biliary salts

30. Demonstration of the biliary system does not need to be performed with the patient in a fasting state because a diseased gallbladder will be well demonstrated without fasting (true or false).

31. The bright linear echo within the liver connecting the gallbladder and the right or main portal vein is the:

    a. right lobar fissure

    b. main lobar fissure

    c. ligamentum teres

    d. left lobar fissure

32. A prominent gallbladder may be seen in some patients. Name the conditions these patients would have:

    a.

    b.

    c.

33. An extrahepatic mass compressing the common bile duct can produce an enlarged gallbladder. This sign is:

    a. Murphy's sign

    b. Christian's sign

    c. Courvoisier's sign

    d. compressed tissue sign

34. The common duct lies _____ and to the _____ of the portal vein in the region of the porta hepatis and gastrohepatic ligament.

    a. posterior; left

    b. posterior; right

   c. anterior; right

   d. anterior; left

35. On a transverse scan, the common duct, hepatic artery, and portal vein have been referred to as the "Mickey Mouse sign."

   a. common duct, left; hepatic artery right; portal vein inferior

   b. common duct, right; hepatic artery left; portal vein posterior

   c. common duct, inferior; hepatic artery right; portal vein right

   d. common duct, anterior; hepatic artery left; portal vein inferior

36. On the sagittal scan, the hepatic artery passes _____ to the common duct.

   a. posterior

   b. anterior

   c. lateral

   d. medial

37. The _____ branch of the hepatic artery can be seen between the duct and the portal vein as a small circular structure.

   a. left

   b. middle

   c. right

38. Classic symptoms of gallbladder disease include all but:

   a. right upper quadrant pain

   b. right shoulder pain

   c. nausea and vomiting

   d. hematuria

39. Some gallbladders may be so packed with inspissated bile that it becomes difficult to separate the gallbladder from the liver parenchyma (true or false).

40. (Choose 2 answers) Two common echographic features of gangrene are:

   a. the presence of diffuse medium to coarse echogenic densities filling the gallbladder lumen in the absence of bile duct obstruction

   b. no shadowing

   c. diffuse shadowing

   d. layering effect

41. Thickening of the gallbladder wall may be caused by all but:

   a. hepatitis

   b. pancreatitis

   c. adenomyomatosis

   d. cholecystitis

42. The most common sign for carcinoma of the gallbladder is:

   a. shadowing posterior to the gallbladder

    b. gallbladder wall thickening

    c. irregular fungating mass that contains low-intensity echoes within the gallbladder

    d. mass will change with position changes

43. A polyp appears sonographically as a low-level echogenic mass attached to the wall of the gallbladder (true or false).

44. Dilated ducts are always associated with jaundice (true or false).

45. The second part of the CBD is _____ to the first part of the duodenum.

    a. anterior

    b. posterior

    c. lateral

    d. medial

46. The third part of the duct lies in a groove on the _____ surface of the head of the pancreas.

    a. anterior

    b. posterior

    c. lateral

    d. medial

47. The common bile duct is joined by the main pancreatic duct. Together they open through the _____ into the duodenal wall.

    a. ampulla of Water

    b. ampulla of Vater

    c. ampulla of Oddi

    d. ampulla of Vauter

48. The end parts of both ducts and the ampulla are surrounded by circular muscle fibers called the:

    a. sphincter of Odi

    b. sphincter of Vater

    c. sphincter of Oddi

    d. sphincter of ampullae

49. The _____ crosses between the common bile duct and the portal vein.

    a. right hepatic artery

    b. left hepatic artery

    c. middle hepatic artery

    d. splenic artery

50. A fusiform dilation of the common bile duct that causes obstruction is known as:

    a. choledochal cyst

    b. adenomyomatosis

    c. cholangitis

    d. phrygian cap

51. Inflammation of the gallbladder is:

    a. cholecystitis

    b. choledocholithiasis

    c. cholesterosis

    d. adenomyomatosis

52. The condition of having gallstones in the gallbladder or biliary tree is:

    a. cholelithiasis

    b. choledocholithiasis

    c. adenomyomatosis

    d. cholesterosis

53. A condition causing RUQ pain in which small polypoid masses arise from the gallbladder wall is:

    a. adenomyomatosis

    b. choledocholithiasis

    c. cholesterosis

    d. pruritus

54. The normal length of the gallbladder is:

    a. 2 to 4 cm

    b. 5 to 7 cm

    c. 7 to 10 cm

    d. 10 to 13 cm

55. The normal width of the gallbladder is:

    a. 1 to 3 cm

    b. 2 to 4 cm

    c. 4 to 6 cm

    d. 5 to 8 cm

56. Gallstones are more common in females than in males (true or false).

57. Factors affecting formation of gallstones include all but:

    a. abnormal bile composition

    b. stasis

    c. infection

    d. low saline levels

58. Gallstone appearance on ultrasound examination is:

    a. dependent, mobile, echogenic

    b. dependent, immobile, echogenic

    c. dependent, float, immobile

    d. independent, mobile, hypoechoic

59. Typical of gallstones is the shadow beyond the stone. This is characterized as:

    a. fuzzy margins

    b. low-level echoes beyond the stone

    c. shaggy borders of the margin

    d. clean shadow with distinct margins

60. A reverberation within the shadow would indicate stones containing calcium (true or false).

61. In the case of a porcelain gallbladder, all of the following facts would be true except:

    a. 90% associated with stones

    b. higher incidence in females than in males

    c. dense wall without shadowing

    d. hyperechoic semilunar structure with shadowing

62. Nonshadowing, low-amplitude echoes in a dependent gallbladder is most characteristic of:

    a. stones

    b. porcelain gallbladder

    c. cholecystitis

    d. sludge

63. In cholecystitis, the following factors may be found:

    a. female

    b. over 40 years of age

    c. gallbladder wall shows "halo"

    d. smaller volume

    e. no RUQ pain

    f. gallstones

    g. positive Murphy's sign

64. In patients with acalculous cholecystitis, the ultrasound findings would include:

    a. small gallbladder

    b. enlarged gallbladder

    c. localized wall thickening

    d. diffuse or focal wall thickening

    e. pericholecystic fluid

    f. positive Murphy's sign

    g. diffuse homogeneous echogenicity

65. Gangrenous cholecystitis occurs in diabetic patients and in patients with gallstones. The sonographic findings include all but:

    a. hypoechoic internal structure

    b. diffuse intraluminal echoes

    c. no layer or shadow

    d. right upper quadrant pain

66. Gallbladder perforation may appear in patients with the following diseases except for:

    a. acute cholecystitis

    b. negative Murphy's sign

    c. gangrenous cholecystitis

    d. chronic cholecystitis

67. (Choose 2 answers) The sonographic findings of a gallbladder perforation are:

    a. hydrops

    b. pericholecystic fluid

    c. intramural mass

    d. intraperitoneal collection

68. (Choose 3 answers) Which of the following relates to patients with AIDS?

    a. 55% have gallbladder wall thickening

    b. many patients have ductal abnormalities

    c. no ductal dilation

    d. extrabiliary CMV

69. The ultrasound appearance of a gallbladder neoplasm is:

    a. hydrops

    b. wall thickening, wall mass

    c. normal wall, internal echoes

    d. wall thickening

70. Malignant neoplasms are frequently associated with stones (true or false).

71. The physiologic effect of a fatty meal includes all except:

    a. stimulation of CCK

    b. contraction of gallbladder

    c. decrease of bile flow to liver

    d. relaxation of sphincter of Oddi

72. In intrahepatic ductal dilation there is acoustic enhancement (true or false).

73. The most common level of obstruction is:

    a. intrahepatic

    b. pancreatic head

    c. cystic duct

    d. sphincter of Oddi

74. The second most common level of obstruction is:

    a. porta hepatis

    b. suprapancreatic

    c. pancreatic head

    d. cystic duct

75. The most common primary biliary neoplasm is:

   a. adenocarcinoma

   b. metastatic

   c. lymphoma

   d. rhabdomyoma

76. Ultrasound findings in a primary neoplasm include all except:

   a. marked dilation in presence of normal pancreas

   b. abrupt termination or stricture

   c. normal duct

   d. mass involving duct

77. The most frequent cause of metastatic disease to the biliary system is:

   a. pancreatitis

   b. pancreatic carcinoma

   c. lymphoma

   d. sarcoma

78. The common bile duct may be found anterior and lateral to the portal vein (true or false).

79. The right and left hepatic ducts emerge from the right lobe of the liver in the porta hepatis and unite to form the:

   a. cystic duct

   b. common hepatic duct

   c. common bile duct

   d. common pancreatic duct

Case Reviews

1. A 59-year-old male comes to the hospital with clinical signs of hepatomegaly. No significant laboratory values are noted during his physical evaluation. Evaluate the ultrasound findings (Figure 5-5).

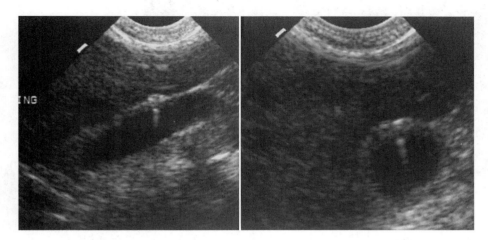

2. Look at Figure 5-6, **A, B, C,** and **D.** Describe the ultrasound findings of each. Are these findings consistent with a normal or a pathologic process in the gallbladder?

   A. _____

   B. _____

   C. _____

   D. _____

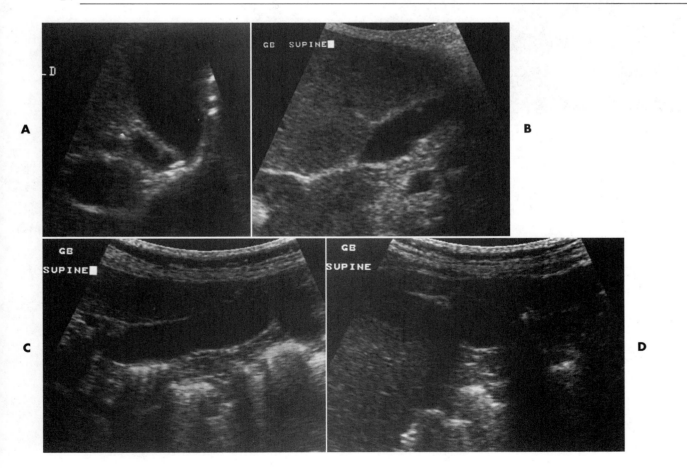

3. A 39-year-old mother of five children complains of right upper quadrant pain that has been intermittent during her last two pregnancies. What are your ultrasound findings (Figure 5-7)?

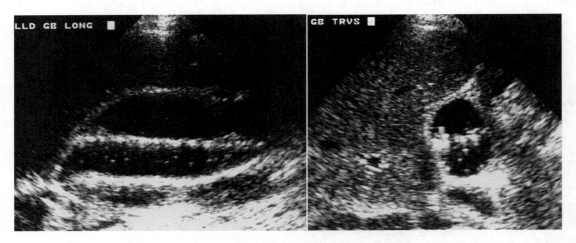

4. A 2-year-old male has abdominal pain, palpable mass, and jaundice. The laboratory values show increased bilirubin. What areas should the sonographer evaluate and what ultrasound findings are noted (Figure 5-8)?

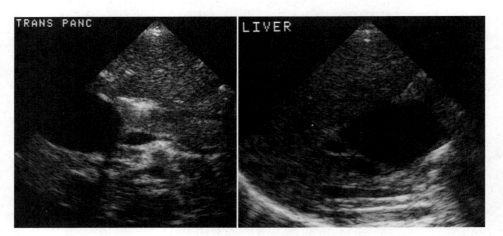

5. Thickening of the gallbladder wall is found in various medical conditions. What is the definition for gallbladder wall thickening? How much should it measure? What other modalities should be used to make sure it is gallbladder wall thickening? What are your findings (Figure 5-9)?

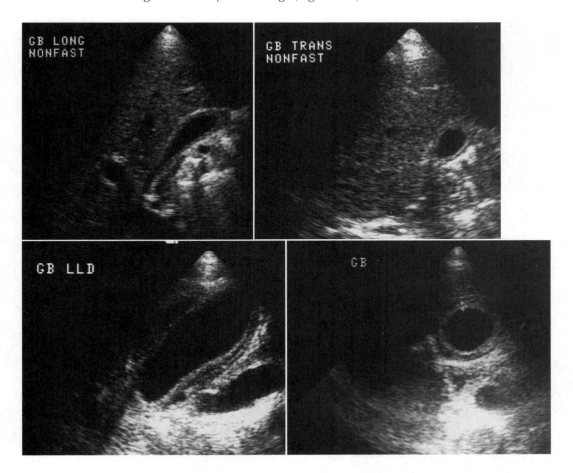

6. A 45-year-old obese female complains of persistent right upper quadrant pain radiating to the right shoulder. Historically this patient has come to the hospital on numerous occasions with similar symptoms. She has had nausea and vomiting for the past 5 days. What would you expect to find on ultrasound examination? Describe the ultrasound findings (Figure 5-10).

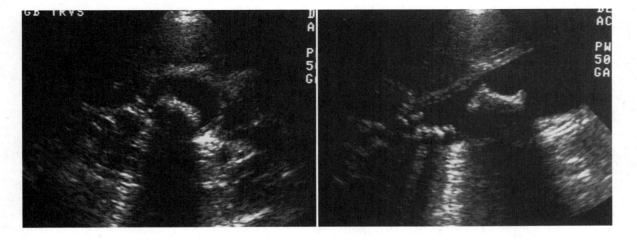

7. A young patient with AIDS has been hospitalized for several days. His bilirubin is elevated, and he is experiencing abdominal pain. What is your diagnosis, based on the ultrasound findings (Figure 5-11)?

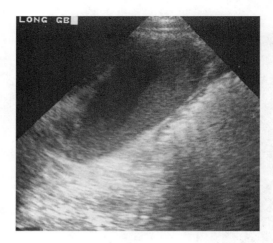

8. A 66-year-old female has abdominal pain, weight loss, and jaundice. She is known to have gallstones from previous ultrasound findings. What are your ultrasound findings (Figure 5-12)?

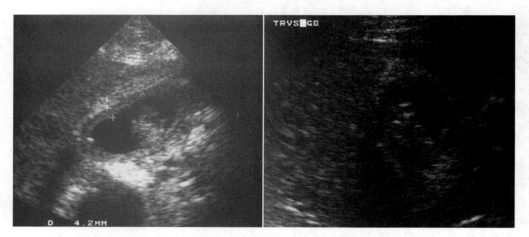

9. A young female arrives at the emergency room with intense right upper quadrant pain. The pain radiates to the back and right shoulder. The young woman has had nausea and vomiting for 3 days. What are the ultrasound findings (Figure 5-13)?

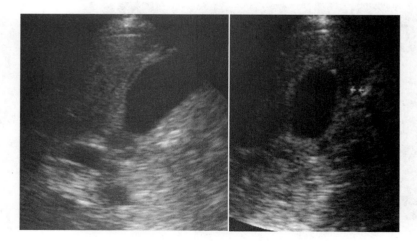

10. A 62-year-old male presents with vague right upper quadrant pain. What are your ultrasound findings (Figure 5-14)?

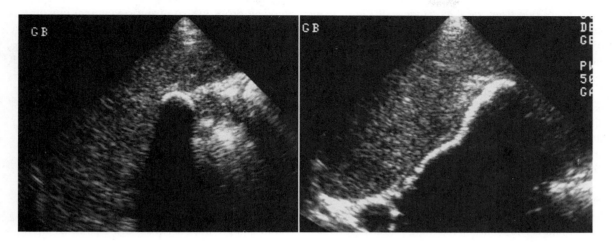

Answers to Review Exercise A

1. The primary functions of the extrahepatic biliary tract are the transportation of bile from the liver to the intestine and the regulation of its flow. Since the liver secretes approximately 1 to 2 liters of bile per day, this is an important function.

2. When the gallbladder and bile ducts are functioning normally, they respond in a fairly uniform manner during various phases of digestion. Concentration of bile in the gallbladder occurs during a state of fasting. It is forced into the gallbladder by an increased pressure within the common bile duct that is produced by the action of the sphincter of Oddi at the distal end of the gallbladder.

3. During the fasting state, very little bile flows into the duodenum. Stimulation produced by the influence of food causes the gallbladder to contract, resulting in an outpouring of bile into the duodenum.

   When the stomach is emptied, duodenal peristalsis diminishes, the gallbladder relaxes, the tonus of the sphincter of Oddi increases slightly, and thus very little bile passes into the duodenum. Small amounts of bile secreted by the liver are retained in the common duct and forced into the gallbladder.

4. When the gallbladder is removed, there is loss of tonus of the sphincter of Oddi, and pressure within the common bile duct drops to that of intraabdominal pressure. Bile is no longer retained in the bile ducts but is free to flow into the duodenum during fasting and digestive phases.

   Dilation of the extrahepatic bile ducts, which is usually less than one centimeter, occurs after cholecystectomy. Secretion is largely caused by a bile salt–dependent mechanism, and ductal flow is controlled by secretion. Bile salts form micelles, and solubilize triglyceride fat and assist in its absorption, together with calcium, cholesterol, and fat-soluble vitamins from the intestine.

5. Bile is the principle means of excretion of bilirubin and cholesterol. The products of steroid hormones are also excreted in the bile. It is also the way drugs and poisons (such as salts of heavy metals) are excreted. The bile salts from the intestine stimulate the liver to make more bile. Bile salts activate intestinal and pancreatic enzymes.

6. Some of the clinical signs and symptoms of gallbladder disease are fat intolerance, mid-epigastric pain, jaundice, abdominal pain, and chills and fever.

Answers to Review Exercise B

1. Adenomyomatosis: small polypoid masses arising from gallbladder wall; causes RUQ pain

2. Biliary atresia: a condition in which the bile ducts become narrowed; affects infants a few months old

3. Bilirubin: yellowish pigment in the bile formed by red cell breakdown. Causes jaundice if present in increased amounts and is elevated in all types of jaundice. Can be measured in the urine and serum. Direct elevation of the bilirubin level is usually caused by obstructive jaundice

4. Choledochal cyst: fusiform dilation of the common duct that causes obstruction

5. Cholangitis: inflammation of a bile duct

6. Cholecystitis: inflammation of the gallbladder

7. Choledochojejunostomy: surgical procedure in which the bile duct is anastomosed to the jejunum; food and air may reflex into the bile ducts

8. Choledocholithiasis: gallstone in the bile duct

9. Cholelithiasis: gallstones in the gallbladder or the biliary tree

10. Cholesterosis: a variant of adenomyomatosis, in which cholesterol polyps arise from the gallbladder wall

11. Cirrhosis: diffuse disease of the liver with fibrosis; causes portal hypertension

12. Collaterals: dilated veins that appear when portal hypertension is present; seen in the region of the porta hepatis and pancreas

13. Courvoisier's sign: An RUQ mass with painless jaundice implies that there is a carcinomatous mass in the head of the pancreas causing biliary duct obstruction. (A palpable mass indicates a hydroptic gallbladder)

14. Fatty infiltration: diffuse involvement of the liver with fat; associated with ETOH, obesity, diabetes mellitus, steroid overadministration, jejunoileal bypass, and malnutrition

15. Glisson's capsule: layer of fibrous tissue that surrounds the bile ducts, hepatic arteries, and portal veins within the liver as they travel together; also surrounds the liver

16. Hartmann's pouch: portion of the gallbladder that lies nearest the cystic duct where stones often collect

17. Hepatitis: inflammation of the liver as a result of viral infections transmitted by fecal-oral (type A) route or hematogenous (type B) route; disease may be acute or may become chronic after an acute episode

18. Jaundice: yellow pigmentation of the skin caused by excessive bilirubin accumulation. The severity of disease is best judged by the appearance of the sclerae

19. Phrygian cap: variant gallbladder shape in which the fundus of the gallbladder is tilted and has a partial septum

20. Portal hypertension: increased portal venous pressure usually caused by liver disease; leads to dilation of the portal vein with splenic and superior mesenteric vein enlargement, splenomegaly, and formation of collaterals; may be caused by portal vein thrombosis

21. Pruritus: Itching, which may be caused by an excessive amount of bilirubin, is found in patients with obstructive jaundice

22. Serum enzymes. SGOT, SGPT, LDH, alkaline phosphatase are liver enzymes released from damaged hepatic cells. They are elevated with both obstructive and intrinsic liver disease. The alkaline phosphatase is higher in obstruction, whereas the others are higher in intrinsic liver disease.

23. Sphincter of ODDI: opening of the CBD and pancreatic duct into the duodenum

Answers to Review Exercise C

1. jaundice
2. adenomyomatosis
3. portal hypertension
4. cholecystitis
5. Courvoisier's sign
6. phyrygian cap
7. choledochojejunostomy
8. choledocholithiasis
9. cholelithiasis
10. cholesterosis
11. Hartmann's pouch
12. biliary atresia
13. fatty infiltration
14. hepatitis
15. pruritus
16. jaundice
17. choledochal cyst
18. Glisson's capsule
19. collaterals
20. cirrhosis
21. true
22. true
23. true
24. false
25. false
26. a, c, e, h, i

Answers to Review Exercise D

1. True benign tumors of the gallbladder are very rare. An adenoma is the most common type. This tumor occurs as a flat elevation located in the body of the gallbladder. Adenomas almost always occur in or near the fundus and must be distinguished pathologically from adenomyomatosis.

2. Adenomyomatosis is a hyperplastic change in the gallbladder wall. Papillomas may occur singly or in groups and may be scattered over a large part of the mucosal surface of the gallbladder. These are not precursors to cancer. Compression and various patient positions show that the lesion is not freely moveable within the gallbladder.

3. On ultrasound examination, benign tumors appear as small elevations in the gallbladder lumen. These elevations maintain their initial location during position changes, and there is no acoustic shadow behind a papillomatous elevation.

4. Malignant tumors are encountered in three clinical situations:
   1. Rarely, malignancy may appear during a screening examination of the abdomen as an irregular mass within the gallbladder. (Small intravesicular tumors appear either as polypoid masses without acoustic shadowing, or as areas of localized wall thickening.)
   2. More commonly, malignancy is found after palpation of a right upper quadrant mass.
   3. In most cases, malignant tumors are found during the evaluation of a jaundiced patient.
   Gallbladder carcinoma is almost never detected at a resectable stage. Obstruction of the cystic duct by the tumor or lymph nodes occurs early in the course of the disease.

5. The causes of a fixed filling defect include cholesterosis, adenomyomatosis, adherent gallstone, adenoma, papilloma, carcinoid, carcinoma, metastases, mucosal hyperplasia, inflammatory polyp, varices, and arterial tortuosity and aneurysm.

6. The term porcelain gallbladder is used when extensive calcification of the wall of the gallbladder occurs. It is found in less than 1% of gallbladders removed at surgery. It is caused by long term cholecystitis. Patients have an increased incidence of cancer. This is twice as common as cancer of bile ducts and occurs most frequently in women 60 years of age and older.
   On ultrasound the appearance of calcification of the gallbladder wall is a hyperechoic semilunar area with posterior acoustic shadowing.

7. Carcinoma of the gallbladder arises in the body and rarely in the cystic duct. The tumor infiltrates the gallbladder locally or diffusely, and causes thickening and rigidity of the wall. The adjacent part of the liver is often invaded by direct spread of the tumor, extending through tissue spaces, the ducts of Luschka, and/or the lymph channels. Obstruction of the cystic duct is caused by direct extension of the tumor or extrinsic compression by involved lymph nodes that occurs early.

8. Metastatic cancer of the gallbladder is usually a result of melanoma. It may be accompanied by liver metastases. Most patients have no symptoms that relate to the gallbladder unless there is complicating acute cholecystitis.

9. Tumors arising from the CBD and ampullar cancer have the same ultrasonic features as pancreatic

tumors. A specific pattern exists when the ampulloma bulges inside a dilated common bile duct. Cancer of the biliary convergence or of the hepatic duct usually infiltrates the ductal wall without bulging outside. It may be difficult to image these tumors; diagnosis is indirect, with biliary dilation above the tumor.

10. Tumors from the intrahepatic bile ducts have the same features as primary tumors of the liver (infiltrative or nodular). They are associated with dilation of intrahepatic ducts.

Answers to Self-Test

1. c
2. 1. common bile duct
   2. cystic duct
   3. cystic artery
   4. common hepatic duct
   5. middle hepatic artery
   6. left hepatic artery
   7. proper hepatic artery
   8. portal vein
   9. common hepatic artery
   10. pancreas
   11. duodenum
   12. gallbladder
   13. liver
   14. stomach
3. Hartmann's pouch is an outpouch near the neck of the gallbladder.
4. false
5. true
6. cystic artery
7. a. AIDS
   b. adenomyomatosis
   c. cholecystitis
   d. obstructive disease
   e. hepatitis
   f. ascites
   g. drugs
8. Jaundice is the presence of bile in the tissues, which results in yellow pigmentation of the skin, sclerae, and body secretions caused by excessive bilirubin accumulation. The severity of the disease is best judged by the appearance of the sclerae.
9. Pneumobilia is air in the biliary tract. It may occur after endoscopy or surgery, or it may result from a biliary enteric fistula complicating cholelithiasis.
10. CCK is a hormone, cholecystokinin. It is released from the duodenum into the blood. The gallbladder activity is mediated through CCK. It stimulates contraction of the gallbladder and the secretion of pancreatic enzymes.

11. Fatty foods cause the greatest CCK reaction.
12. A porcelain gallbladder is a calcification in the gallbladder wall.
13. Acute cholecystitis is an acute inflammation of the gallbladder. It usually results from obstruction of the cystic duct by gallstones. It occurs more commonly in women in their forties.
14. When scanning a patient with acute cholecystitis, the sonographer may find the following characteristics:
    a. dilation and rounding of the gallbladder as a result of cystic duct obstruction
    b. a positive Murphy's sign
    c. an anteroposterior diameter of the gallbladder exceeding 5 cm
    d. associated gallstones (in 95% of patients)
    e. echogenic bile
    f. thickened gallbladder wall with edema
15. b, c, d, e, f
16. Klatzkin's tumor occurs at the junction of the right and left hepatic ducts, near the portal triad. The intrahepatic ducts would be dilated because the bile would not be able to drain from the liver to the gallbladder.
17. a
18. b
19. b
20. c
21. c
22. b
23. false
24. c
25. c
26. b
27. c
28. b
29. c
30. false
31. b
32. a. prolonged fasting
    b. pancreatic mass compressing the common bile duct
    c. obstruction of the cystic duct

33. c
34. c
35. b
36. a
37. c
38. d
39. true
40. a, b
41. b
42. c
43. true
44. false
45. b
46. b
47. b
48. c
49. a
50. a
51. a
52. a
53. a
54. c
55. b
56. true
57. d
58. a
59. d
60. true
61. c
62. d
63. a, b, c, f, g
64. b, d, e, f, g
65. a
66. b
67. b, d
68. a, b, d
69. b
70. true
71. c
72. true
73. c
74. c
75. a
76. c
77. b
78. true
79. b

Answers to Case Reviews

1. (Figure 5-5) The ultrasound shows the distended gallbladder with focal polyp–type lesions attached to the wall. This most likely represents adenomyomatosis of the gallbladder. The typical "comet tail ring down" of echoes is seen beyond the lesion. Often these patients are asymptomatic, and the finding is incidental.

2. (Figure 5-6)
   A. Septated gallbladder—normal variant
   B. Polyp of the gallbladder wall.
   C & D. Phrygian cap—located at the fundus of the gallbladder within normal limits

3. (Figure 5-7) The ultrasound shows a distended gallbladder with layered stones within. The sludge is so viscous that the stones appear to float within the gallbladder.

4. (Figure 5-8) A choledochal cyst is more commonly seen in the neonate and pediatric population. A palpable mass in a young child would bring a Wilms' tumor into focus; however, the increased bilirubin would lead the sonographer toward the analysis of the biliary system.

   The choledochal cyst is a derivative from the anomalous insertion of the common duct into the proximal pancreatic duct. On ultrasound examination, the mass appears cystic, which is closely related to the normal gallbladder. Often the dilated duct can be seen as it enters the cyst.

5. (Figure 5-9) The common conditions that cause thickening of the gallbladder wall include acute cholecystitis, chronic cholecystitis, hepatic dysfunction, congestive heart failure, hepatitis, AIDS, nonfasting gallbladder, polyps, and ascites.

   The gallbladder wall measures 2 mm, with 3 mm upper normal. The sonographer should use color Doppler to make sure the wall is thick and that pericholecystic fluid, or varices, does not appear to surround the gallbladder.

6. (Figure 5-10) The patient has typical clinical signs of cholecystitis. On ultrasound examination, you would look for signs of chronic cholecystitis because the patient has had these symptoms for many months. The gallbladder may be somewhat small for a nonfasting status. The sonographer should look for calculi along the posterior border of the gallbladder.

   On ultrasound examination, the gallbladder is completely packed with stones (This is otherwise is known as a "packed bag," or the WES sign: wall-echo-shadow). Only the anterior wall of the gallbladder is shown with a clean shadow posterior. The best way to locate the gallbladder in this case is with the longitudinal scan over the right lobe of the liver. The portal vein and main lobar fissure should be identified. This linear structure from the fissure leads directly to the neck of the gallbladder. The clean shadow beyond the anterior wall demarcates the multiple stones within the organ.

7. (Figure 5-11) This patient shows hepatosplenomegaly. The gallbladder is distended, and the presence of sludge is seen to layer along the posterior border. Sludge is seen frequently in patients on long-term intravenous feeding. Findings to look for in a patient with AIDS include gallbladder wall thickening, cholecystitis with pericholecystic fluid, and sclerosis of the common duct.

8. (Figure 5-12) This ultrasound shows a diffuse solid mass that fills the lumen of the gallbladder. It is usually seen to arise from the wall of the gallbladder and is generally associated with stones. Focal wall thickening may be present. The differential diagnosis among gallbladder carcinoma and sludge within the gallbladder is sometimes difficult; however, the clinical evaluation of the patient is usually helpful in the differential. The patient may be rescanned the following day if the diagnosis is not definitive. If the gallbladder is filled with sludge, the shape will change; if it is tumor, the shape will be unchanged.

9. (Figure 5-13) The sonographer should be careful to ask the patient specifically where the pain is and to note if a positive Murphy's (pain over the area of the gallbladder) sign is present during the examination of the gallbladder. The gallbladder is usually enlarged and edematous. The gallbladder wall is thickened. Careful analysis should include the evaluation of pericholecystic fluid surrounding the gallbladder. Often gallstones are present.

10. (Figure 5-14) The ultrasound shows a well-defined anterior border of the gallbladder with posterior shadowing. This could represent a packed bag, indicating chronic cholecystitis, or a porcelain gallbladder.

CHAPTER

6

The Pancreas

OBJECTIVES

At the completion of this chapter, students will show orally, in writing, or by demonstration that they will be able to:

1. Describe the various positions and size of the normal pancreas.
2. Define the internal, surface, and relational anatomy of the pancreas.
3. Illustrate the cross-sectional anatomy of the pancreas and adjacent structures.
4. Describe congenital anomalies affecting the pancreas.
5. Identify the enzymes and secretions by explaining the functions of the pancreas.
6. Select the pertinent laboratory tests and other diagnostic procedures.
7. Explain the use of laboratory tests in evaluating the function of the pancreas.

8. Differentiate between sonographic appearances by explaining the clinical significance of the pathologic processes as related to the pancreas in the following diseases:
   a. acute pancreatitis
   b. acute hemorrhagic pancreatitis
   c. chronic pancreatitis
   d. pancreatic cysts
   e. benign tumors of the pancreas
   f. neoplasms of the pancreas

To further enhance learning, students should use marking pens to color the anatomic illustrations that follow.

PANCREAS

FIGURE 6-1

Pancreas and Its Surrounding Relationships

The pancreas is a retroperitoneal gland bounded anteriorly by the stomach and duodenum and posteriorly by the prever-tebral vessels (Figure 6-1). It is located deep in the epigastrium and left hypo-chondrium behind the lesser omental sac. The pancreas is generally found in a horizontal-oblique line, extending from the concavity of the duodenum to the hilum of the spleen. It is approximately 12 cm long and 2 cm thick. The gland is divided into three major areas: head, neck/body, and tail (Figures 6-2 and 6-3).

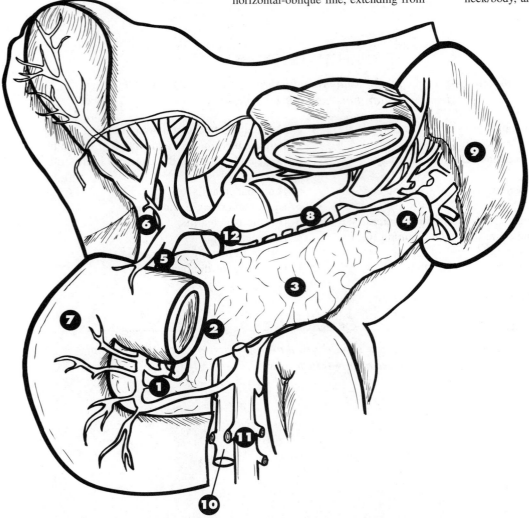

1	head of the pancreas	7	duodenum
2	neck of the pancreas	8	splenic artery
3	body of the pancreas	9	spleen
4	tail of the pancreas	10	superior mesenteric vein
5	gastroduodenal artery	11	superior mesenteric artery
6	common bile duct	12	celiac axis

FIGURE 6-2

Arterial Supply Surrounding the Pancreas

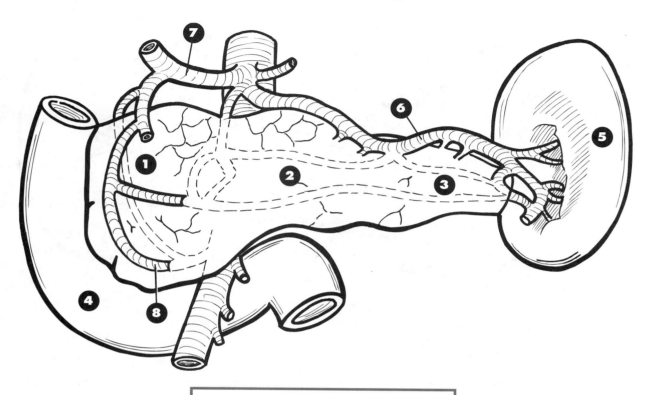

1	head of the pancreas
2	body of the pancreas
3	tail of the pancreas
4	duodenum
5	spleen
6	splenic artery
7	hepatic artery
8	pancreaticoduodenal arteries

FIGURE 6-3
Pancreas and Its Main Arteries

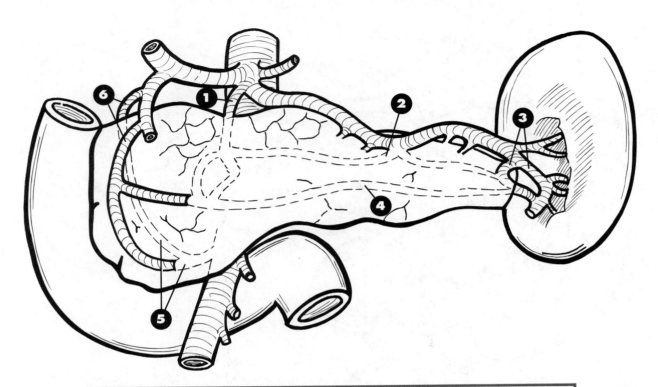

1	dorsal pancreatic artery
2	great pancreatic artery
3	caudal pancreatic artery
4	inferior pancreatic artery
5	posterior and anterior inferior pancreaticoduodenal arteries
6	posterior and anterior superior pancreaticoduodenal arteries

FIGURE 6-4
Blood Supply to the Pancreas and Duodenum

Head (FIGURE 6-4)

The head of the pancreas is anterior to the inferior vena cava and left renal vein, inferior to the caudate lobe of the liver and the portal vein, and lateral to the second portion of the duodenum. It lies in the "lap" of the duodenum. These structures pass posterior to the superior mesenteric vessels and antrum of the stomach. The uncinate process is posterior to the superior mesenteric vessels. The common bile duct passes through a groove posterior to the pancreatic head, and the gastroduodenal artery serves as the anterolateral border.

Neck/Body

The neck/body is the largest part of the gland and lies on an angle from caudal right to cephalad left, posterior to the stomach and anterior to the origin of the portal vein. It rests posteriorly against the aorta, the origin of the superior mesenteric artery, the left renal vessels, the left adrenal glands, and the left kidney. The tortuous splenic artery is usually the superior border of the pancreatic body. The anterior surface is separated by the omental bursa from the posterior wall of the stomach. The inferior surface, below the attachment of the transverse mesocolon, is adjacent to the duodenojejunal junction and the splenic flexure of the colon.

Tail

The tail of the pancreas lies anterior to the left kidney, close to the spleen and the left colic flexure. The splenic artery forms the anterior border, the splenic vein forms the posterior border, and the stomach forms the superoanterior border.

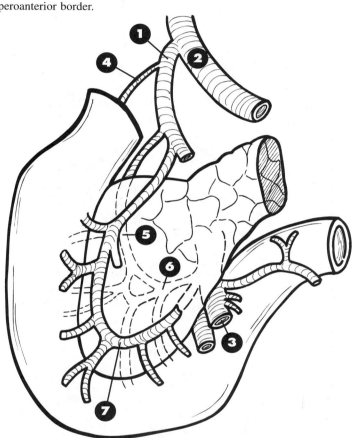

1	**gastroduodenal artery**
2	**hepatic artery**
3	**first jejunal artery**
4	**superior mesenteric artery**
5	**supraduodenal artery**
6	**anterior superior pancreaticoduodenal artery**
7	**posterior and anterior inferior pancreaticoduodenal arteries**

FIGURE 6-5
Anterior View of the Pancreas and Duodenum

Pancreatic Ducts (FIGURE 6-5)

The Wirsung's duct is a primary duct extending the entire length of the gland. It receives tributaries from lobules at right angles and enters the medial second part of the duodenum with the common bile duct at Vater's ampulla (guarded by the sphincter of Oddi).

Santorini's duct is a secondary duct that drains the upper anterior head. It enters the duodenum at the minor papilla approximately 2 cm proximal to Vater's ampulla.

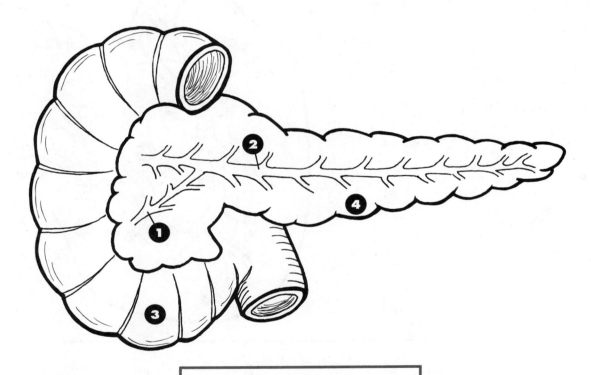

1	accessory pancreatic duct
2	main pancreatic duct
3	duodenum
4	pancreas

FIGURE 6-6

Relationship of the Splenic-Portal Vein to the Pancreas as Viewed from Posterior

Relational Anatomy
(FIGURE 6-6)

Structures related to the posterior surface include the inferior vena cava, the aorta, the superior mesenteric vessels, the splenic and portal veins, and the common bile duct. The splenic artery and stomach lie along the superior border of the pancreas, and the hilum of the spleen lies in contact with the tail of the gland. The anterior pancreatic surface is bounded by the stomach and the lesser peritoneal cavity, whereas the inferior surface lies along the greater peritoneal cavity.

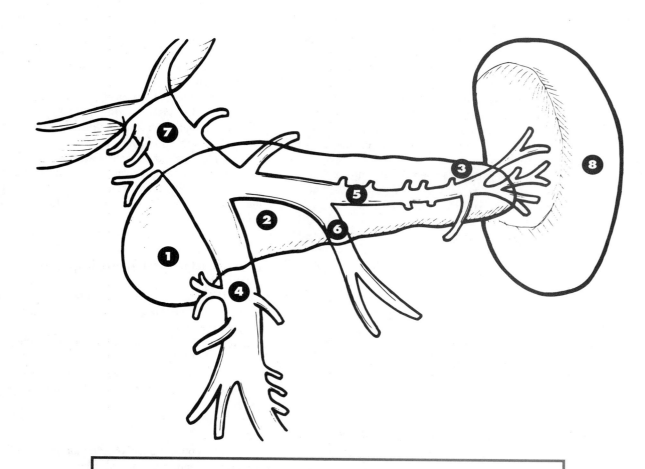

1	head of the pancreas	5	splenic vein
2	body of the pancreas	6	inferior mesenteric vein
3	tail of the pancreas	7	portal vein
4	superior mesenteric vein	8	spleen

Pancreas Review Notes

ULTRASOUND TECHNIQUE

- The pancreas is the most difficult abdominal organ to image.
- The patient should fast 6 to 8 hours.
- Fasting promotes dilation of the gallbladder and ducts and ensures an empty stomach.
- Fasting causes less bowel gas.
- Realtime allows visualization of peristalsis, duodenum, and stomach.
- In adults, use 3 MHz to 5 MHz transducer with mid-focal zone.
- In pediatric patients, use 5 MHz to 7.5 MHz.

Scan Technique

- Identify the head, neck, body, and tail in longitudinal and transverse planes.
- Evaluate shape, contour, lie, and texture (compare with characteristics in liver).
- The prone position may allow visualization of the pancreatic tail when ascites is present. (Do not confuse splenic flexure and distal transverse colon as they cross anterior to left kidney—the colon is usually caudal to the tail of the pancreas.)
- Most scans are taken with the patient in the supine position.
- Coronal scans may improve visualization of the pancreas and peripancreatic region.
- Identify the surrounding structures:
  - SMA: superior mesenteric artery
  - SMV: superior mesenteric vein
  - PV: portal vein
  - SV: splenic vein
  - AO: aorta
  - IVC: inferior vena cava
  - CBD: common bile duct
  - GDA: gastroduodenal artery
  - LRV: left renal vein
  - Duodenal bulb
  - Posterior wall of stomach
  - Pancreatic duct
- Windows for visualization include the following:
  - Left lobe of liver
  - Stomach
  - Colon
  - Water technique—The patient drinks 32 to 300 ml of water through a straw in the erect or left lateral decubitus position. With the patient in an upright position, use the stomach as the window; if the patient is unable to sit up, the examination can be performed in the decubitus position.
- Other ingestions for pancreatic visualization include the following:
  - Glucagon (inhibits peristalsis)
  - Fatty meal (not for patients with pancreatitis or gallbladder disease)
  - Methylcellulose (aqueous suspension that fills stomach)

NORMAL ANATOMY

- Arises from two duodenal buds (dorsal and ventral), which fuse.
- Ventral bud grows slowly and swings around the gut to join the dorsal bud.
- The entire body and tail are the dorsal anlage, and the remainder are from the ventral bud.
- The duct drainage system anatomoses with the major duct.
- The major dorsal duct, Wirsung's duct, drains into the duodenum. (In 60% of adults, this duct empties into the common bile duct.)
- The ventral duct usually disappears; if it persists, it is an accessory duct, Santorini's duct.
- The normal pancreas in the adult is 15 cm in length.
- It weighs 60 to 100 g.
- It is usually located near the level of L1 or L2.
- The pancreas is a nonencapsulated multilobular gland located in the retroperitoneal space extending from the second portion of the duodenum to the splenic hilum.
- This is an exocrine and endocrine gland.
- As an exocrine gland, numerous small glands (acini) aggregate into lobular acini and are separated by connective tissue.
- The ductal system begins with fine radicles in secretor acini, which eventually drain into Wirsung's duct by progressive anastomosis.
- The endocrine function is represented by the islets of Langerhans.
- Regulation of pancreatic secretion is complex and is related to humoral, vagal, and local neurogenic reflexes.
- Secretin is the most important humoral agent (produced in duodenum).
- Fats and alcohol are active stimulators of secretin.
- Pancreatic secretory activity is correlated with the ingestion of food.
- Proteolytic enzymes, trypsin and chymotrypsin, are secreted as inactive precursors and are important in protein-digesting ferments.
- The proteases—amylase, lipase, phospholipase, and elastases—are all elaborated by the pancreas and activated in the duodenum.
- The main hormones produced by the endocrine portion include insulin and glucagon.

VASCULAR SUPPLY

- Blood supply is from the splenic artery, gastroduodenal artery, and superior mesenteric artery.
- Venous drainage is through tributaries of the splenic and superior mesenteric veins.

VASCULAR AND DUCTAL LANDMARKS

Portal Vein and Tributaries

- The portal vein and tributaries are formed behind the neck of the pancreas by the junction of the SMV and SV.
- The SV runs from the splenic hilum along the posterior superior aspect of the pancreas.
- The SMV runs posterior to the lower neck of the pancreas and anterior to the uncinate process.
- The PV courses superiorly at various obliquity.

Splenic Artery

- The splenic artery arises from the celiac artery and runs along the superior margin of the gland, slightly anterior and superior, to follow its vein.

Common Hepatic Artery

- The common hepatic artery arises from the celiac artery.
- It courses along the superior margin of the first portion of the duodenum and divides into the proper hepatic artery and GDA, usually when it crosses onto the front of the portal vein.
- It is seen in 75% of patients as it proceeds superiorly along the anterior aspect of the portal vein with the CBD lateral to it.
- The GDA is seen in 30% of patients as it travels a short distance along the anterior aspect of the head just to the right of the neck before it divides into the superior pancreaticoduodenal branches; they join with the inferior pancreaticoduodenal, which arises from the SMA.
- In 14% of patients, the RHA arises from the SMA and courses posterior to the medial portions of the SV and runs along the aspect of the PV.

Superior Mesenteric Artery

- The superior mesenteric artery arises from the aorta behind the lower portion of the body.
- It courses anterior to the third portion of the duodenum to enter the small bowel mesentery.

Common Bile Duct

- The common bile duct crosses the anterior aspect of the portal vein to the right of the proper hepatic artery.
- The portal vein crosses anterior to the IVC; the duct passes off the front of the portal vein and travels behind the first portion of the duodenum to course inferior and somewhat posterior in the parenchyma of the head

of the pancreas, where it is close to the second portion of the duodenum.
- It joins the pancreatic duct close to the ampulla.

ANATOMY OF THE PANCREAS

Head

- The head is located to the right of the SMV.
- The right lateral border is the second portion of the duodenum.
- The IVC is posterior.
- The GDA is the anterior lateral border.
- The CBD is anterior and lateral to the GDA.
- The PV is cranial to the head.
- The uncinate process is directly posterior to the SMV.
- The head measurements are as follows: AP—2.1 to 2.5 cm; longitudinal AP—2.0 to 2.4 cm.

Neck

- The neck is directly anterior to the SMV.
- The PV is formed behind the neck by the junction of the SMV and SV.
- Measures over the SMV as follows: longitudinal—1.0 to 1.3 cm; AP—0.95 to 1.1 cm.

Body

- The body is the largest section of the pancreas.
- It is anterior to the SMA.
- The anterior border is the posterior wall of the antrum of the stomach.
- The right lateral border is the neck.
- The left lateral border is indefinite.
- The SV courses along the posterior surface.
- The tail begins to the left lateral margin.
- The body measures are as follows: longitudinal—1.2 to 1.5; AP—1.1 to 1.4 cm.

Tail

- The tail is the most difficult to image.
- It begins to the left of the left lateral border of the vertebral body and extends to the splenic hilum.
- It may be at a higher level (41%), the same level (51%), or an inferior level (2%).
- The SV courses along the posterior surface of the body and tail.
- The tail is anterior to the left kidney, posterior to the stomach, and medial to the spleen.
- Measurements are as follows: 0.7 to 2.8 cm.

Shape

- Sausage, dumbbell, tadpole, and comma

Texture

- The texture depends on the amount of fat between the lobules and to a lesser extent on interlobular fibrous tissue.

- Internal echoes of the pancreas consist of regularly and closely spaced elements of uniform intensity, with uniformly distributed variation throughout the gland.
- The pancreas is either equally as dense as the liver or more dense than the liver.

Pancreatic Duct

- The pancreatic duct is seen more in the body than in the tail.
- It appears as an echogenic line or a lucency bordered by two echogenic lines.
- The main duct passes steeply cephalad from Vater's ampulla obliquely to the left, then transversely and upward across the midline to the left of the spine, and then upward more steeply in the tail.
- It measures 2 mm.
- It decreases toward the tail
- Do not confuse it with vascular structures.

CONGENITAL ABNORMALITIES

- Congenital abnormalities are uncommon.
- Agenesis or hypoplasia is seen.
- Annular pancreas (persistence of the dorsal and ventral pancreas, with the head encircling the duodenum) is another congenital abnormality.
- Congenital cysts result from anomalous development of the pancreatic ducts; they are usually multiple—range from small to 3 to 5 cm in size.

Cystic Fibrosis

- Incidence is 1:2000; 1:20 are genetic carriers.
- Problems with the liver, biliary, and pancreas increase with age.
- Exocrine glands secrete increased amounts of abnormal mucus.
- In the pancreas, there is precipitation or coagulation of secretions in the small pancreatic ducts that form obstructing eosinophilic concretions.
- Proximal distention of ductules and acini leads to their degeneration and replacement by small cysts.
- Atrophy of glandular elements and replacement of altered architecture by fibrosis or fat are late changes.
- Increased echoes in pancreas are caused by fibrosis and fat infiltration.
- Do not compare with an abnormal liver pattern.

ACUTE PANCREATITIS

- An attack of pancreatitis is related to biliary tract disease and alcoholism.
- Gallstones are present in 40% to 60% of patients.
- Acute pancreatitis is the initial symptom in 5% of patients with gallstones.

- Other causes include trauma, inflammation from adjacent peptic ulcer or abdominal infection, vascular thrombosis and embolism, and drugs.
- Pancreatic enzymes—proteases, lipase, and elastase—are keys to pancreatic destruction.

Production of Acute Pancretitis

1. Bile reflex
2. Hypersecretion and obstruction (rupture of ducts by pancreatic hypersecretion possibly potentiated by partial duct obstruction)
3. Alcohol-induced changes
4. Duodenal reflux

Morphologic Changes in Acute Pancreatitis

1. Proteolytic destruction of pancreatic substance
2. Necrosis of blood vessels, with subsequent hemorrhage
3. Necrosis of fat by lipolytic enzymes
4. Accompanying inflammatory reaction

- The process may be severe, with damage to the acinar tissue and duct system producing damage by the exudation of pancreatic juice into the interstitium of the gland, leakage of secretions into the peripancreatic tissues, or both.
- After the acini or duct disrupt, the secretions migrate to the surface of the gland.
- A common course is for fluid to break through the pancreatic connective tissue layer and thin posterior layer of the peritoneum and enter the lesser sac.
- Pancreatic juice enters the anterior pararenal space by breaking through the thin layer of the fibrous connective tissue; the fluid may migrate to the surface of the gland and remain within the confines of the fibrous connective tissue layer.
- Collections of fluid in the peripancreatic area generally retain communication with the pancreas.
- Dynamic equilibrium is established, so fluid is continuously absorbed from the collection and replaced by additional pancreatic secretions.
- Drainage of juices may cease as the pancreatic inflammatory response subsides and the rate of pancreatic secretions returns to normal.
- Collections of extrapancreatic fluid should be reabsorbed or, if drained, should not recur with recovery of proper drainage through the duct.

Clinical Signs

- Persistent abdominal pain
- Fever
- Leukocytosis beyond the 5 days of the usual attack of acute pancreatitis
- Risk for abscess and hemorrhage

Clinical Course

- Pain begins with severe pain that usually occurs after large meal or ETOH binge.
- The pain is constant and intense.
- The serum amylase level increases within 24 hours, and the serum lipase level increases within 72 to 94 hours.
- Approximately 5% of patients die from acute effects of peripheral vascular collapse and shock during the first week of the clinical course.

Other Complications

- Pseudocyst formation (10%)
- Phlegmon (18%)
- Abscess (1% to 9%)
- Hemorrhage (5%)
- Duodenal obstruction

Ultrasound Findings

- Normal pancreas (29%)
- Increase in size (52%) with loss of normal texture (28%)
- Hypoechoic to anechoic and less echogenic than liver
- Borders possibly indistinct but smooth
- Loss of distinction of splenic vein

HEMORRHAGIC PANCREATITIS

- A sudden, more or less diffuse enzymatic destruction of the pancreatic substance is caused by the sudden escape of active pancreatic enzymes into the glandular parenchyma.
- Enzymes cause focal areas of fat necrosis in and about the pancreas, which leads to rupture of the pancreatic vessels and hemorrhage.
- Approximately 45% of patients have sudden necrotizing destruction of pancreas after an alcoholic debauch or excessively large meal.

Clinical Signs

- Decreased hemocrit and serum calcium levels
- Hypotension despite volume replacement
- Metabolic acidosis
- Adult RDS

Complications

- Hemorrhagic necrosis of the pancreatic parenchyma
- Deposition of hemorrhagic fluid into the retroperitoneal tissue or peritoneal cavity
- Hemorrhage into a pancreatic pseudocyst
- Incidence of 2% to 33%
- Mortality of 25% to 100%

Ultrasound Findings

- Findings depend on the age of the hemorrhage.

- Hemorrhage is seen as a well-defined homogeneous mass.
- At 1 week, the mass may appear cystic with solid elements or septation.
- After several weeks the hemorrhage may appear cystic.

PHLEGMONOUS PANCREATITIS

- A phlegmon is a spreading diffuse inflammatory edema of soft tissues that may proceed to necrosis and suppuration.
- Extension outside the gland occurs in 18% to 20% of patients with acute pancreatitis.
- The phlegmon appears hypoechoic with good through transmission.
- It does not represent extrapancreatic fluid.
- It usually involves the lesser sac, left anterior pararenal space, and transverse mesocolon.
- Less commonly, it involves the small bowel mesentery, lower retroperitoneum, and pelvis.

LIQUEFACTIVE NECROSIS

- A necrotis pancreas may become an excavated necrotis sac surrounded by a shell of tissue forming a sac that conforms to the axis and contour of the pancreas.
- It is best defined by direction injection into the pancreatic duct.
- On ultrasound a debris containing a cystic structure is seen in the region of the pancreas without a definite extrapancreatic pseudocyst being found.
- It appears hypoechoic and resembles a diffusely edematous gland or cyst.

ACUTE PANCREATITIS IN CHILDREN

- More easily seen, less body fat
- Left lobe liver more prominent
- Gland more isosonic than hyperechoic
- Gland increased in size
- Hypoechoic
- Indistinct outline

Causes

- Trauma
- Drugs
- Infection
- Congenital anomalies
- Familial or idiopathic origin

COMPLICATIONS OF PANCREATITIS
Aneurysms Secondary to Pancreatitis

- The splenic artery is the most common site.
- The pancreatic arteries are pancreaticoduodenal arcades and dorsal and transverse pancreatic arteries.

Abscess

- Incidence of 1% to 9%
- Related to degree of tissue necrosis
- 40% related to postoperative pancreatitis
- 4% with ETOH binge
- 7% with biliary disease
- High mortality, 32 to 65%; untreated, 100%
- Development due to superinfection of necrotic pancreatic and retroperitoneal tissues and less commonly due to superinfection of a pseudocyst
- Occurrence caused by hematogenous, lymphatic, or transmural spread of enteric organisms from the adjacent GI tract
- Possibly unilocular or multilocular and can spread superiorly into the mediastinum, inferiorly into the transverse mesocolon, or down the retroperitoneum into the pelvis

Clinical Patterns

- Persistent fever and leukocytosis
- Development 7 to 14 days after onset of symptoms in acute necrotizing pancreatitis
- Chills, hypotension, and a tender abdomen with a growing mass
- Bacteremia

Ultrasound Findings

- Hypoechoic mass with smooth walls
- Little internal echoes
- Possible irregular walls with internal echoes
- Echo free to echo dense

PSEUDOCYSTS

- Pseudocysts are a collection of fluid that arises from loculation of inflammatory processes, necrosis, or hemorrhage.
- They are usually associated with pancreatitis.
- They are usually single, oval to round, and vary in size.
- They arise in any portion of the pancreas and can cause dilation of the pancreatic duct.
- They lie within the pancreas or adjacent to the pancreas—especially in the tail.
- The wall may be thin or quite thick and fibrosis.
- No epithelial lining is present.
- No communication with the duct occurs.
- A marked inflammatory reaction is seen.
- Fluid may accumulate in the lesser sac or extend down into the retroperitoneal soft tissue planes in any direction.
- Locations include the following:
  - The most common is lesser sac anterior to the pancreas and posterior to the stomach.
  - The second most common location is the anterior pararenal space (posterior to lesser sac, bounded by

Gerota's fascia). The spleen is the lateral border of the anterior, pararenal space on the left. Fluid occurs more commonly in the left pararenal space than the right.
  - Sometimes the posterior pararenal space is fluid filled. Fluid spreads from the anterior pararenal space to the posterior pararenal space on the same side.
  - Fluid may enter the peritoneal cavity via Winslow's foramen or by disrupting the peritoneum in the anterior surface of the lesser sac.
  - The pseudocyst may extend into the mediastium by extending through an esophageal or aortic hiatus.
  - It may extend into small bowel mesentery or down into the retroperitoneum into the pelvis and groin.
- It may simulate splenic, renal, duodenal, and mediastinal pathologic processes.
- Many pseudocysts regress, with a 20% rate of spontaneous regression.
- Some decompress into pancreatic duct, others into the GI tract; Some rupture into the GI or peritoneal cavity (70% mortality).
- It usually takes 4 to 6 weeks for cyst wall maturation.
- Pseudocysts in the lesser sac tend to reaccumulate.
- Drainage is more successful if the cyst is mature.

Ultrasound Findings

- Sharply defined smooth walls
- Usually acoustic enhancement
- Possibly multiple septations
- Internal echoes
- Mimicking of cystadenoma or cystadenocarcinoma

Confusion with Other Structures

- Fluid-filled stomach
- Dilated pancreatic duct (look for continuity of cyst with duct)
- Left renal vein varix

CHRONIC PANCREATITIS

- Chronic pancreatitis represents progressive destruction of the pancreas by repeated flare ups of a mild or subclinical type of acute pancreatitis.
- Hypercalcemia and hyperlipidemia predispose to chronic pancreatitis.
- It is more common in males.

Morphologic Changes

- Chronic calcifying changes
- Atrophy of acini
- Increases in interlobular fibrous tissue and chronic inflammatory infiltration
- Stones of calcium carbonate located inside the ductal system
- Pseudocysts common

- Chronic obstructive pancreatitis:
  - Lesions in the lobules
  - Ductal epithelium less involved
  - Stenosis of the sphincter of Oddi most common
- Recurrent bouts of pain at intervals of months to years

Ultrasound Findings

- An increased echogenicity of the pancreas beyond the normal is caused by fibrotic and fatty changes.
- Calcification, ductal dilation, and irregular outline are present.
- Focal or diffuse enlargement of the gland may be associated with an irregular outline.
- Pancreatic lithiasis is associated with alcoholic pancreatitis.
- The duct may be dilated secondary to a stricture or as a result of an extrinsic stone from the smaller pancreatic duct into the major duct.
- Shadowing may be present.
- The most common site of obstruction is at the papilla and the site of origin of the main duct.
- The incidence of carcinoma with pancreatic calcification is 25%.

Complications

- Pseudocysts in 20% of patients
- Thrombosis of the splenic and/or portal vein

PANCREATIC NEOPLASMS
Pancreatic Cysts

- True cysts are lined by a mucous epithelium and may be congenital or acquired.
- Congenital cysts result from anomalous development of the pancreatic duct.
- They are usually single but are sometimes multiple and without septation.
- Acquired cysts are retention cysts, parasitic cysts, and neoplastic cysts.

CYSTADENOMA AND CYSTADENOCARCINOMA
Macrocystic Adenoma

- Uncommon
- Slow-growing tumor
- Arising from ducts as cystic neoplasm
- Composed of large cyst with or without septations
- Significant malignant potential
- Epigastric pain or palpable mass usual initial symptom
- Concurrent diseases: diabetes, calculous disease of biliary tract, and arterial hypertension
- Occurring more in middle-aged women
- Tail, 60%; head, 5%
- Body and tail most frequent sites
- Frequent foci of calcification

Microcystic Adenoma

- Tiny cysts
- Lined by flattened or cuboidal cells that contain glycogen and little to no mucin
- Benign lesions
- Occurring more in females
- Body and tail, 60%; head, 30%

CYSTIC NEOPLASMS

- Similar appearance to pseudocysts
- Four ultrasound patterns:

  1. Anehoic mass with posterior enhancement and irregular margins
  2. Anechoic mass with internal homogeneous echoes, stratified supine and mobile decubitus
  3. Anechoic mass with irregular internal vegetations protruding into the lumen and showing no movement
  4. Completely echogenic mass with nonhomogeneous pattern

ADENOCARCINOMA

- Fatal tumor
- Involvement of the exocrine portion of the gland
- 95% of all malignant pancreatic tumors
- Usually occurring in 60 to 80 year olds
- Males more common
- Carcinoma occurring in head of gland in 60% to 70% of cases; 20% to 30% of cases in body; and 5% to 10% of cases in tail
- 21% are diffuse
- Tumors in head seen early

Clinical Course

- Weight loss
- Abdominal pain
- Back pain
- Anorexia
- Nausea and vomiting
- Generalized malaise and weakness
- Time from symptoms until diagnosis—4 months, with death occurring after 8 months to 1.6 years

Ultrasound Findings

- The lesions represent localized change in the echodensity of the pancreas.
- The echopattern is hypoechoic (less dense than that of the pancreas or liver).
- Approximately 95% are found to be hypoechoic.
- The borders are irregular.
- Pancreatic enlargement may occur.
- Masses in the head are smaller than in the tail (compression of CBD).
- Dilation of the pancreatic duct occurs.

- Liver mets, nodal mets, portal venous system involvement, splenic vein enlargement, SMA displacement, and ascites are seen.
- SM vessels may be displaced posteriorly by the pancreatic mass.
  - Anterior displacement occurs when the carcinoma is in the uncinate process.
  - Posterior displacement occurs when the tumor is in the head or body.
- Soft tissue thickening caused by neoplastic infiltration of perivascular lymphatics may be seen surrounding the celiac axis or SMA (occurs more with CA of the body and tail).
- Most patients have obstructive jaundice.
- It can compress the splenic vein, producing secondary splenic enlargement.
- The tumor may displace or invade the splenic or portal vein or produce thrombosis.
- A mass in the head may compress the anterior wall of the IVC.

ISLET CELL TUMORS

- There are several types of islet cell tumors, including functional and nonfunctional tumors.
- These represent benign adenomas or malignant tumors.
- Nonfunctioning islet cell tumors comprise one third of all islet cell tumors—92% are malignant.
- The most common functioning islet cell tumor is **insulinoma** (60%) followed by the **gastrinoma** (18%).
- The tumors occur mostly in the body and tail where there is the greatest concentration of islets of Langerhans.
- The tumors are small and difficult to detect.

METASTATIC DISEASE TO PANCREAS

- Intraabdominal lymphomas cause a hypoechoic mass in the pancreas.

- Superior mesenteric vessels are displaced anteriorly instead of posteriorly as seen with a primary pancreatic mass.
- Multiple nodes are seen along the pancreas, duodenum, porta, and superior mesenteric vessels; they may be difficult to distinguish from a pancreatic mass.
- The nodes appear hypoechoic.

PANCREATIC CARCINOMA

Carcinoma of the head of the pancreas is a rather loose term including carcinoma of Vater's ampulla, the lower end of the bile duct, and the acini of the pancreas. In its diagnosis and differential from gallstone obstruction, there are several helpful pointers:

1. Patients are more often men over 50 years old.
2. Onset is insidious, often with weight loss and malaise preceding the onset of jaundice. The jaundice progresses steadily compared with the more acute and intermittent pattern seen with gallstones.
3. Back pain is common. Pruritus may occur.
4. An enlarged gallbladder may be present.
5. An associated thrombophlebitis may occur in the adjacent splenic vein, resulting in congestive splenomegaly.
6. There may be evidence for metastases
7. Stools may contain occult blood. Their fat content may be elevated.
8. There may be changes in the duodenal mucosal pattern and motility. Dilation of the second part of the duodenum may be seen.

Review Exercise A • The Pancreas

1. Describe the shape of the pancreas and position the pancreas occupies in the abdominal cavity. _____

_____

_____

_____

2. Describe the physiology of the pancreas as an exocrine and endocrine gland. _____

_____

_____

_____

3. What are the islets of Langerhans? _____

_____

_____

_____

_____

4. What role does insulin play in the pancreas? _____

_____

_____

_____

5. What is the principal action of glucagon in the pancreas? _____

_____

_____

_____

_____

6. What controls the regulation of insulin and glucagon secretion? _____

_____

_____

_____

7. Define direct bilirubin and its influence on pancreatic function. _____

_____

_____

_____

_____

_____

8. There are two enzymes that are specific for pancreatic disease. Name them and describe their role. _____

_____

_____

_____

_____

_____

Review Exercise B • The Pancreas

1. Describe the texture of the pancreas. _____

_____

_____

_____

2. Discuss the causes, clinical signs, symptoms, and ultrasound appearance of acute pancreatitis. _____

_____

_____

_____

_____

3. What is hemorrhagic pancreatitis? _____

_____

_____

_____

_____

4. Describe the term *phlegmonous pancreatitis.* _____

_____

_____

_____

_____

5. What are the causes and findings of acute pancreatitis in children? _____

_____

_____

_____

6. What is a pancreatic pseudocyst? _____

_____

_____

_____

_____

_____

_____

7. What other structures may cause confusion with a pancreatic pseudocyst in the left upper quadrant? _____

_____

_____

_____

_____

8. What are the causes, clinical signs and symptoms, and ultrasound findings in chronic pancreatitis? _____

_____

_____

_____

_____

9. Discuss the findings in a cystadenoma of the pancreas. _____

_____

_____

_____

_____

10. Discuss the clinical signs, symptoms, and ultrasound findings of adenocarcinoma. _____

_____

_____

_____

_____

11. What are the types of islet cell tumors of the pancreas? _____

_____

_____

_____

12. What is the occurrence and ultrasound findings in metastatic disease to pancreas? _____

_____

_____

_____

_____

Self-Test • The Pancreas

1. The pancreas is a _____ gland.
   a. intraperitoneal
   b. extraperitoneal
   c. retroperitoneal
   d. peritoneal

2. The pancreas is bounded anteriorly by the _____ and _____ and

   posteriorly by the _____ .
   a. stomach, duodenum, and prevertebral vessels
   b. liver, jejunum, and SMA
   c. stomach, jejunum, and SMV
   d. liver, duodenum, and SMV

3. The pancreas is found behind the _____ omental sac.
   a. greater
   b. lesser
   c. inferior
   d. superior

Which statements are true, and which are false?

4. _____ The head of the pancreas is anterior to the IVC.

5. _____ The head of the pancreas is superior to the caudate lobe.

6. _____ The head of the pancreas is posterior to the portal vein.

7. _____ The head of the pancreas is lateral to the second portion of the duodenum.

8. _____ The uncinate process is posterior to the superior mesenteric vessels.

9. _____ The gastroduodenal artery is the anterolateral border of the head.

10. _____ The body is the largest part of the pancreas.

11. _____ The splenic artery is the superior border of the body.

12. _____ The tail of the pancreas lies anterior to the left kidney in the hilus of the spleen.

13. Wirsung's duct is the primary pancreatic duct (true or false).

14. The pancreas is most commonly found in what "lie" in the abdomen?
    a. horseshoe
    b. horizontal oblique
    c. vertical
    d. horizontal

15. The head of the pancreas lies in the:
    a. lap of the liver
    b. lap of the gallbladder, CBD
    c. lap of the duodenum
    d. lap of the lesser omentum

16. The head of the pancreas is anterior to the:

    a. SMA, AO, SV

    b. SMV, IVC, RRV

    c. PV, IVC, SMA

    d. HA, SMA, IVC

17. The head of the pancreas is inferior to the:

    a. caudate lobe of liver

    b. right lobe of liver

    c. right lateral fissure of liver

    d. left lateral fissure of liver

18. The uncinate process is anterior to the superior mesenteric vessels (true or false).

19. The _____ passes through a groove posterior to the pancreatic head.

    a. common bile duct

    b. gastroduodenal artery

    c. hepatic duct

    d. superior mesenteric vein

20. The _____ is the anterolateral border of the pancreas.

    a. common bile duct

    b. gastroduodenal artery

    c. hepatic duct

    d. superior mesenteric vein

21. What part of the pancreas is anterior to the aorta, SMA, LRV, and left adrenal?

    a. head

    b. neck and body

    c. tail

22. The vessel that is the upper border of the pancreas body is the:

    a. superior mesenteric artery

    b. superior mesenteric vein

    c. splenic artery

    d. splenic vein

23. The anterior surface of the body is separated by the:

    a. lesser sac

    b. duodenum

    c. omental bursa from the posterior wall of the stomach

    d. lesser sac from the jejunum

24. The tail of the pancreas is found:

    a. posterior to the left kidney, near the splenic hilum

    b. anterior to the left kidney, near the splenic hilum

    c. posterior to the right kidney, near the liver hilum

    d. anterior to the right kidney, near the liver hilum

25. The splenic vein forms the:

    a. anterior border

    b. superior border

    c. posterior border

    d. inferior border

26. _____ is the primary pancreatic duct.

    a. Santorini's duct

    b. Ampulla's duct

    c. Vater's duct

    d. Wirsung's duct

27. The duct receives tributaries from lobules at right angles and enters the medial second part of the duodenum with the CBD at the:

    a. Santorini junction

    b. Wirsung ampulla

    c. Vater's ampulla

    d. pancreatic ampulla

28. The portal triad is composed of:

    a. right and left portal veins, CBD

    b. right and left hepatic ducts, portal vein

    c. portal vein, CBD, hepatic artery

    d. right and left hepatic artery, CBD

29. The arterial supply to the gallbladder is via the:

    a. hepatic artery

    b. superior mesenteric artery

    c. cystic artery

    d. gastroduodenal artery

30. The portal vein drains blood:

    a. from the GI tract from the lower end of the esophagus to the upper end of the anal canal

    b. from the adrenal

    c. from the kidneys

    d. from the gallbladder

31. The splenic vein runs along the _____ margin of the pancreas.

a. inferior

b. medial

c. lateral

d. superior

32. What vessel passes anterior to the third part of the duodenum and posterior to the neck of the pancreas?

a. superior mesenteric artery

b. superior mesenteric vein

c. inferior mesenteric vein

d. splenic vein

33. The hepatic artery arises from the celiac trunk and courses to the right of the aorta at almost a 90-degree angle (true or false).

34. The head of the pancreas, the duodenum, and parts of the stomach are supplied by the:

a. hepatic artery

b. gastroduodenal artery

c. splenic artery

d. superior mesenteric artery

35. The _____ runs posterior to the neck of the pancreas.

a. superior mesenteric artery

b. splenic artery

c. hepatic artery

d. gastroduodenal artery

36. The distribution of the superior mesenteric artery is to the (2 answers):

a. distal half of colon

b. small intestine

c. large intestine

d. proximal half of colon

37. The left renal artery passes posterior to the aorta (true or false).

38. The pancreas is a retroperitoneal gland (true or false).

39. Santorini's duct is a:

a. small accessory duct to the gallbladder

b. accessory duct to the pancreas

c. accessory duct to the cystic duct

d. small opening in the duodenum

40. The hepatic artery may course along the upper margin of the pancreatic head (true or false).

41. The normal pancreas is larger in adults than in young children (true or false).

42. Generally speaking, the normal pancreas is shown to be:

    a. more echogenic than the liver

    b. less echogenic than the liver

    c. the same echogenicity of the liver

    d. variable

43. The pancreas may be divided into several segments except:

    a. tail and body

    b. tail, body, head, neck

    c. tail, body, head, neck, uncinate process

    d. tail, body, head, uncinate process

44. The normal dimension of the pancreatic head is usually less than:

    a. 3 mm

    b. 2 cm

    c. 2.4 cm

    d. 1 cm

45. The normal dimension of the pancreatic body is generally larger than the pancreatic head (true or false).

46. Visualization of the tail of the pancreas is usually quite easy because of its relationship to the hilus of the spleen (true or false).

47. It is possible to have acute pancreatitis with a coexisting pseudocyst (true or false).

48. The normal size of the pancreatic duct is less than:

    a. 1 mm

    b. 3 mm

    c. 5 mm

    d. 6 mm

49. The enzyme that is the most sensitive in the laboratory tests for the diagnosis of acute pancreatitis is:

    a. SGOT

    b. SCPT

    c. amylase

    d. lipase

50. The pancreas is both an _____ and an _____ gland.

51. The _____ function of the pancreas secretes hormones directly into the blood. These secretions include insulin, glucagon, and gastrin.

52. The _____ function of the pancreas includes lipase, trypsine, and amylase.

53. What is the microscopic collection of cells numbering 1 to 2 million imbedded within tissue throughout the gland?

a. glucagon cells

b. islets of Langerhans

c. insulin

d. amylase cells

54. The splenic vein is considered to be the:

a. superior posterior border of the pancreas

b. superior border of the pancreas

c. medial posterior border of the pancreas

d. inferior posterior border of the pancreas

55. If the celiac axis is well visualized, the sonographer should move the transducer in which direction to image the pancreas?

a. superior

b. anterior

c. inferior

d. posterior

56. The splenic artery is considered to be the:

a. superior border of the pancreas

b. lateral border of the pancreas

c. anterior border of the pancreas

d. inferior posterior border of the pancreas

57. The main pancreatic duct joins the _____ before entering the second part of the duodenum.

a. common bile duct

b. Santorini's duct

c. cystic duct

d. accessory duct

58. Clinical signs and symptoms for acute pancreatitis include all except:

a. severe abdominal pain radiating to the back

b. severe abdominal pain radiating to the right shoulder

c. elevated amylase

d. nausea and vomiting

59. What can cause obstruction of the pancreatic duct?

a. cystic fibrosis

b. chronic pancreatitis with fibrosis

c. carcinoma of the pancreas

d. calculi

60. Common causes of acute pancreatitis are:

   a. alcohol intake

   b. calculi

   c. cholecystitis

   d. colitis

61. How can one sonographically distinguish acute pancreatitis from chronic?

62. Describe the difference between a true cyst and a pseudocyst of the pancreas.

63. What is the most common type of primary neoplasm of the pancreas?

64. What are the clinical symptoms of pancreatic carcinoma?

65. The ventral duct of the pancreas usually disappears; if it persists, it is called:

   a. Wirsung's duct

   b. Warsaw's duct

   c. Santorini's duct

   d. duct of Langerhans

66. The reason the pancreas is reflective in its sonographic appearance is because of the multiple:

   a. islets of Langerhans

   b. Cooper's ligaments

   c. small glands or acini

   d. fat between the lobules

67. Blood supply to the pancreas is via the:

   a. splenic artery

   b. gastroduodenal artery

   c. superior mesenteric artery

   d. a and c

   e. all of the above

68. The _____ runs posterior to the lower neck of the pancreas and anterior to the uncinate process.

   a. splenic vein

   b. superior mesenteric vein

   c. gastroduodenal artery

   d. hepatic artery

69. The _____ courses along the superior margin of the first portion of the duodenum and divides into two branches.

   a. common hepatic artery   c. gastroduodenal artery

   b. proper hepatic artery   d. superior mesenteric artery

70. In many patients, the _____ arises from the superior mesenteric artery.

    a. left hepatic

    b. inferior mesenteric

    c. renal artery

    d. right hepatic artery

71. The _____ courses anterior to the third portion of the duodenum to enter the small bowel mesentery.

    a. superior mesenteric artery

    b. inferior mesenteric artery

    c. gastroduodenal artery

    d. inferior pancreatic artery

72. The _____ crosses anterior to the portal vein to the right of the hepatic artery.

    a. hepatic duct

    b. common bile duct

    c. splenic vein

    d. superior mesenteric artery

73. The pancreatic duct is seen more in the tail than in the body (true or false).

74. The persistence of the dorsal and ventral pancreas with the head encircling the duodenum is called:

    a. hypoplasia

    b. cystic fibrosis

    c. agenesis

    d. annular pancreas

75. A condition that causes increased secretion of abnormal mucus by the exocrine glands is:

    a. cystic fibrosis

    b. lipimucosa

    c. diabetes

    d. cystic mucosal disease

76. Gallstones are present in 40% to 60% of patients with:

    a. chronic pancreatitis

    b. annular pancreas

    c. cystic fibrosis

    d. acute pancreatitis

77. A common course of enzyme destruction via the pancreas is to accumulate in the:

    a. greater omentum

    b. lesser omentum

    c. lesser sac

    d. greater sac

78. Clinical signs of acute pancreatitis include all but:

    a. persistent abdominal pain

    b. diarrhea

    c. fever

    d. leuokocytosis

79. On ultrasound, acute pancreatitis may appear:

    a. echogenic

    b. calcified

    c. hypoechoic

    d. homogeneous

80. A patient on a binge who has presented with acute pancreatitis now presents with decreased hemocrit and hypotension. Your differential would include:

    a. pancreatic hemorrhage

    b. cholecystitis

    c. pseudocyst

    d. chronic pancreatitis

81. The spreading of diffuse inflammatory edema of soft tissues that may proceed to necrosis and suppuration is:

    a. chronic pancreatitis

    b. hemorrhagic pancreatitis

    c. phlegmon

    d. pseudocyst

82. The most common cause of acute pancreatitis in children is:

    a. surgery

    b. drinking

    c. baseball

    d. trauma

83. Which statements are true regarding pseudocyst formation?

    a. _____ usually not associated with pancreatitis

    b. _____ usually single, oval to round

    c. _____ may cause pancreatic duct to dilate

    d. _____ no epithelial lining

    e. _____ fluid may only accumulate in the pancreatic area

    f. _____ has sharp, smooth walls

    g. _____ may have internal echoes

    h. _____ most common in lesser sac

    i. _____ can mimic cystadenoma

    j. _____ most all rupture into the duodenum

84. Calcification of the pancreatic duct is at the:

a. papilla and site of origin of the main duct

b. Santorini's duct

c. common bile duct

d. head

85. Cystadenoma is a fast growing tumor (true or false).

86. Most frequent sites for cystadenoma growth are the body and tail (true or false).

87. Cystadenomas on ultrasound may appear as what?

88. Where do most malignant tumors occur?

a. head

b. neck

c. body

d. tail

89. Why is jaundice a common clinical finding in a patient with pancreatic CA?

90. Why is pancreatic cancer so fatal?

91. What type of tumor occurs mostly in the body and tail?

a. islet cell

b. adenoma

c. adenocarcinoma

d. lymphoma

Case Reviews

1. A 35-year-old man comes to the hospital with persistent epigastric pain radiating to the back. On his admittance to the emergency room, laboratory values reveal increased amylase levels. What would you look for and what are the ultrasound findings (Figure 6-7)?

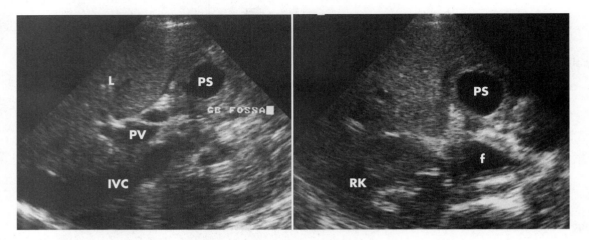

2. The normal pancreas has many different appearances when compared with the normal liver texture. Describe these appearances and distinguish which image shows a normal pancreatic texture. What are your findings (Figure 6-8)?

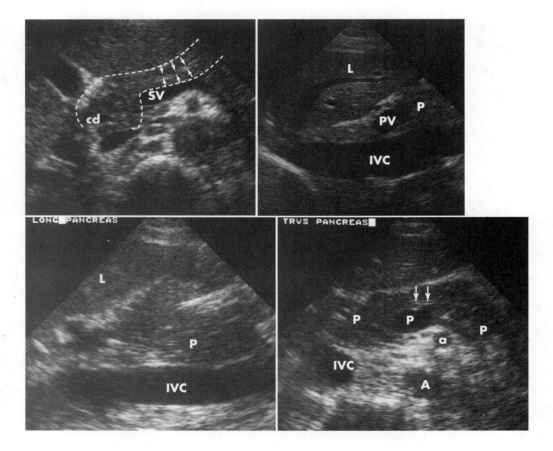

3. A 63-year-old man is seen with a 35-pound weight loss over the past several months, midepigastric pain radiating to the back, and nausea and vomiting symptoms. He has a palpable mass in the midepigastrium and appears jaundiced. On his admission to the hospital, laboratory values show increased bilirubin and amylase levels. What is your preliminary diagnosis and what structures would you want to image carefully in your ultrasound examination (Figure 6-9)?

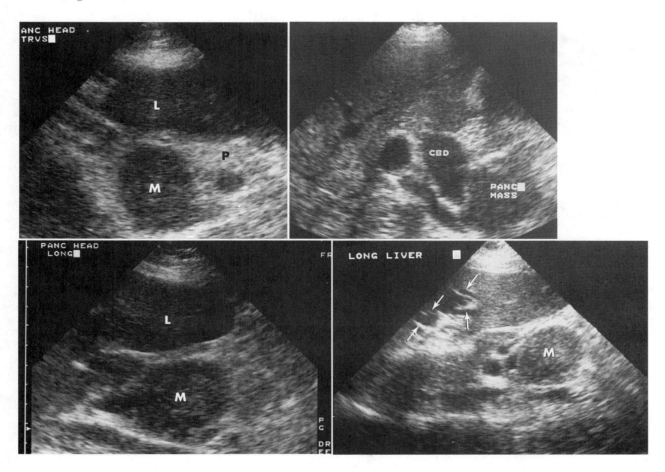

4. A patient with vague back pain and intermittent episodes of nausea and vomiting was seen by his family physician. Laboratory values showed a mild elevation in serum amylase levels. He did not have a fever, and his physician thought it was probably a viral infection. He was sent home and 1 week later reappeared in the emergency room with intense abdominal pain. On examination, he appeared intoxicated, with pain in the midepigastric area. Laboratory values showed increased levels in serum lipase and serum calcium levels. An ultrasound was ordered to evaluate the pancreas. What would you expect to find (Figure 6-10)?

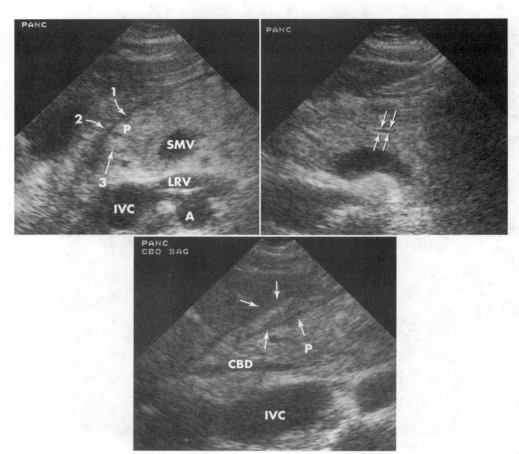

5. The normal pancreas may consistently be identified by numerous anatomic landmarks. Name, describe, and identify these landmarks (Figure 6-11):

a. _____

b. _____

c. _____

d. _____

e. _____

f. _____

g. _____

h. _____

i. _____

j. _____

k. _____

l. _____

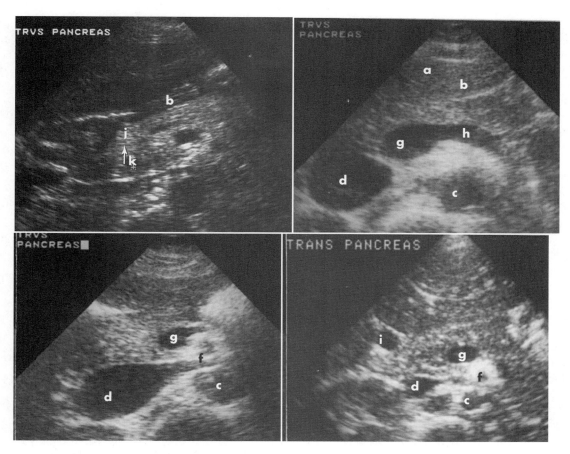

6. This 55-year-old woman had a previous history of cirrhosis and heavy alcohol abuse. She came to the emergency room with constant midepigastric back pain, nausea, and vomiting. Her laboratory values show increased levels of serum amylase and lipase. What would you expect to find on her ultrasound examination? What areas should the sonographer closely evaluate (Figure 6-12)?

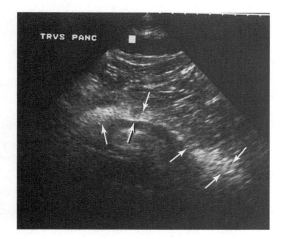

7. What is one of the difficulties in examining a patient with pancreatitis?

Answers to Review Exercise A

1. The pancreas is a large, elongated gland that lies in the abdomen inferior to the stomach; its head is embraced by the C-shaped curve of the duodenum. The pancreatic duct joins the bile duct coming from the liver, forming a single duct that passes into the duodenum. An accessory pancreatic duct is frequently present.

2. The pancreas is a rather complex gland because it has both endocrine and exocrine functions. Its endocrine function, in which hormones are secreted directly into the bloodstream, consists of the production of the hormones insulin and glucagon.

   Insulin exerts a major control over carbohydrate metabolism, and glucagon aids in this metabolic process. These hormones are produced in clusters of cells called the *islets of Langerhans*. These clusters consist of two major cell types: the beta cells, which produce insulin, and the alpha cells, which secrete glucagon.

   To perform its exocrine gland duties, the pancreas also contains tubuloacinar units that consist of acinar cells, each connected to tiny tubules uniting to form larger tributaries (ducts) that eventually join Wirsung's duct.

   The acinar cells secrete the pancreatic enzymes trypsin, lipase, and amylase, which are released into the duodenum to aid in the digestion of proteins, fats, and starches, respectively.

3. More than a million small clusters of cells known as the *islets of Langerhans* are scattered throughout the pancreas. About 70% of the islet cells are beta (β) cells that produce the hormone insulin. Alpha (α) cells secrete the hormone glucagon.

4. Insulin is a protein hormone that exerts widespread influence on metabolism. Its principal action is to facilitate diffusion and storage of glucose into most cells, especially muscle and fat cells. By stimulating cells to take up glucose from the blood, insulin lowers the blood-sugar level.

   Insulin reduces the use of fatty acids as fuel and instead stimulates their storage in adipose tissue. It affects protein metabolism by increasing active transport of amino acids into cells and by stimulating protein synthesis.

5. Glucagon's principal action is to raise the blood-sugar level. It does this by stimulating liver cells to convert glycogen to glucose and by stimulating the liver cells to make glucose from noncarbohydrates.

   Glucagon also promotes release of fat stores from adipose tissue, thereby raising fatty acid levels in the blood and providing nutrients for glucose production. Note that all these actions are opposite to those of insulin.

6. The secretion of insulin and glucagon is directly controlled by the blood-sugar level. After a meal, when the blood-glucose level rises as a result of absorption of nutrients from the intestine, the beta cells are stimulated to increase insulin secretion. Then as the cells remove glucose from the blood, decreasing its concentration, insulin secretion decreases accordingly.

   Insulin and glucagon work together but in opposite ways to keep the blood-sugar level within normal limits. When the glucose level rises, insulin release brings it back to normal; when it falls, glucagon acts to raise it again. The insulin-glucagon system is a powerful, fast-acting mechanism for keeping the blood-sugar level normal.

7. Various pancreatic pathologic conditions cause obstruction of Vater's ampulla and/or the common bile duct, and this obstruction is reflected in the bilirubin levels. The conjugated, or direct, bilirubin levels are elevated in patients with carcinoma of the head of the pancreas and acute pancreatitis that causes obstruction.

8. Amylase is a digestive enzyme produced in the pancreas that aids in converting starches to sugars. (This enzyme is also produced in the salivary glands, liver, and fallopian tubes.) Increased amylase levels in the blood are seen in cases of inflammation of the pancreas.

   In acute pancreatitis, the amylase levels are greatly increased starting 3 to 6 hours after the first signs of clinical symptoms. The levels remain elevated for approximately 24 hours after the acute episode and then start to decrease.

   Elevated amylase values also occur in chronic pancreatitis (acute attack), partial gastrectomy, obstruction of the pancreatic ducts, perforated peptic ulcer, alcoholic poisoning, acute cholecystitis, and intestinal obstruction with strangulation.

   Decreased amylase levels occur in hepatitis and cirrhosis of the liver. Because of the nonspecificity of this test for acute pancreatitis, some authorities believe that the diagnosis of acute pancreatitis should be based on clinical symptoms.

   Lipase is an enzyme produced by the pancreas that changes fats to fatty acids and glycerol. Serum lipase levels are increased after damage has occurred to the pancreas.

   In acute pancreatitis, lipase levels may not be elevated until 24 to 36 hours after the onset of the acute attack. However, the lipase level remains elevated for a longer period (up to 14 days) than amylase levels. Therefore this test may be quite helpful because some patients may not seek medical attention until several days after the onset of their clinical symptoms.

   Increased lipase levels are also seen in obstruction of the pancreatic duct, pancreatic carcinoma, acute cholecystitis, cirrhosis, and severe renal disease.

Answers to Review Exercise B

1. The texture depends on the amount of fat between the lobules and to a lesser extent on the interlobular fibrous tissue. Internal echoes of the pancreas consist of regularly and closely spaced elements of uniform intensity with uniformly distributed variation throughout the gland.

   On ultrasound examination, the pancreas is either equally as dense as the liver or more dense than the liver.

2. An attack of pancreatitis is related to biliary tract disease and alcoholism. Gallstones are present in 40% to 60% of patients. A small percentage of patients with gallstones present with acute pancreatitis. Other causes include trauma, inflammation from adjacent peptic ulcer or abdominal infection, vascular thrombosis and embolism, and drugs.

   The process may be severe, with damage to the acinar tissue and duct system producing damage by the exudation of pancreatic juice into the interstitium of the gland, leakage of secretions into the peripancreatic tissues, or both.

   Clinical signs include persistent abdominal pain, fever, leukocytosis beyond the 5 days of the usual attack of acute pancreatitis. The patient is at risk for abscess and hemorrhage.

   The clinical course is as follows: Pain begins with severe pain that usually occurs after a large meal or an ETOH binge and is constant and intense. The serum amylase level increases within 24 hours, and the serum lipase level increases within 72 to 94 hours. Approximately 5% of patients die from acute effects of peripheral vascular collapse and shock during the first week of the clinical course.

   Other complications include pseudocyst formation, phlegmon, abscess, hemorrhage, and duodenal obstruction.

   Ultrasound shows a normal pancreas that increases in size with loss of normal texture. The gland is hypoechoic to anechoic and less echogenic than the liver. The borders may be indistinct but smooth. There is loss of distinction of the splenic vein.

3. Hemorrhagic pancreatitis is an enzymatic destruction of the pancreatic substance caused by a sudden escape of active pancreatic enzymes into the glandular parenchyma.

   The enzymes cause focal areas of fat necrosis in and around the pancreas, which leads to a rupture of the pancreatic vessels and subsequent hemorrhage.

   Clinical signs include decreased hemocrit and serum calcium levels, hypotension despite volume replacement, metabolic acidosis, and adult RDS.

   Complications include hemorrhagic necrosis of the pancreatic parenchyma, deposition of hemorrhagic fluid into the retroperitoneal tissue or peritoneal cavity, and hemorrhage into a pancreatic pseudocyst. The incidence is 2% to 33% and mortality is 25% to 100%.

   Ultrasound findings depend on the age of the hemorrhage. At first the hemorrhage is a well-defined homogeneous mass; at one week, the mass may appear cystic with solid elements or septation. At several weeks the hemorrhage may appear cystic.

4. A phlegmon is spreading diffuse inflammatory edema of soft tissues that may proceed to necrosis and suppuration. An extension outside the gland occurs in 18% to 20% of patients with acute pancreatitis.

   The phlegmon appears hypoechoic, with good through transmission. It usually involves the lesser sac, left anterior pararenal space, and transverse mesocolon. Less commonly, it involves the small bowel mesentery, lower retroperitoneum, and pelvis.

5. The pancreas is more easily seen because of less body fat, the left lobe of the liver is more prominent, and the gland is more isosonic than hyperechoic. In acute pancreatitis the gland is increased in size and hypoechoic with an indistinct outline.

   Causes include trauma, drugs, infection, congenital anomalies, and familial or idiopathic causes.

6. A pancreatic pseudocyst is a collection of fluid that arises from a loculation of inflammatory processes, necrosis, or hemorrhage. The condition is usually associated with pancreatitis.

   The pseudocyst is usually single, oval to round, and varies in size. It may cause dilation of the pancreatic duct. The pseudocyst may lie within the pancreas or adjacent to the pancreas, with extension into the lesser sac or anterior or posterior pararenal space. The walls may be thin or quite thick with fibrosis.

   The difference between a cyst and a pseudocyst is that there is no epithelial lining.

   Ultrasound findings include sharply defined smooth walls, usually with acoustic enhancement. There may be multiple septations and internal echoes. The pseudocyst can mimic cystadenoma or cystadenocarcinoma.

7. Other structures that may be mistaken for a pseudocyst in the left upper quadrant are a fluid-filled stomach, a dilated pancreatic duct (look for continuity of cyst with duct), or a left renal vein varix.

8. Chronic pancreatitis represents progressive destruction of the pancreas by repeated flare-ups of a mild or subclinical type of acute pancreatitis. Hypercalcemia and hyperlipidemia predispose to chronic pancreatitis. Patients experience recurrent bouts of pain at intervals of months to years.

   Ultrasound findings include increased echogenicity of pancreas beyond the normal resulting from fibrotic and fatty changes, calcification, ductal dilation, and irregular outline. Focal or diffuse enlargement of the gland may be associated with irregular outline. Pancreatic lithiasis is associated with alcoholic pancreatitis. (Shadowing may be present.)

9. There are two classifications of adenomas: macrocystic and microcystic.

    A macrocystic adenoma is an uncommon, slow-growing tumor that arises from ducts as a cystic neoplasm. It is composed of a large cyst with or without septations. It has significant malignant potential. Patients are seen with epigastric pain or a palpable mass and may also have concurrent diseases such as diabetes, calculous disease of biliary tract, and arterial hypertension. Macrocystic adenoma occurs more in middle-aged women, with 60% occurring in the tail and 5% in the head. The body and tail are the most frequent sites. There is frequently foci of calcification.

    A microcystic adenoma consists of tiny cysts lined by flattened or cuboidal cells that contain glycogen and little to no mucin. Microcystic adenomas are benign lesions that occur more frequently in females. They involve the body and tail in 60% of cases and the head in 30% of cases.

10. Adenocarcinoma is a fatal tumor that involves the exocrine portion of the gland. At least 95% of all malignant pancreatic tumors are adenocarcinoma. It usually occurs in 60 to 80-year-old men. The tumor is found most often in the head of the gland in 60% to 70% of cases, then in the body, and last in the tail. The tumors in the head present early with obstructive symptoms.

    The clinical course includes weight loss, abdominal pain radiating to the back, anorexia, nausea and vomiting, and generalized malaise and weakness. The time from symptoms until diagnosis is 4 months, to death 8 months to 1.6 years.

    Ultrasound findings include lesions that represent localized change in echodensity of the pancreas. The echopattern is hypoechoic (less dense than that seen in the pancreas or liver.) Approximately 95% are found to be hypoechoic. Borders are irregular, and there may be pancreatic enlargement. Masses in the head are smaller than in the tail (compression of CBD) and there is dilation of the pancreatic duct. Liver mets, nodal mets, portal venous system involvement, splenic vein enlargement, SMA displacement and ascites may be seen. Superior mesenteric vessels may be displaced posteriorly by the pancreatic mass. Soft tissue thickening caused by neoplastic infiltration of perivascular lymphatics may be seen surrounding the celiac axis or SMA (occurs more with CA of body and tail). Most patients have obstructive jaundice. The tumor can compress the splenic vein, producing secondary splenic enlargement. The tumor may displace or invade the splenic or portal vein or produce thrombosis. The mass in the head may compress the anterior wall of the IVC.

11. There are several types of islet cell tumors and are classified as functional or nonfunctional. These tumors represent benign adenomas or malignant tumors. The nonfunctioning islet cell tumors comprise one third of all islet cell tumors—92% are malignant. The most common functioning islet cell tumor is insulinoma followed by gastrinoma.

    The tumors occur mostly in the body and tail, where there is greatest concentration of islets of Langerhans. Islet cell tumors are small and difficult to detect with ultrasound.

12. The intraabdominal lymphomas may cause a hypoechoic mass in the pancreas. The superior mesenteric vessels are displaced anteriorly instead of posteriorly as seen with a primary pancreatic mass.

    Multiple nodes are seen along the pancreas, duodenum, porta, and superior mesenteric vessels; the nodes may be difficult to distinguish from a pancreatic mass. On ultrasound the nodes appear hypoechoic.

Answers to Self-Test

1. c	**12.** true	**23.** c
2. a	**13.** true	**24.** b
3. b	**14.** b	**25.** c
4. true	**15.** c	**26.** d
5. false	**16.** b	**27.** c
6. false	**17.** a	**28.** c
7. false	**18.** false	**29.** c
8. true	**19.** a	**30.** a
9. true	**20.** b	**31.** b
10. true	**21.** b	**32.** b
11. true	**22.** c	**33.** true

34. b
35. a
36. b, d
37. false
38. true
39. b
40. true
41. false
42. d
43. a
44. c
45. false
46. true
47. true
48. b
49. d
50. endocrine; exocrine
51. endocrine
52. exocrine
53. b
54. c
55. c
56. a
57. a
58. b

59. a
60. a
61. Acute pancreatitis is an inflammation of the entire gland. The borders become irregular; the gland is hypoechoic. Chronic pancreatitis shows a smaller gland, with calcifications and a hyperechoic glandular pattern.
62. A true cyst has an epithelial lining; a pseudocyst does not.
63. adenocarcinoma
64. weight loss, vomiting and nausea, back pain, jaundice
65. c
66. d
67. d
68. b
69. a
70. d
71. a
72. b
73. false
74. d

75. a
76. d
77. c
78. c
79. c
80. a
81. c
82. d
83. b, c, d, g, h, i
84. a
85. false
86. true
87. anechoic cysts with acoustic enhancement and internal septations
88. a
89. because the tumor is usually located in the head of the gland and blocks the common bile duct
90. Pancreatic carcinoma is located near the celiac axis, which allows a rapid spread of invasive cells to other parts of the body.
91. a

Answers to Case Reviews

1. (Figure 6-7) On ultrasound, you should look for pancreatitis (acute or chronic), abnormal liver patterns, ascites, and a pseudocyst formation. This patient had a pseudocyst located near the head of the pancreas. A pseudocyst is a "sterile" abscess (collection of amylase that has escaped from the pancreas). It may have walled itself off and collected anywhere in the mediastinum and abdomen, although most frequently it is related to the area of the pancreas. It may be any size and usually takes the available space surrounding it. The borders are usually smooth, with debris located along the posterior wall. Transmission of the ultrasound is increased posterior to the mass.

   Patients with a pseudocyst collection usually have a heavy drinking history and frequent episodes of acute pancreatitis. Pancreatitis may or may not be present at the time the pseudocyst is seen on ultrasound.

2. (Figure 6-8) The pancreas is usually slightly more hyperechoic than the liver texture. This is because of the fat accumulation interspersed between the islets of Langerhans. The pancreas has also been reported to be slightly hypoechoic in comparison to the liver parenchyma. Careful analysis of the size of the gland should be assessed when the gland is hypoechoic. The normal head measures 2.4 cm, the body and tail 2.0 cm. In patients with acute pancreatitis the gland may swell

from edema in the tissues (causing the pancreas to appear enlarged and hypoechoic).

3. (Figure 6-9) Your preliminary diagnosis should be pancreatic carcinoma with obstructive jaundice and hydrops of the gallbladder. You would want to document the pancreas, common bile duct, gallbladder, and liver (dilated intrahepatic ducts and metastases) and search for the presence of celiac adenopathy.

   Pancreatic lesions on ultrasound are usually quite large, 2 to 3 cm. If they are located in the head of the gland, progressive enlargement may cause compression of the common bile duct, leading to hydrops of the gallbladder and subsequent intrahepatic ductal dilation. If the tumor has been present for some time, metastases to the liver and retroperitoneum should be considered.

   The appearance of a pancreatic tumor on ultrasound usually shows an ill-defined mass lesion with poorly marginated walls, hypoechoic internal texture, and decreased transmission.

   The pancreatic duct may be enlarged; the common bile duct is enlarged when the mass is located in the head of the gland. Associated ascites may be present, with liver metastases or paraortic adenopathy.

4. (Figure 6-10) This patient has a classic case of acute pancreatitis. The pancreas may appear enlarged and

hypoechoic secondary to edema and swelling. The borders may be somewhat irregular and shaggy. The sonographer should search for extrapancreatic fluid collections (pseudocyst formation, fluid in the lesser sac or anterior pararenal space secondary to pancreatitis).

5. a. (Figure 6-11) Left lobe of liver: The liver should measure at least 3 cm to aid the sonographer in identifying the body and tail of the pancreas.

b. Collapsed wall of the antrum of the stomach: the stomach can be seen anterior to the body of the pancreas and posterior to the left lobe of the liver. With ingested fluid, the stomach may be filled to outline the pancreas. The duodenum is the lateral landmark of the head of the gland.

c. Aorta: This vessel is the posterior border of the body of the pancreas.

d. Inferior vena cava: This is the posterior border of the body and head of the pancreas.

e. Splenic artery: This is the left branch of the celiac trunk that demarcates the superior border of the pancreas.

f. Superior mesenteric artery: This vessel is best seen on the transverse view as the posterior border of the body of the gland.

g. Superior mesenteric vein: This vessel demarcates the posterior border of the body and anterior border of the uncinate process of the pancreas.

h. Splenic vein: This vessel marks the medial posterior border of the body of the pancreas.

i. Right branch of the portal vein: The right branch of the portal vein is superior to the head on the pancreas on the longitudinal scan.

j. Gastroduodenal artery: This vessel marks the antero-lateral border of the head of the gland.

k. Common bile duct: This structure is seen as the posterior border of the pancreas.

6. (Figure 6-12) The sonographer should expect to see ascites; the liver should show signs of chronic cirrhosis (echogenic, decreased vascular markings, small size). The pancreas should be evaluated for signs of chronic pancreatitis with dilation and/or calcification of the pancreatic duct. The overall gland texture will probably be hyperechoic, and the size may be reduced. The margins will appear irregular. Associated pseudocyst formation should be considered.

7. The patient with pancreatitis generally presents with GI symptoms and a developing ileus. This ileus formation makes it extremely difficult to image the midline structures surrounding the pancreas. Sometimes the patient may be scanned in an upright position or given several glasses of fluid to provide an adequate window to scan the pancreatic area.

Acute pancreatitis may exist with a phlegmon extension. Mittelstaedt states that a phlegmon is a spreading diffuse inflammatory edema of soft tissues that may proceed to necrosis and even suppuration. It usually appears as a hypoechoic area with poorly defined margins. Most commonly it involves the lesser sac, the left anterior pararenal space, and the transverse mesocolon.

CHAPTER

7

The Gastrointestinal Tract

OBJECTIVES

At the completion of this chapter, students will show orally, in writing, or by demonstration that they will be able to:

1. Describe the various positions and size of the normal gastrointestinal (GI) tract.
2. Define the internal, surface, and relational anatomies of the gastrointestinal tract.
3. Illustrate the cross-sectional anatomy of the gastrointestinal tract and adjacent structures.
4. Describe congenital anomalies affecting the gastrointestinal tract.
5. Identify the enzymes and secretions of the gastrointestinal tract by explaining its functions.
6. Select pertinent laboratory tests and other diagnostic procedures.
7. Differentiate among sonographic appearances of each of the following diseases by explaining the clinical significance of the pathologic processes as related to the gastrointestinal tract:
   a. gastric abnormalities

   b. gastritis and ulcer disease
   c. gastric wall abnormalities
   d. benign tumors
   e. malignant tumors
   f. small bowel abnormalities
   g. duodenal obstruction or dilation
   h. hematoma
   i. meconium cyst and peritonitis
   j. appendiceal abnormalities
   k. colonic abnormalities
8. Create high-quality diagnostic scans demonstrating the appropriate anatomy in all planes pertinent to the gastrointestinal tract.
9. Select the correct equipment settings appropriate to individual body habitus.
10. Distinguish among the normal and abnormal sonographic appearances of the gastrointestinal tract.

To further enhance learning, students should use marking pens to color the anatomic illustrations that follow.

GASTROINTESTINAL TRACT

FIGURE 7-1
Parts of the Duodenum

Esophagus and Stomach

The tubular esophagus descends from the thorax to enter the right side of the stomach through an opening in the right crus of the diaphragm. It is posterior to the left lobe of the liver and the left crus of the diaphragm.

The stomach lies under the ribs in the left upper abdomen. It extends from the left hypochrondriac region into the epigastric and umbilical regions. Its J-shaped structure has two openings (the cardiac and pyloric orifices), two curvatures (lesser and greater), and two surfaces (anterior and posterior).

The stomach is usually divided into the following parts: the fundus, body, pyloric antrum, and pyloris.

Duodenum and Small Intestine

Most of the digestion and absorption of food takes place in the small intestine. The small intestine is divided into three parts: the duodenum, the jejunum, and the ileum. The first section of the small intestine is the duodenum. The duodenum leads into the middle portion, the jejunum, and the small intestine then terminates in the ileum. The entire small intestine is about 23 feet long and 1 inch in diameter.

Duodenum

The duodenum, a C-shaped tube, curves around the head of the pancreas. The first few centimeters are covered with peritoneum; while the remainder lies retroperitoneally. The duodenum is divided into four parts for anatomic study (Figure 7-1).

The first part begins at the pylorus and runs upward and backward on the right side of the first lumbar vertebra. It is related to the quadrate lobe of the liver and the gallbladder anteriorly; the lesser sac, the gastroduodenal artery, the common bile duct, the portal vein, and the inferior vena cava posteriorly; the epiploic foramen superiorly; and the head of the pancreas inferiorly.

The second part runs anterior to the left kidney on the right side of the second and third lumbar vertebrae. It is related to the fundus of the gallbladder, the right lobe of the liver, the transverse colon, and the small intestine anteriorly; the hilum of the right kidney posteriorly; the ascending colon, the right colic flexure, and the right lobe of the liver laterally; and the head of the pancreas medially. The common bile duct and main pancreatic duct pierce the duodenal wall midway down its posterior aspect.

The third part of the duodenum runs horizontally to the left, following the inferior margin of the pancreatic head. It is related to the root of the mesentery of the small intestine (and the superior mesenteric vessels) and the jejunum anteriorly; the right ureter, right psoas muscle, inferior vena cava, and aorta posteriorly; the head of the pancreas superiorly; and the jejunum inferiorly.

The fourth part of the duodenum runs upward and to the left, then runs forward at the duodenojejunal junction. (The ligament of Treitz ascends to the right crus and holds the junction in position.) It is related to the root of the mesentery and jejunum anteriorly and the left margin of the aorta and the medial border of the left psoas muscle posteriorly.

The upper half of the duodenum is supplied by the superior pancreaticoduodenal artery, and the lower half is supplied by the inferior pancreaticoduodenal artery. The veins of the duodenum drain into the portal circulation.

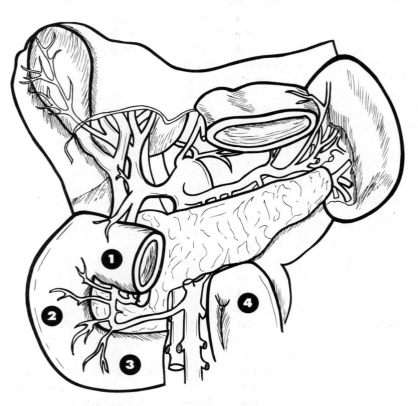

1	**first part of the duodenum (superior part)**
2	**second part of the duodenum (descending part)**
3	**third part of the duodenum (horizontal part)**
4	**fourth part of the duodenum**

Gastrointestinal Tract Review Notes

ULTRASOUND TECHNIQUES AND APPEARANCES OF GI STRUCTURES

- To view the upper GI tract, the patient should drink 10 to 40 oz. of water through a straw.
- To view the lower GI tract, usually no preparation is necessary; however, if needed, a patient may have a water enema.

Stomach

- In the stomach, if there is a cystic mass in the left upper quadrant (LUQ), the sonographer should define if it is the stomach or another mass.
- The sonographer may give the patient a carbonated drink to see bubbles.
- An NG tube should be used for drainage.
- The sonographer should check for changes in shape or size with the intake of fluids.
- The patient should be upright for the sonographer to view the LLD and RLD.
- Peristalsis may be seen.
- The patient should drink water to enable the sonographer to see a possible swirling effect.
- On sagittal scan, the esophagogastric (EG) junction will be seen to the left of the midline as a "bull's-eye" or target structure anterior to the aorta and posterior to the left lobe of the liver, next to the hemidiaphragm. The left lobe of the liver must be large enough to project anterior to the EG junction.
- The gastric antrum can be seen as a target in the midline.
- The remainder of the stomach is usually not visualized unless it is dilated with fluid.
- For the sonographer to get an image with fluid ingestion, the patient should drink in the LLD position. The sonographer should scan the patient in the LLD position, when the patient is supine, and in the RLD position.
- The wall of the stomach is thin and uniform.
- Peristalsis is seen.

Duodenum

- For the sonographer to view the duodenum, the patient should ingest water.
- The patient may change position to help fill the duodenum.

Small Bowel

- The sonographer should look for peristalsis, air movement, or movement of intraluminal fluid contents in the small bowel.
- Usually, peristalsis is seen.

Appendix

- The patient should have an empty bladder for the sonographer to examine the right upper quadrant (RUQ).
- A high-resolution linear array transducer should be used.
- Graded compression over the area of maximum tenderness will help to delineate the area of the appendix.
  - Anterior and posterior abdominal walls may be approximated by displacing the bowel contents and compressing fat and soft tissues to bring the appendix and bowel loops into the focal zone of the transducer.
  - Visibility of retrocecal and paracecal areas is improved by displacing gas and other bowel loop contents from the scanning field.
  - The pliability of the appendix and other bowel loops in the RLQ may be assessed.

Colon

- A colon filled with fluid may appear as a mass.
- Administration of a water enema may help the sonographer to image the colon.
  - The patient should have a full bladder.
  - The enema should be lukewarm water, and the patient should be in the LLD position.
  - The water should follow the rectum and rectosigmoid colon.
- Normal wall thickness is approximately 4 mm.
- Layers of the colon are 1 and 2, mucosa; 3, submucosa; 4, mucularis propria; and 5, serosa and subserous fatty tissue.

Normal Anatomy

- Intraluminal air is echogenic and is usually associated with an incomplete or mottled distal acoustic shadow produced by the scattering effect of gas contained within the GI tract.
- The rim of lucency represents the GI tract wall, which is formed by the intima, media, and serosa layers, and its periserosal fat produces the outer echogenic border of the tract wall.
- The wall of the GI tract should measure less than 5 mm, and when distended should measure less than 3 mm.
- The sonographer should measure from the edge of the echogenic core where the intraluminal gas is located, to the outer border of the anechoic halo, where the bowel wall is located.
- If the bowel wall is dilated, the sonographer should measure from the fluid to the outside of the wall or distention. It is considered adequate if the stomach is

greater than 8 cm, the small bowel is greater than 3 cm, and the lower bowel is greater than 5 cm; the entire halo should measure less than 2 cm. These measurements on ultrasound appear as a target sign.

PATHOLOGIC PROCESS

- When a pathologic process is present, the serosal layer of the normal gastric wall running toward the serous side of a tumor allows distinction between intramural and extraserosal tumors.
- If serosal bridging layer is present (e.g., three layers seen on the mucosal side of the tumor, with at least two of them continuous with layers 1 and 2 of the normal gastric wall), the tumor lies within the gastric wall instead of external to the gastric wall.
- If mucosal bridging that is continuous with mucosal layers of the normal gastric wall is present, intramucosal or deeply infiltrated carcinoma can be excluded.
- The sonographer should orient the transducer vertically to view the area of transition between the lesion and the stomach wall.

Duodenum

- When a pathologic process is present in the duodenum, usually only a duodenal cap filled with gas is seen to the right of the pancreas.
- The duodenum is divided into four sections for viewing:
  1. The superior section courses anteroposteriorly from the pylorus to the level of the neck of the gallbladder.
  2. This section takes a sharp bend into the descending section, which runs along the IVC at the level of the fourth layer of the colon.
  3. The transverse section passes right to left, with slight inclination in front of the great vessels and crura.
  4. The fourth, or ascending, section rises to the right of the aorta and reaches the upper border to the second layer of the colon, where at the duodenojejunal flexure, it turns forward to become the jejunum, which is usually not seen on ultrasound examination.

Small Bowel

- A tumor in the small bowel usually can't be seen on ultrasound examination; however, if fluid has been ingested, the **valvulae conniventes** may be seen as linear echodensities spaced 3 to 5 mm apart. This appearance is known as a keyboard sign, and may be seen in the duodenum and the jejunum.
- The ileum has a smooth wall.
- The small bowel wall is less than 3 mm thick.

Appendix

- In the appendix, the terminal ileum may be identified by its medial location to the cecum, its tubular appearance, its small caliber, its thin hypoechoic muscular wall (1 to 2 cm), active peristalsis, and fluid content mixed with air bubbles.
- If seen, the terminal ileum appears thin (<6 mm in caliber), is 8 to 10 cm long, is fusiform, and appears as a blind-ended structure without peristalsis.

Colon

- When filled with fluid, the colon is identified with haustral markings 3 to 5 cm apart in the ascending and transverse colon. The descending colon appears as a tubular structure with an echogenic border.

Gastric Abnormalities

Gastroesophageal Reflux

- This condition is common among newborns.
- The patient is examined in the supine position 45 minutes after gavage feeding (cardiac suprasternal and right subclavicular).
- The sonographer should image the length of the esophagus between the diaphragm and larynx.
- Morphologic findings associated with significant reflux include a short intraabdominal part of the esophagus; rounded gastroesophageal angle; and a "beak" at the EG junction.
- The ability of the diaphragmatic crura to hold the distal esophagus in place during esophageal hiatus prevents the esophagus from sliding upward.
- A sliding hiatal hernia of the distal esophagus leading to LES incompetency can be identified.

Dilation

- A stomach filled with fluid may be the result of:
  - pylorospasm
  - inflammation
  - intrinsic or extrinsic tumor
  - electrolyte imbalance
  - diabetes
  - amyloidosis
  - neurologic disease
  - medication
- When dilated, the stomach is a pear-shaped cystic structure in the LUQ.
- The characteristic configuration includes discrete thin walls, movement of strong echoes caused by food particles when light pressure is applied, gas-fluid level, and compressibility.

Bouveret Syndrome

- Bouveret syndrome is a gastric outlet obstruction that is secondary to a gallstone impacted within the duodenal bulb.

- Stones larger than 2.5 cm may produce obstruction in the intestine, particularly in the distal ileum.
- An eroding stone will pass spontaneously in 80% to 90% of cases.
- A gallstone in the duodenum may produce the double-arc sign on ultrasound examination. The duodenal wall produces the anterior arc, which is similar to what is commonly seen with gallbladder disease.
- The sonographer should look for pneumobilia.

Duplication

- Duplication cysts are embryologic mistakes; they cause symptoms depending on their size, location, and histology.
- The criteria for a duplication cyst include the following:
    1. a cyst lined with alimentary tract epithelium
    2. a well-developed muscular wall
    3. contiguity with the stomach
- These cysts may arise from the pancreas or duodenum.
- They occur more often in female infants than in males.
- The cysts are usually on the greater curvature of the stomach.
- The patient may have symptoms of high intestinal obstruction; e.g., distention, vomiting, and abdominal pain; also possibly hemorrhage and fistula formation may occur.
- The solid component is caused by hemorrhage and inspissated material within the cyst
- On ultrasound examination, a duplication cyst is anechoic with a thin inner echogenic rim, which is the mucosa, and wider outer hypoechoic rim, which is the muscle layer.
- The differential diagnosis may be mesenteric or omental cyst, pancreatic cyst or pseudocyst, enteric cyst, renal cyst, splenic cyst, congenital cyst of LLL, or gastric distention.

Hypertrophic Pyloric Stenosis

- This condition is hereditary, with a ratio of four males to one female.
- There is an occurrence rate of 6% in children whose parents had HPS.
- A mother with HPS has a four times greater chance of having affected offspring than a father who has HPS.
- Newborns experience projectile vomiting in the second or third week of life.
- Another physical sign is a palpable abdominal mass.
- Hypertrophy and hyperplasia of circular muscle result in elongation of the pylorus and constriction of the canal; narrowing may lead to edema or inflammatory changes.
- On ultrasound examination, the sonographer should check the volumetric measurement of NG aspirate, pyloric diameter, pyloric muscle thickness, pyloric

length, and check for the cervix sign and the double track sign.

Volumetric Measurement

- Patients with NG aspirate of 10 ml or greater should be referred for further ultrasound evaluation, while those with less should be referred for fluroscopy to determine the possibility of gastroesophageal reflux.

Pyloric Diameter

- The target lesion associated with HPS is usually located by orienting the transducer in the sagittal plane.
- A measurement of 15 mm or more is abnormal for pyloric diameter; normal is less than 10 mm.
- A normal adult pylorus is 3.8 mm to 8.5 mm; abnormal is greater than 9 mm.

Pyloric Muscle Thickness

- The wall, or hypoechoic rim, of the target represents the hypertrophied muscle, which is greater than 4 mm thick.
- The HPS is greater than 5 mm on longitudinal view.

Pyloric Length of Channel

- The echogenic central line of mucosa indicates the pyloric length.
- The elongated pyloric channel is a mucosal double-track sign.
- The normal length is 18 mm; abnormal is 2.1 mm or more.

Cervix Sign

- The cervix sign is hypertrophied muscle that has gone into the antrum.

Double Tract Sign

- This sign is produced with fluid-aided real-time ultrasonography, and it is seen as a result of pyloric fluid that has been compressed into smaller tracks as it impinges circumferentially by thickened circular muscle.

Antropyloric Muscle Thickness

- Antropyloric muscle thickness is measured in the mid-longitudinal plane of the fully distended, fluid-filled antrum.
- A normal measurement is 2 mm or less; abnormal is 3 mm or greater.

General

- Direct signs of HPS on ultrasound examination include an obstructed stomach, exaggerated peristaltic waves, failure of fluid to pass from the stomach into the duodenum, and failure to image the descending duodenum.

Gastritis and Ulcer Disease

- The patient should be examined in various positions, especially upright for good distention of the gastric wall.
- Benign gastric ulcers are associated with gastric wall thickening and loss of the five-layer structure of the gastric wall.
- Signs of gastritis or ulcer disease on ultrasound examination include gastric wall edema associated with ulcer crater, gastric wall edema, increased wall thickness with a mean of 12.88 mm, asymmetric thickening of the mucosa and muscularis, and spasm and deformity of the gastric wall.

Complications

- The most common complications of peptic ulcer disease are obstruction, hemorrhage, penetration, and perforation.
- The distal stomach and proximal duodenum are the most frequent locations of peptic ulcer disease. Focal peritonitis caused by perforation is usually located in the RUQ; the localized exudate does not change shape or location when the patient's position is altered.
- On ultrasound examination, the sonographer may see free air in perforated peptic ulcers; visualization of an interference echo with shifting phenomenon is a strong indication of the presence of free air in the abdominal cavity.
- The differential diagnosis of Chilaiditi syndrome, in which the colon is interposed between the right hemidiaphragm and the liver, producing typical interference echopattern, may be made.
- Other findings include subphrenic and/or subhepatic fluid collection, thickening of the gallbladder wall, and presence of an inflammatory mass in the upper abdomen.

Pediatric Gastric Ulcer Disease

- Ultrasound signs of pediatric gastric ulcer disease include thickening of the mucosa (greater than 4 mm) in the antropyloric region, elongation of the antropyloric canal, persistent spasm, and delayed gastric emptying.
- Measurements are made at three sites along the antrum from the distal end to a point where the gastric lumen becomes normal. Normal is 2.5 mm to 3.5 mm; abnormal is 4 mm to 7.5 mm

Gastric Phytobezoar

- Bezoars are divided into the following three categories:
  1. Trichobezoars are hair balls found in young women.
  2. Phytobezoars are composed of vegetable matter, such as unripe persimmons.
  3. Concretions are composed of inorganic materials, such as sand, asphalt, and shellac.

Gastric Bezoars

- Gastric bezoars are movable, intraluminal masses of congealed ingested materials that are seen on examination of the upper GI tract.
- Patients experience nausea, vomiting, and abdominal pain.
- A gastric bezoar may simulate a tumor in appearance.
- On ultrasound examination, the sonographer may see a complex mass with internal mobile echogenic components in a fasting patient; a broad band of high-amplitude echoes or a hyperechoic curvilinear dense strip at the anterior margin is seen superior, with a complete clean shadow posterior.

Miscellaneous Gastric Wall Abnormalities

Gastric Wall Abnormalities in Children

- In children, normal wall thickness is greater than 3 mm; abnormal is 5 mm to 15 mm.
- An abnormal wall is seen in varioliform gastritis, gastric ulcers, lymphoid hyperplasia, and gastric hamartomas.

Menetrier's Disease

- Menetrier's disease is characterized by giant hypertrophy of the gastric mucosa.
- Predominantly, it affects middle-aged men, and there is a 10% risk of complicating carcinoma.
- Clinical symptoms include edema occasionally associated with ascites, pleural effusions, anorexia, vomiting, abdominal pain, and diarrhea.
- On ultrasound examination, the sonographer will see edema, hypoproteinemia, and thickening and hypertrophy of the gastric folds, especially in the fundus and corpus.
- In the fasting state, an ultrasound study of an empty stomach shows polypoid mucosal hypertrophy, especially in the fundus and corpus. The stomach wall may be thickened and poorly echogenic. The rugae will become flattened after ingestion of fluid, but the wall will remain thick.

Gastric Amyloidosis

- Gastric amyloidosis is classified into two groups:
  1. Fibrils that consist mainly of amyloid light-chain (AL) protein originate from light chains of immunoglobulins.
     - This type of fibrils is primary amyloidsis.
     - There is concentric narrowing of the gastric antrum.
     - On ultrasound examination, homogeneous hypoechogenicity of the thickened gastric wall cannot be distinguished from malignant processes and other benign causes of gastric wall thickening. The walls of the stomach and colon are markedly thickened.

2. Fibrils that consist primarily of amyloid protein A originate from serum amyloid A protein.
   • This type of fibril is secondary amyloidosis.

Hematoma

• Intramural hemorrhage into the GI tract is a rare complication in hemophiliacs. It can be a result of other problems, such as bleeding diathesis, anticoagulant therapy, blunt trauma, or leukemia.
• A hematoma in the GI tract may be associated with signs of obstruction and may appear as an LUQ mass.
• On ultrasound examination, the hematoma appears as a large complex mass consisting of coagula and blood, when symptoms of obstruction appear.
• After several weeks, the ultrasound waves of the mass change to anechoic as a result of liquefication of the hematoma.

Benign Tumors

Polyps

• Polyp lesions are seen with fluid distension of the stomach; they may appear as solid masses adherent to the gastric wall.
• A polyp has variable echogenicity.
• On ultrasound examination, a large polyp may be inhomogeneous; contours may be sharply or not sharply delineated, depending on the nature of the surface; detection of a pedicle may be possible.

Leiomyomas

• A leiomyoma is the most common tumor of the stomach.
• On ultrasound examination, it is seen as a mass, similar to carcinoma, and is usually small and asymptomatic.
• A leiomyoma is often associated with other GI abnormalities, such as cholelithiasis, peptic ulcer disease, adenocarcinoma, and leiomyosarcoma.
• On ultrasound examination, wave patterns are seen as a hypoechoic mass continuous with the muscular layer of the stomach.
• In addition, the sonographer may see a circular or oval lesion, with homogeneous echopattern and hemispheric bulging into the lumen. Frequently, the lesion is separated from the lumen by two or three layers that are continuous with those of the normal wall.
• A leiomyoma may appear as a solid mass with cystic areas that represent necrosis.

Malignant Tumors

Gastric Carcinoma

• 90% to 95% of malignant tumors of the stomach are carcinomas.
• Gastric carcinoma is the sixth leading cause of death in older males.

• Half of the tumors occur in the pylorus, and one fourth in the body and fundus.
• Lesions may be fungating, ulcerated, diffuse, polypoid, or superficial.
• An ultrasound study will show a target or pseudokidney sign, and possibly gastric wall thickening.

Lymphoma of the Stomach

• Lymphoma can occur as a primary tumor of the GI tract. Three percent of lymphomas are stomach tumors.
• In desseminated lymphoma, a primary tumor occurs as multifocal lesions in the GI tract.
• Lymphoma is characterized by enlarged and thickened mucosal folds, multiple submucosal nodules, ulceration, and a large extraluminal mass.
• Physical symptoms of lymphoma are nausea and vomiting, and weight loss.
• On ultrasound examination, lymphoma appears as a large and poorly echogenic (hypoechoic) mass. In addition, there is thickening of the gastric walls, and a spoke-wheel pattern within the mass.

Leiomyosarcoma

• Leiomyosarcoma is the second most common gastric sarcoma, making up 1 to 5% of malignant tumors.
• Leiomyosarcoma usually affects people who are 50 to 70 years of age.
• The tumor is generally globular or irregular and may become huge, outstripping the blood supply with central necrosis leading to cystic degeneration and cavitation.
• An ultrasound study will show a target lesion with a variable pattern. Hemorrhage and necrosis may occur, causing irregular echoes or a cystic cavity.

Metastatic Disease

• Metastatic disease is rare to the stomach; it originates as melanoma or lung or breast cancer.
• It is found within the submucosal layer of the stomach, forming circumscribed nodules or plaques.
• An ultrasound study will show a target pattern with circumscribed thickening or uniform widening of the wall, with an absence of layering.

Small Bowel Abnormalities

Obstruction or Dilation

• Small bowel obstruction is associated with dilation of the bowel loops proximal to the site of the obstruction.
• In 6% of cases, the dilated loops are filled with fluid and can be mistaken for a soft tissue mass on x-ray examination.
• Dilated loops may have a tubular or round echo-free appearance.
• In an adynamic ileus, a dilated bowel has normal to

somewhat increased peristaltic activity; there is less distension than with a dynamic ileus.

- In a dynamic ileus, the loops are round with minimal deformity at the interfaces with adjacent loops of distended bowel; valvulae conniventes and peristalsis are seen.
- Fluid-filled loops are not always associated with obstruction; they can also occur with gastroenteritis and a paralytic ileus.
- Demonstrate pliability and compressibility of bowel wall.

Closed-Loop Obstruction or Volvulus

- With volvulus, the involved loop is doubled back on itself abruptly so a U-shaped appearance is seen on sagittal scan and a C-shaped anechoic area with dense center is seen on transverse scan; the dense center represents medial bowel wall and mesentery.

Duodenal Obstruction and/or Dilation

Midgut Volbulus

- This condition constitutes an acute medical emergency.
- The patient has acute onset of vomiting.
- On ultrasound examination, to-and-fro hyperperistaltic motion is seen in the obstructed duodenal loop.
- The sonographer will see the fluid-filled proximal duodenum ending in a twist or arrowhead configuration; the duodenum does not cross the midline, and the more distal duodenum is not seen to fill with fluid. By following the fluid in the duodenum from the antrum to Treitz's ligament, the normal rotation can be seen. Malrotation without volvulus and subtle abnormalities in the course of the duodenum can be seen even when the duodenum crosses from right to left.

Midgut Malrotation

- Midgut malrotation is the incomplete rotation and fixation of the gut in a fetus.
- Midgut volvulus may be a complication.
- Symptoms are produced by obstructing peritoneal bands that cross over the descending duodenum or occasionally the cecum, which may lie on top of the duodenum.
- Physical symptoms are vomiting, abdominal distention, and bloody stools.
- On ultrasound examination, the sonographer will see a fluid-filled, distended duodenum; dilated, thick-walled bowel loops to the right of the spine and peritoneal fluid; a distended proximal duodenum, an extrinsic arrowhead compression of duodenum over the spine, an abnormal relationship of SMA and SMV with SMV on the left; distended, thick-walled loops of bowel below the duodenum and to the right of the spine in association with peritoneal fluid.

Duodenal Stenosis

- Obstruction or relative stenosis may cause dilation of the more proximal duodenal bulb and pyloric channel.
- The patient will experience nausea and vomiting.
- An ultrasound study will show a fluid-filled bowel and an epigastric mass that is solid or has a heterogeneous pattern or targetlike structure; lesions have high-level central echoes and hypoechoic peripheries.

Superior Mesenteric Artery Syndrome

- The stomach and the duodenum may be dilated to a point in the third portion of the duodenum where the SM vessels press on the duodenum.
- This condition can be seen when a patient is supine, and disappears when the patient is prone.
- This condition is more common in thin patients, and in those with extensive burns, rapid weight loss, acute pancreatitis, severe trauma, or a body cast.

Matted Bowel Loops

- Matted bowel loops may be caused by adhesions, peritoneal implants, or intraperitoneal inflammatory processes.
- The loops are tortuous, echo free tubular structures; they consist of a complex of masslike lesions with echo-free areas and areas with weak or strong echoes; irregular lesions with weak echoes are similar to a solid mass.

Hematoma

- Intramural hemorrhage may occur from a hematoma in the following conditions: bleeding diatheses, hemophilia, anticoagulant therapy, blunt trauma, leukemia, and lymphoma.
- Hematomas are sometimes found in victims of child abuse.
- Abdominal pain precedes skin lesions.
- Internal hematomas may occur at any portion of the intestinal tract, but are most common in areas adjacent to relatively fixed portions of the intestine.
- When the duodenum is affected, there may be secondary effects of gastric outlet obstruction of the biliary tree and extrinsic compression on the IVC.
- A lesion in the duodenum produces thickening of the duodenal wall; a target sign or echogenic mass may be seen on ultrasound examination.
- A hematoma produces eccentric thickening of the bowel wall.

Intussusception

- Intussusception is the most common cause of obstruction in children.
- When it is located in the colon, 50% of these obstructions are malignant, whereas most lesions in the small bowel are benign.

- Patients affected are most often children between 6 months and 2 years of age.
- In adults intussusception is chronic, and the patients experience minimal pain, diarrhea, and vomiting.
- Categories of enterocolic intussusception include the following:
  1. enteric (small bowel invaginates into the small bowel)
  2. ileocolic (ileum invaginates through the stationary ileocecal valve)
  3. ileocecal (ileocecal valve itself leads to intussusception)
  4. colocolic (the colon invaginates into the colon)
- On ultrasound examination, intussusception appears as a target, bull's eye, doughnut or pseudokidney; or, it may appear as a concentric ring sign, with a highly reflective intussusceptum and an unstructured wave pattern corresponding to a solid tumor.
- With the doughnut, target, or pseudokidney pattern, there is a thickened hypoechoic rim that represents the edematous intussuscipiens that surround the hyperechoic center as a result of multiple interfaces of compressed mucosal and serosal surfaces of the intussusceptum.
- The concentric ring sign occurs when there are lesser degrees of edema; the various layers of mucosa and serosa are less stretched and thinned, thereby becoming echogenic and resulting in formation of concentric rings or layering.
- Ultrasound findings of two mixed hypoechoic-echogenic oval structures within the large hyperechoic center suggest the presence of an ileocecal type of intussusception.
- Intussusception is a known complication in patients who have cystic fibrosis.

Meckel's Diverticulum

- Meckel's diverticulum is located on the antimesenteric border of the ileum, approximately 2 ft from the ileocecal valve.
- This condition affects approximately 2% of the population.
- Adults may have intestinal obstruction, rectal bleeding, and diverticular inflammation.
- Acute appendicitis and acute Meckel's diverticulum may not be distinguished clinically.
- The wall of Meckel's diverticulum is composed of mucosal, muscular, and serosal layers.
- Noncompressibility of the obstructed inflamed diverticulum indicates that the intraluminal fluid is trapped.
- The area of maximum tenderness is evaluated with its distance from the cecum.

Intestinal Lymphangiectasia
Small Bowel Bezoar

- Small bezoars are more common in the stomach; they may pass into the small bowel.

- On ultrasound examination, these bezoars appear as a large, echogenic intraluminal mass with complete acoustic shadowing so the bezoars mimic a heavily calcified lesion.

Intestinal Ascaris

- On ultrasound examination, intestinal ascaris is identified by the worms that are seen within fluid-filled, small bowel loops.

Crohn's Disease

- Crohn's disease, or regional enteritis, is a recurrent granulomatous inflammatory disease that affects the terminal ileum and/or any level of the colon.
- Reaction involves entire thickness of bowel wall.
- Physical symptoms include diarrhea, fever, and RLQ pain.
- Ultrasound findings include the following:
  - Symmetrically swollen bowel
  - Targetlike wave pattern with preserved parietal layers around the stenotic, hyperdense lumen
  - Findings are most prominent in ileocolonic disease, with uniformly increased wall thickness involving all layers, but especially the mucosa and submucosa
  - Matted-loop wave pattern is found in late states
  - Rigidity to pressure exerted from transducer
  - Absent or sluggish peristalsis
  - Dilation with hyperperistalsis and water and air stasis

Meconium Cyst and Peritonitis

- Meconium peritonitis is a sterile chemical peritonitis resulting from the extrusion of meconium from the fetal gut into the peritoneal cavity.
- Causes of these conditions include bowel perforation proximal to obstruction, meconium ileus, volvulus, hernia, and atresia.

Meconium Cyst

- There are three clinical forms of meconium peritonitis: cystic, fibroadhesive, and generalized.
- A meconium cyst is formed when the bowel perforates in utero.
- Meconium that is extruded into the peritoneal cavity becomes walled off by fibrous adhesions.
- If the perforation remains open, the meconium cyst is in communication with the bowel at the site of perforation.
- On ultrasound examination, a meconium cyst appears as an inhomogeneous mass with several central areas of increased echogenicity and faint posterior shadowing, and a highly echogenic, thick peripheral rim.

Meconium Peritonitis

- Meconium peritonitis is characterized by chemical peritonitis that has an intense fibroplastic reaction to digestive enzymes in the meconium.

- Perforation may persist postnatally, or a dense adherent membrane may be formed on the peritoneal surface, which seals off the site of perforation and leads to fibroadhesive meconium peritonitis.
- On ultrasound examination, echogenic ascites may be visualized with meconium, and peritonitis, thus mimicking liver parenchyma.
- Calcification may be present in the bowel.

Intestinal Tumors

Lymphoma

- Generally, lymphoma occurs in patients who are approximately 65 years of age; however, it is the most common tumor of the GI tract in children under 10 years of age.
- There may be systemic involvement, and lymphoma may cause multiple nodules; arises in the GI tract in 10% to 20% of patients.
- Intraperitoneal masses frequently involve the mesenteric vessels that encase them.
- Signs of lymphoma include intestinal blood loss, weight loss, anorexia, and abdominal pain.
- The patient will have intestinal obstruction and a palpable mass.
- On ultrasound examination, a lymphoma appears as a large discrete mass with a targetlike wave pattern and an exoenteric pattern with a large mass on the mesenteric surface of the bowel, or a small anechoic mass representing subserosal nodes or mesenteric nodal involvement.
- Lymphomatous involvement of the intestinal wall may lead to pseudokidney or hydronephrotic pseudokidney.
- The lumen may be dilated with fluid, which indicates a lack of peristalsis.
- The bowel wall is uniformly thickened, with homogeneous low echogenicity between well-defined mucosal and serosal surfaces that contain a persistent, echofree, wide and long lumen.

Leiomyosarcoma

- Leiomyosarcoma represents 10% of primary small bowel tumors.
- 10% to 30% of these tumors occur in the duodenum; 30% to 45% in the jejunum; and 35% to 55% are located in the ileum.
- It affects patients who are 50 to 60 years of age.
- An ultrasound study will show a large, solid mass containing necrotic areas anterior to solid viscus.

Carcinoid

- Can arise anywhere in the GI tract, bronchi, biliary tree, or pancreas.
- Found in appendix, small bowel, rectum, lower bowel.
- Most lesions are small, (1.5 cm).

- An ultrasound study will show a sharply marginated hypoechoic mass with a strong back wall, and a lobulated contour with lack of acoustic enhancement; both of these patterns are nonspecific.

Peutz-Jeghers Syndrome

- Peutz-Jeghers syndrome is characterized by polyps in the GI tract, particularly in the small bowel.

Associated Mesentery Abnormalities

- The normal mesentery has an elongated shape, with an echogenic surface and small vessels in the center.
- The small bowel mesentery is a fan-shaped structure that connects the convolutions of the jejunum and ileum to the posterior wall of the abdomen. The small bowel mesentery consists of two layers of peritoneum containing blood vessels, nerves, lacteals, lymphatic glands, and a variable amount of fat.
- The normal mesentery is .5 cm to 1.0 cm thick, with a maximum breadth of .7 cm to 1.2 cm.
- An abnormal mesentery may have enlarged lymph nodes, lymphoma, and mesenteric desmoid tumors.

Retractile Mesenteritis

- Retractile mesenteritis is caused by chronic inflammation and fibrosis, and is characterized by focal or diffuse thickening of the mesentery.
- This condition is more commonly found in male children who are 8 years of age.
- On ultrasound examination, the sonographer will see a separation of intestinal loops, kinking or angulation of the small intestine, and narrowing of the colon.

Mesenteric Adenitis and Terminal Ileitis or Bacterial Ileocecitis

- Mesenteric adenitis is a frequent clinical diagnosis in patients with acute appendicitis.
- This condition may cause secondary infection.
- An ultrasound study will show mural thickening of the terminal ileum, cecum, and part of the ascending colon; enlargement of mesenteric lymph nodes; nonvisualization of inflamed appendix.

Appendiceal Abnormalities

- With appendicitis, an ultrasound examination will show a typical target lesion in the RLQ.
- There may be thickening of the bowel wall as a result of edema, and an echogenic core as a result of a necrotic appendix or appendiceal lumen.
- An abnormality may consist of a noncompressible mass.
- There may be fluid or abscess collection.
- Appendiceal diameter is greater than 6 mm.
- Muscular wall thickness is greater than 3 mm.
- Visualization of a complex mass is possible.

Perforation with Acute Appendicitis or Abscess

- On ultrasound examination, the sonographer may see loculated pericecal fluid, prominent pericecal fat, and circumferential loss of the submucosal layer of the appendix.

Postappendectomy Fluid Collections

- On ultrasound examination, the sonographer must be able to distinguish between the colon and fluid collection.

Radiation Appendicitis

- The sonographer may see an inflamed appendix in patients who have received radiation therapy for extensive rectal carcinoma.

Crohn's Appendicitis

- In 25% of patients with Crohn's ileocolitis, the appendix may be involved, with appendicitis being the initial manifestation of this disease.

Mucocele

- A mucocele is a rare lesion.
- If the patient is symptomatic, he or she may experience vague abdominal distress, acute or chronic pain, and intermittent colicky pain caused by intussusception of mucocele into the cecum.
- In addition, the patient may have chronic or acute RLQ pain.
- An ultrasound study will show a cystic mass or well-defined hypoechoic mass with an echogenic solid area in the RLQ; the mass may contain septations and may be echogenic; calcification may be indicated if the walls of the mass are echogenic.

Appendiceal Tumors

- Primary adenocarcinomas of the appendix are rare.
- A primary adenocarcinoma may manifest as acute appendicitis with perforation.

Colonic Abnormalities

Imperforate Anus

- If the pouch of the anus is less than 1.5 cm from the perineum, it is consistent with a low lesion that can be passed through the puborectalis portion of the levator sling.
- If pouch terminates above the base of bladder, it is indicative of a high lesion.

Necrotizing Enterocolitis

- An inflammatory process of the bowel is sometimes seen in newborns and premature infants and is characterized by clinical findings of gastric retention, bilious vomiting, abdominal distension, bloody stools, diarrhea, and erythema of the abdominal wall.
- Complications include bowel perforation.
- On ultrasound examination, necrotizing enterocolitis appears as a tubular structure with a well-defined wall seen across the left upper abdomen and in the left flank.
- In addition, the bowel wall is thickened, and there is portal venous gas.
- Stenosis and acquired atresia are present in both the large and small bowel. Malabsorption, formation of enterocysts, pneumoperitoneum, and abscess are also present.

Diverticular Disease

- Ultrasound findings of diverticular disease include the following:
  1. Focal gut wall thickening (greater than 4 mm with a range of 5 to 15 mm)
  2. Inflamed diverticula with echogenic shadowing foci seen in outpouches of the thickened colon wall or beyond the pericolonic soft tissues
  3. Inflammatory changes in pericolic fat
  4. Intramural or pericoloic inflammatory mass with the presence of fluid or air in a mass or abscess
  5. Intramural fistulae

Review Exercise • Gastrointestinal Tract

1. Describe the technique used to image the gastrointestinal tract. _____
_____
_____

2. What should the sonographer do to define a cystic mass in the left upper quadrant? _____
_____
_____
_____

3. How is the duodenum best imaged on ultrasound? _____
_____
_____
_____
_____

4. Describe the ultrasound technique used to image the small bowel. _____
_____
_____
_____

5. Describe the sonographic technique used to image the appendix. _____
_____
_____
_____

6. What is the ultrasound technique used to define the colon? _____
_____
_____

7. Describe the "bull's eye" or target sign seen on the sagittal scan of the abdomen. _____
_____
_____

8. Describe the ultrasound technique used to determine gastroesophageal reflux. _____
_____
_____
_____

9. What are causes of dilation of the stomach? _____
_____
_____
_____

10. What is Bouveret syndrome? _____

_____

_____

11. Discuss the duplication cyst and its differential diagnosis. _____

_____

_____

12. Discuss hypertrophic pyloric stenosis and the sonographic findings. _____

_____

_____

_____

13. What is the sonographic appearance of a gastric phytobezoar? _____

_____

_____

14. Describe the sonographic appearance of a polyp in the stomach. _____

_____

_____

15. Name the most common tumor of the stomach and describe its ultrasound appearance. _____

_____

_____

16. What is the ultrasound appearance of gastric carcinoma? _____

_____

_____

_____

17. What is the most common cause of GI obstruction in children? _____

_____

_____

18. Describe the anomaly that can be confused with appendicitis. _____

_____

_____

_____

19. Describe the mesentery anatomy and abnormalities. _____

_____

_____

_____

20. Describe the sonographic appearances of the following appendiceal abnormalities?
Appendicitis: _____

_____

_____

_____

Perforation with acute appendicitis/abscess: _____

_____

_____

_____

Postappendectomy fluid collections: _____

_____

_____

_____

Crohn's appendicitis: _____

_____

_____

_____

Self-Test • Gastrointestinal Tract Examination

1. The stomach may be described as a " _____ "-shaped structure with two openings, _____

    and _____ ; two curvatures, _____ and _____ ;

    and two surfaces, _____ and _____ .

2. The stomach is divided into:

    a.

    b.

    c.

    d.

3. Most of the digestion and absorption of food takes place in the _____ .

4. What are the three parts of the above structure?

    _____ _____ _____

5. The duodenum may be considered a peritoneal and retroperitoneal structure (true or false).

6. The duodenum is divided into four parts (1, 2, 3, 4). Place the part of the duodenum that corresponds to the anatomy described below.

    a. _____ runs anterior to the left kidney.

    b. _____ related to the quadrate lobe of the liver and gallbladder.

    c. _____ runs upward and to then left, then forward at the duojejunal junction.

    d. _____ related to the CBD, portal vein, IVC.

    e. _____ follows the inferior margin of the pancreatic head.

    f. _____ related to the fundus of the gallbladder.

7. The upper half of the duodenum is supplied by the _____ .

8. What characteristics of the GI tract are used to help identify it from other abdominal structures?

    a. gas or air accompanied by a shadow

    b. mucus pattern shows echogenicity without a shadow

    c. increased thickness of the wall may indicate an abnormality

    d. fluid within the GI tract shows as hypoechoic, with speckled echoes moving slowly within

9. The structure often seen on a sagittal ultrasound to the left of the midline as a "bulls-eye" or target pattern anterior to the aorta and posterior to the left lobe of the liver is the:

    a. pancreatic duct

    b. common bile duct

    c. ligamentum teres

    d. esophagogastric junction

10. Gastric dilation may be caused by all of the following except:

    a. amyloidoisis   c. extrinsic tumor

    b. cholelithiasis   d. pylorospasm

11. Hypertrophic pyloric stenosis is more commonly found in males than in females (true or false).

12. Characteristics of pyloric stenosis include all of the following except:

    a. hypertrophy of the circular muscle

    b. hypoplasia of the circular muscle

    c. projectile vomiting in second or third week of life

    d. hyperplasia of the circular muscle

13. Which of the following statements are true regarding gastric carcinoma?

    a. _____ Ninety percent of malignant tumors of the stomach are lymphomas.

    b. _____ Ninety percent of malignant tumors of the stomach are carcinomas.

    c. _____ One half of these tumors occur in the pylorus.

    d. _____ One fourth of the tumors occur in the pylorus.

    e. _____ One fourth of the tumors occur in the body and fundus.

    f. _____ Clinical signs are nonspecific.

14. The characteristic signs of lymphoma of the stomach are all of the following except:

    a. relatively large and highly echogenic

    b. relatively large and hypoechoic

    c. marked thickening of the gastric walls

    d. spoke wheel pattern

15. Small bowel obstruction is associated with dilation of the bowel loops distal to the site of obstruction (true or false).

16. The most common cause of obstruction in children is:

    a. duplication cysts

    b. choledochal cyst

    c. lymphoma

    d. intussusception

17. The most common tumor of the GI tract in children under ten years of age is:

    a. lymphoma

    b. carcinoma

    c. Hodgkin's leukemia

    d. Wilms' tumor

18. Acute appendicitis may be seen on ultrasound examination as a:

    a. hypoechoic mass with good transmission

    b. hyperechoic mass with fair transmission

    c. target lesion

    d. hyperechoic mass with good transmission

19. The most common causes of a mucocele of the appendix include all except:

    a. postappendiceal scarring   c. cecal carcinoma

    b. fecalith   d. appendicitis

20. Lymphoma and metastatic disease to the colon are uncommon (true or false).

Case Reviews

1. Figure 7-2 is a transverse scan of the upper abdomen. Name the anatomy as labeled.

a.   c.   e.

b.   d.

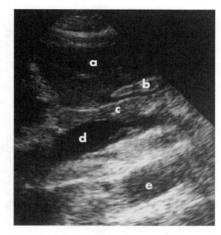

2. Figure 7-3 is a transverse scan of the upper abdomen. Name the anatomy as labeled.

a.   e.   i.

b.   f.   j.

c.   g.   k.

d.   h.

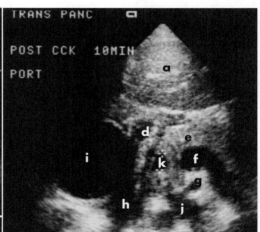

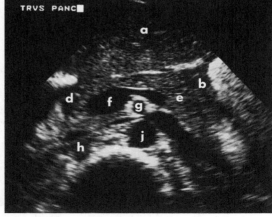

3. Figure 7-4 is a sagittal scan of the upper abdomen slightly to the left of the midline. Name the anatomy as labeled.

a.   c.   e.

b.   d.

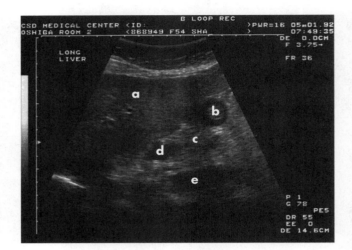

4. Figure 7-5 is a sagittal scan of the left abdomen. A large hypoechoic structure is shown. Describe your findings.

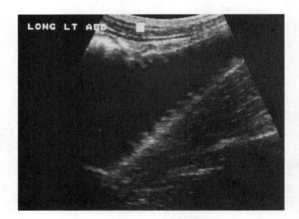

5. A young patient presents with RUQ pain and nausea. Describe the fluid collections seen in the upper abdomen (Figure 7-6).

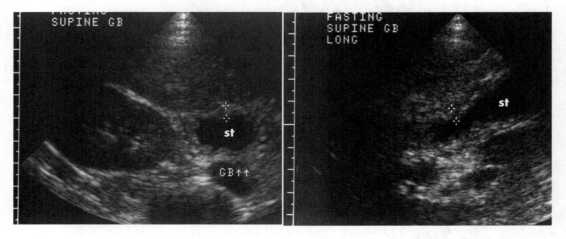

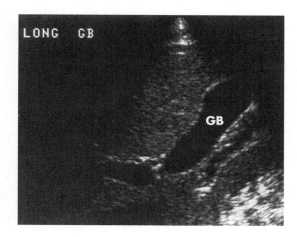

6. A 17-year-old male with cystic fibrosis with meconium ileus equivalent was sent to have an ultrasound examination to rule out abscess. What is your evaluation (Figure 7-7)?

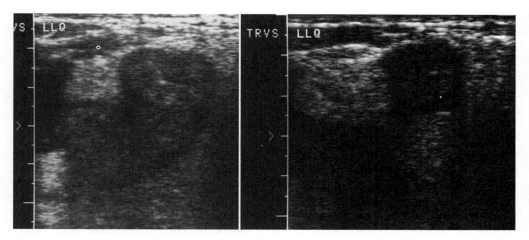

7. A young female arrived at the hospital with severe RLQ cramping pain. Her icon test was negative, and her last menstrual period was three weeks earlier. Blood tests showed an elevated white count. What is your evaluation (Figure 7-8)?

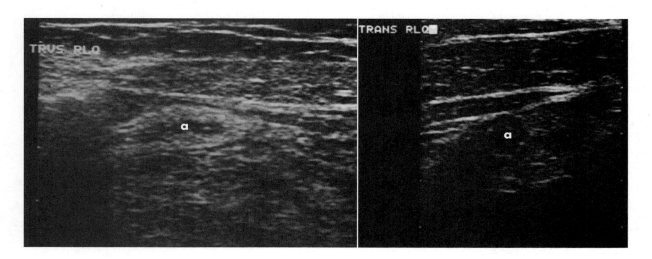

Answers to Review Exercise

1. **Upper GI tract:** The patient drinks 10 to 40 ounces of water through a straw to eliminate air bubbles. **Lower GI tract:** Usually no preparation is needed; however, if needed, the patient may have a water enema to delineate the colon.

2. To define a cystic mass in the LUQ, the sonographer should define if the mass is a fluid-filled stomach or other mass. He/she may give the patient a carbonated drink to see bubbles in stomach. An NG tube should be inserted for drainage of the stomach. The stomach will change in shape or size with fluids. The patient should be scanned in an upright or decubitus position. The sonographer should watch for peristalsis.

3. The duodenum is best imaged on ultrasound with water ingestion to fill the duodenal bulb. The patient may change positions to help fill the duodenum.

4. The sonographer should look for peristalsis, air movement, or movement of intraluminal fluid contents. The normal small bowel wall is under 3 mm.

5. A high resolution, linear array transducer should be used to examine the right lower quadrant with an empty bladder. Gradual graded compression over the area of maximum tenderness is used to displace bowel, fat, and soft tissues to delineate the area of the appendix.

   The visualization of retrocecal and paracecal areas is improved with displacement of gas and other bowel loop contents out of the scan field.

   If the appendix is seen, it appears as a thin tubular structure, less than 6 mm in caliper, 8 mm to 10 cm long.

6. The colon is best imaged with the lukewarm water enema technique with the patient in the left lateral decubitus position. The patient should be scanned with a full bladder to help delineate anatomical structures. The water should follow the rectum and rectosigmoid colon. Normal wall thickness is 4 mm. The five layers of the colon should be defined: 1 and 2, mucosa; 3, submucosa; 4, mucularis propria; 5, serosa and subserous fatty tissue.

7. On sagittal scan, the esophagogastric (EG) junction will be seen to the left of the midline as a "bull's-eye" or target structure anterior to the aorta and posterior to the left lobe of the liver, next to the hemidiaphragm. The left lobe of the liver must be large enough to project anterior to the EG junction.

   The gastric antrum can be seen as a target in the midline also. The remainder of the stomach is usually not visualized unless it is dilated with fluid.

8. Reflux is more common in newborns than in adults. The patient is examined in the supine position 45 minutes after gavage feeding (cardiac suprasternal and right subclavicular).

   It is important to image the length of the esophagus between the diaphragm and larynx.

   Morphologic findings associated with significant reflux include a short intraabdominal part of the esophagus, a rounded gastroesophageal angle, and a "beak" at the EG junction.

   The ability of the diaphragmatic crura to hold the distal esophagus in place during esophageal hiatus prevents it from sliding upward.

9. A fluid-filled stomach may be caused by pylorospasm, inflammation, an intrinsic or extrinsic tumor, electrolyte imbalance, diabetes, amyloidosis, neurologic disease, or medication.

   On ultrasound examination, the stomach appears as a pear-shaped cystic structure in the left upper quadrant. It has a characteristic configuration: discrete thin walls, movement of strong echoes (food particles) when light pressure is applied, gas-fluid level, and compressibility.

10. Bouveret syndrome is a gastric outlet obstruction that is secondary to a gallstone impacted within the duodenal bulb. Stones larger than 2.5 cm may produce obstruction in the intestine, particularly in the distal ileum. An eroding stone will pass spontaneously in most cases.

    A gallstone in the duodenum may produce the double-arc sign on ultrasound examination. The duodenal wall produces the anterior arc, which is similar to what is commonly seen with gallbladder disease. The sonographer should also look for pneumobilia.

11. The duplication cysts are embrylogic mistakes; they cause symptoms depending on their size, location, and histology.

    The criteria for a duplication cyst is a cyst lined with alimentary tract epithelium, a well-developed muscular wall, and contiguity with the stomach.

    These cysts may arise from the pancreas or duodenum. They occur more often in females than in males. They usually occur on the greater curvature of the stomach.

    The patient may have symptoms of high intestinal obstruction—distention, vomiting, and abdominal pain; also possibly vomiting, hemorrhage, and fistula formation. The solid component is caused by hemorrhage and inspissated material within the cyst.

    Ultrasound findings: A duplication cyst appears anechoic with a thin inner echogenic rim (mucosa) and wider outer hypoechoic rim (muscle layer).

    Differential diagnosis: mesenteric or omental cyst, pancreatic cyst or pseudocyst, enteric cyst, renal cyst, splenic cyst, congenital cyst of LLL, or gastric distention.

12. Pyloric stenosis is familial with a 4:1 male/female ratio. There is an occurrence rate of 6% in children whose parents had hypertrophic pyloric stenosis. A mother with HPS has a 4 times greater chance of having affected offspring than a father with HPS.

    Symptoms of projectile vomiting occur in the second or third week of life. The child may have a palpable abdominal mass. Hypertrophy and hyperplasia of circular muscle results in elongation of the pylorus and constriction of the canal; this narrowing may lead to edema or inflammatory changes.

    Ultrasound findings include volumetric measurement of nasogastric aspirate, pyloric diameter, pyloric muscle thickness, pyloric length, cervix sign, or double track sign.

    Volumetric measurement: Patients with NG aspirate of 10 ml or greater should be referred for further ultrasound evaluation, while those with less should be referred for fluroscopy to determine the possibility of gastroesophageal reflux.

    Pyloric diameter: The target lesion associated with HPS is usually located by orienting the transducer in the sagittal plane. A measurement of 15 mm or more is abnormal for pyloric diameter; normal is less than 10 mm. A normal adult pylorus is 3.8 mm to 8.5 mm; abnormal is greater than 9 mm.

    Pyloric muscle thickness: The wall, or hypoechoic rim, of the target represents the hypertrophied muscle, which is greater than 4 mm thick. The HPS is greater than 5 mm on longitudinal view.

    Pyloric length of channel: The echogenic central line of mucosa indicates the pyloric length. The elongated pyloric channel is a mucosal double-track sign. Normal length is 18 mm; abnormal is 2.1 mm or more.

    Cervix sign: a hypertrophied muscle that has gone into the antrum.

    Double track sign: produced with fluid-aided real time ultrasonography; seen as a result of pyloric fluid compressed into smaller tracks as it is impinged circumferentially by thickened circular muscle.

    Antropyloric muscle thickness: measured in the mid-longitudinal plane of the fully distended, fluid-filled antrum. A normal measurement is 2 mm or less; abnormal is 3 mm or greater.

13. A gastric bezoar consists of movable, intraluminal masses of congealed ingested materials that are seen on the upper gastrointestinal exam. Clinically, patients have nausea, vomiting, and pain. The mass may simulate a tumor.

    Ultrasound findings include a complex mass with internal mobile echogenic components in a fasting patient; a broad band of high-amplitude echoes or hyperechoic curvilinear dense strip at anterior margin is seen superior, with a complete clean shadow posterior.

14. A polyp lesion is seen with fluid distension of the stomach; they may appear as solid masses adherent to the gastric wall. The polyp has variable echogenicity. A large polyp may be inhomogeneous; contours may be sharply or not sharply delineated, depending on the nature of the surface; detection of a pedicle may be possible.

15. A leiomyoma is the most common tumor of the stomach. It is seen as a small mass similar to carcinoma. The patient is often asymptomatic. The leiomyoma is often associated with other GI abnormalities, such as cholelithiasis, peptic ulcer disease, adenocarcinoma, and leiomyosarcoma.

    Ultrasound findings: A leiomyoma is seen as a hypoechoic mass continuous with the muscular layer of the stomach. It may be a circular or oval lesion with a homogeneous echopattern and hemispheric bulging into the lumen. Frequently, the lesion is separated from the lumen by two or three layers that are continuous with those of the normal wall. It may also appear as a solid mass with cystic areas that represent necrosis.

16. At least 90% to 95% of malignant tumors of the stomach are carcinomas. Gastric carcinoma is the sixth leading cause of death, occurring more often in older males. One half of the tumors occur in the pylorus, and one fourth in the body and fundus. The lesions may be fungating, ulcerated, diffuse, polypoid, or superficial.

    Ultrasound findings include a target or pseudokidney sign, and possibly gastric wall thickening.

17. Intussusception is the most common cause of obstruction in children. When located in the colon, 50% of these obstructions are malignant, whereas most lesions in the small bowel are benign. Patients affected are most often children between 6 months and 2 years of age. In adults intussusception is chronic, and the patients experience minimal pain, diarrhea, and vomiting.

    Ultrasound findings include a target sign, bull's eye, doughnut or pseudokidney; or it may appear as a concentric ring sign, with a highly reflective intussusceptum and an unstructured pattern corresponding to a solid tumor.

18. Meckel's diverticulum is present in 2% of the population. In adults the disease may cause intestinal obstruction, rectal bleeding, or diverticular inflammation.

    Acute appendicitus and acute Meckel's diverticulum may not be distinguished clinically.

    The wall of Meckel's diverticulum is composed of mucosal, muscular, and serosal layers. The noncompressibility of the obstructed inflamed diverticulum indicates that the intraluminal fluid is trapped. The area of maximum tenderness is evaluated with its distance from the cecum.

19. The normal mesentery has an elongated shape, with an echogenic surface and small vessels in the center.

The small bowel mesentery is a fan-shaped structure that connects the convolutions of the jejunum and ileum to the posterior wall of the abdomen.

The mesentery consists of two layers of peritoneum containing blood vessels, nerves, lacteals, lymphatic glands, and a variable amount of fat. The mesentery is 0.5 cm to 1.0 cm thick, with a maximum breadth of 0.7 cm to 1.2 cm.

Abnormalities of the mesentery include: enlarged lymph nodes, lymphoma, and mesenteric desmoid tumors.

20. **Appendicitis:** Ultrasound findings include a typical target lesion in RLQ, thickening of the bowel wall as a result of edema and an echogenic core as a result of necrotic appendix or appendiceal lumen, noncompressable mass, fluid or abscess collection. Appendiceal diameter is greater than 6 mm, muscular wall thickness is greater than 3 mm, and there is visualization of a complex mass.

Perforation with acute appendicitis/abscess: Ultrasound findings include loculated pericecal fluid, prominent pericecal fat, and circumferential loss of the submucosal layer of the appendix

Postappendectomy fluid collections: Ultrasound findings: on ultrasound examination, the sonographer must be able to distinguish between the colon and fluid collection

Crohn's appendicitis: Patient presents with clinical signs of acute appendicitis. Cannot differentiate Crohn's appendicitis from acute appendicitis.

Answers to Self-Test

1. J; cardiac and pyloric; lesser and greater; anterior and posterior
2. a. fundus
   b. body
   c. pyloric antrum
   d. pyloris
3. small intestine
4. duodenum
   jejunum
   ileum
5. true
6. a. 2
   b. 1
   c. 4
   d. 1
   e. 3
   f. 2
7. pancreatic artery
8.
9. d
10. b
11. true
12. b
13. b, c, e, f
14. a
15. false
16. d
17. a
18. c
19. d
20. true

Answers to Case Reviews

1. (Figure 7-2)
   a. left lobe of the liver
   b. transverse view of the collapsed gastric antrum
   c. body of the pancreas
   d. confluence of splenic and portal veins
   e. aorta
2. (Figure 7-3)
   a. left lobe of the liver
   b. transverse views of the fluid-filled stomach
   c. fluid-filled first part of the duodenum as it outlines the body and head of the pancreas
   d. second part of the duodenum
   e. body of the pancreas
   f. splenic vein
   g. superior mesenteric artery
   h. third part of the duodenum
   i. gallbladder
   j. aorta
   k. common bile duct
3. (Figure 7-4)
   a. left lobe of the liver
   b. longitudinal scan of the typical bulls-eye appearance of the transverse colon
   c. body of the pancreas
   d. superior mesenteric vein
   e. abdominal aorta
4. (Figure 7-5) This is a sagittal scan of a fluid-filled loop of colon. The tiny cilla may be seen to move on the real-time ultrasound examination.
5. (Figure 7-6) The collection anterior to the gallbladder was originally thought to be a thick-walled gallbladder. However, with real-time observation and fluid ingestion, the stomach was filled and clearly separate from the gallbladder.
6. (Figure 7-7) A large, hyperechoic structure is seen just to the left of the umbilicus in the region of the palpable abnormality. This represents a bowel loop with inspissated stool.
7. (Figure 7-8) Complete scans of the right lower quadrant and pelvic area should be made for diagnostic evaluation. Ask the patient specifically where the pain is before starting the exam. In this case, the pelvic ultrasound was normal. However, longitudinal and transverse scans show the thick-walled appendix that does not collapse with compression. At surgery, an inflamed appendix was removed.

CHAPTER
8
The Urinary System

OBJECTIVES

At the completion of this chapter, students will show orally, in writing, or by demonstration that they will be able to:

1. Describe the various positions and the sizes of the normal kidneys and adrenal glands.
2. Define the internal, surface, and relational anatomies of the renal and adrenal glands.
3. Illustrate the cross-sectional anatomies of the renal and adrenal glands and adjacent structures.
4. Describe the congenital anomalies affecting the renal glands.
5. Explain the function of the kidneys.
6. Select pertinent laboratory tests and other diagnostic tests for renal evaluation.
7. Explain the function of each laboratory and diagnostic test for renal evaluation.
8. Differentiate among sonographic appearances of each of the following diseases by explaining the clinical significance of masses that affect the kidney:
   a. sinus lipomatosis
   b. obstruction
   c. cystic disease of the kidneys
   d. medullary cystic disease
   e. hematoma
   f. renal cell carcinoma
   g. metastasis
   h. infection
   i. Wilms' tumor
   j. angiomyolipoma
   k. infarct
   l. trauma
   m. sarcoma
   n. lymphoma
9. Create high-quality diagnostic scans demonstrating the appropriate anatomy in all planes pertinent to the pancreas.
10. Select the correct equipment settings appropriate to individual body habitus.
11. Distinguish between the normal and abnormal sonographic appearances of the kidneys.

To further enhance learning, students should use marking pens to color the anatomic illustrations that follow.

FIGURE 8-1
Anterior Relationships of the Kidneys
(Stomach and Liver Removed)

Kidneys

The kidneys lie on the psoas and quadratus lumborum muscles in the retroperitoneal space under cover of the costal margin. The right kidney lies slightly lower than the left because of the right lobe of the liver. The left kidney contacts the spleen, pancreas, colon, and jejunum, and the superiomedial pole holds the adrenal gland. The right kidney contacts the liver, colon, and adrenal gland (Figure 8-1).

The kidneys are protected posteriorly by the eleventh and twelfth ribs. The inferior poles are not well protected except for that protection provided by the quadratus lumborum muscle. On the medial surface of the kidney are the hilum, the point of exit of the renal vein, and the point of entrance of the renal artery (Figure 8-2). The renal pelvis is also at the hilum and forms the ureter, which narrows to run posteriorly into the bladder.

The kidneys are approximately 12 cm long, 2.5 cm to 3 cm thick, and 4 cm to 5 cm wide.

The kidney is surrounded by a fibrous capsule, called the true capsule, which is closely applied to the renal cortex (Figure 8-3). Outside this capsule is a covering of perinephric fat. The perinephric fascia surrounds the perinephric fat and encloses the kidney and adrenal glands. The renal fascia (Gerota's fascia) surrounds the true capsule and the perinephric fat.

The ureter is 25 cm long and resembles the esophagus in that it has three constrictions along its course: (1) where it joins the kidney; (2) where it is kinked as it crosses the pelvic brim; and (3) where it pierces the bladder wall. The pelvis of the ureter is funnel-shaped at its upper end. It lies within the hilum of the kidney and receives the major calyces. The ureter emerges from the hilum and runs down-

ward along the psoas, which separates it from the tips of the transverse processes of the lumbar vertebrae. It enters the pelvis by crossing the bifurcation of the common iliac artery in front of the sacroiliac joint. It then runs along the lateral wall of the pelvis to the region of the ischial spine and turns forward to enter the lateral angle of the bladder.

On the medial border of each kidney is the renal hilum, which contains the renal vein, two branches of the renal artery, the ureter, and the third branch of the renal artery.

The kidney is composed of an internal medullary portion and an external cortical substance. The medullary substance consists of a series of 8 to 18 striated conical masses, called the renal pyramids. Their bases are directed toward the outer circumference of the kidney. Their apices converge toward the renal sinus, where their prominent papillae project into the lumina of the minor calyces.

Within the kidney's upper, expanded end (or pelvis), the ureter divides into two or three major calyces, each of which divides into two or three minor calyces. The 4 to 13 minor calyces are cup-shaped tubes that usually come into contact with at least one renal papilla. The minor calyces unite to form two or three short tubes, the major calyces; these, in turn, unite to form a funnel-shaped sac, the renal pelvis. Spirally arranged muscles surround the calyces and may exert a milking action on these tubes, aiding in the flow of urine into the renal pelvis. As the renal pelvis leaves the renal sinus, it rapidly becomes smaller and ultimately merges with the ureter.

The kidney is supplied with blood by the renal arteries. The arteries divide into two primary branches, a larger anterior branch and a posterior branch. The arteries finally break down into minute arterioles and are called interlobar arteries. In the portion of the kidney between the cortex and medulla, these arteries are called arcuate arteries.

The renal veins also break down into these categories. Five or six veins join to form the renal vein, which merges from the hilum anterior to the renal artery. The renal vein drains into the inferior vena cava. Further breakdown of the veins and arteries leads to the afferent and efferent glomerular vessels.

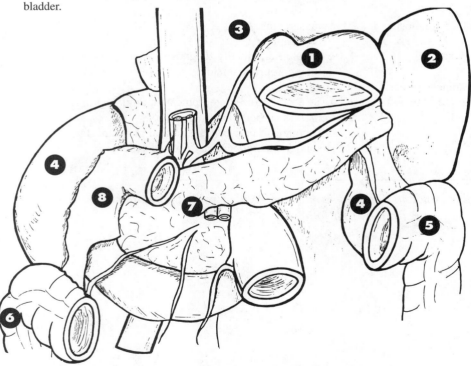

1	stomach	5	descending colon
2	spleen	6	ascending colon
3	diaphragm	7	pancreas
4	kidney	8	duodenum

FIGURE 8-2
Kidneys, Adrenal Glands, and Their Vascular Relationships

Adrenal Glands

The adrenal glands are retroperitoneal organs that lie on the upper pole of each kidney. They are surrounded by perinephric fascia and are separated from the kidneys by perinephric fat. Each gland has a cortex and a medulla.

The right adrenal gland is triangular or pyramidal and caps the upper pole of the right kidney. It lies posterior to the right lobe of the liver, extends medially behind the inferior vena cava, and rests posteriorly on the diaphragm.

The left adrenal gland is semilunar and extends along the medial border of the left kidney (from the upper pole to the hilum). The left adrenal gland lies posterior to the pancreas, the lesser sac, and the stomach, and rests posteriorly on the diaphragm.

There are three arteries supplying each gland: the suprarenal branch of the inferior phrenic artery, the suprarenal branch of the aorta, and the suprarenal branch of the renal artery. A single vein arises from the hilum of each gland and drains into the inferior vena cava on the right and into the renal vein on the left.

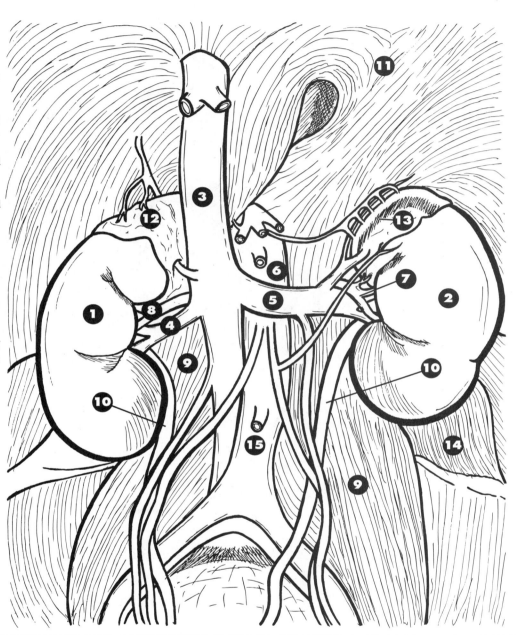

1	**right kidney**	**6**	**aorta**	**11**	**diaphragm**
2	**left kidney**	**7**	**left renal artery**	**12**	**right adrenal gland**
3	**inferior vena cava**	**8**	**right renal artery**	**13**	**left adrenal gland**
4	**right renal vein**	**9**	**psoas muscle**	**14**	**quadratus lumborum muscle**
5	**left renal vein**	**10**	**ureter**	**15**	**aorta**

FIGURE 8-3
Kidney

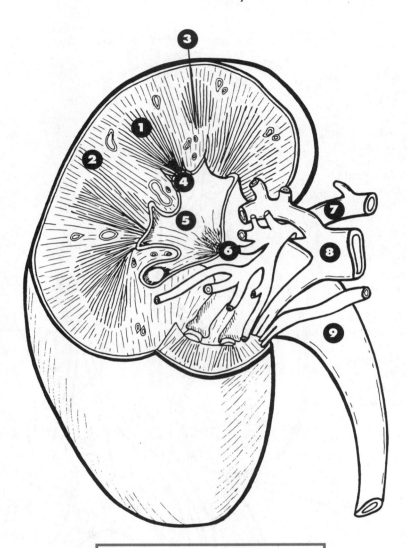

1	renal medulla (pyramid)
2	renal cortex
3	renal papilla
4	minor calyx
5	major calyx
6	renal pelvis
7	renal artery
8	renal vein
9	ureter

Urinary System Review Notes

EXCRETION

- The active life of cells is accompanied by production of waste materials.
- Waste products must be removed quickly.
- Some end products may accumulate and disturb the sequence of essential reactions if they are not removed.
- The process of excretion consists of separation and removal of substances that are harmful to the body.
- Excretion is carried out by the skin, the lungs, the liver, the large intestine, and the kidneys.
- There are two principal functions of the urinary system:
  - Excretion of wastes
  - Regulation of the composition of blood
- Blood composition must not be allowed to vary beyond tolerable limits, or the conditions in tissues that are necessary for cellular life will be lost.
- Regulation of the composition of blood involves not only the removal of harmful waste products but also the conservation of water and metabolites in the body.
- The urinary system consists of the following organs:
  - two large kidneys that secrete urine
  - ureters (ducts leading from the kidneys)
  - bladder (urinary reservoir)
  - urethra (tube from the bladder to the surface of the body)

NORMAL ANATOMY
The Kidneys

- Retroperitoneal location.
- The right kidney is slightly lower than the left because of the liver.
- With respiration, both kidneys move downward approximately 1 inch.
- On the medial surface of each kidney is a vertical slit called the *hilus.*
- The hilus transmits from the front to the back via the following organs:
  1. the renal vein
  2. two branches of the renal artery
  3. ureter
  4. third branch of renal artery
  5. lymph vessels and sympathetic fibers
- The hilus is surrounded by a fibrous capsule that is closely applied to the cortex.
- Outside of the fibrous capsule is a covering of perinephric fat.
- Perinephric fascia surrounds the perinephric fat.
- Within the kidney, the upper expanded end of the ureter, which is the pelvis of the ureter, divides into two or three major calices, each of which divides into two or three minor calices.
- Each minor calyx is indented by the apex of a medullary pyramid called the renal papilla.

- Arterial supply is via the renal artery, which is a branch of the aorta.
- Each artery divides into three branches to enter the hilus of the kidney (two in front and one behind the pelvis of the ureter).
- Five or six veins join to form the renal vein, which emerges from the hilus in front of the renal artery.
- The renal vein drains into the IVC.
- The lymph vessels follow the renal artery to the lateral aortic lymph nodes around the origin of the renal artery.
- Nerves originate in the renal sympathetic plexus and are distributed along the branches of the renal vessels.
- Each kidney is a dark red, bean-shaped organ. Each measures approximately 12 cm long, 5 cm wide, and 2.5 cm thick.
- The inner surface of the medulla is folded into projections, the pyramids, which empty their contents into the collecting space called the *renal pelvis.*
- Numerous collecting tubules bring the urine from its sites of formation in the cortex to the pyramids, where it is discharged into the pelvis. The ureter is an extension of the funnel-shaped pelvis.
- The renal tubules, or nephrons, are the functional units of the kidney. Man has more than one million nephrons.
- Each nephron tubule is approximately 12 mm long, and it has thin walls that are made up of epithelial cells.
- The nephron is open at one end, where it connects with a collecting tubule; at the closed end, the wall forms a cup-shaped concavity known as Bowman's capsule.
- The capsule drains into the proximal convoluted tubule, which is followed by a straighter portion called Henle's loop.
- Henle's loop enters the medulla of the kidney and continues as the distal convoluted tubule, which joins other similar tubules to form the collecting tubes.
- Blood supply to nephrons begins at the renal artery.
- The artery subdivides within the kidneys, and a small vessel, the afferent arteriole, enters Bowman's capsule, where it forms a tuft of capillaries, the glomerulus, which entirely fills the concavity of the capsule.
- Blood leaves the glomerulus via the afferent arteriole, which subdivides into a network of capillaries that surround the proximal and distal tubules and eventually unite as veins that become the renal vein.
- The renal vein returns the cleansed blood to the general circulation.
- By movements of substances between the nephron and the capillaries of the tubules, the composition of the blood filtrate that moves along in the tubules is changed.
- From the nephrons, the fluid moves to collecting tubules and into the ureter, which leads to the bladder, where urine is stored.

Ureter

- The ureter is approximately 10″ long.
- The ureter has three constrictions, which are in the following locations:
  1. the point at which the pelvis of the ureter joins the ureter
  2. the point at which the ureter is kinked as it crosses the pelvic brim
  3. the point at which the ureter pierces the bladder wall
- The pelvis is the funnel-shaped, expanded upper end of the ureter. It lies within the hilus of the kidney and receives the major calices.
- The ureter emerges from the hilus of the kidney and runs vertically downward behind the parietal peritoneum on the psoas muscle, which separates it from the tips of the transverse processes of the lumbar vertebrae.
- The ureter enters the pelvis by crossing the bifurcation of the common iliac artery in front of the sacroiliac joint.
- The ureter runs down the lateral wall of the pelvis to the region of the ischial spine and turns forward to enter the lateral angle of the bladder.
- The arterial supply to the ureter is from the:
  - renal artery
  - testicular or ovarian artery
  - superior vesical artery

The Urinary Bladder

- The urinary bladder is a large, muscular bag.
- The bladder has three openings: two that are posterior and lateral for the ureters, and one that is anterior for the urethra.
- The interior of the bladder is lined with highly elastic transitional epithelium.
- When the organ is full, the lining is smooth and stretched; when it is empty, the lining is a series of folds.
- In the middle layer of the bladder a series of smooth muscles distends as urine collects, and the muscles contract to expel urine through the urethra.
- Urine is produced almost continuously and accumulates in the bladder until the increased pressure stimulates the organ's nervous receptors.

The Urethra

- The urethra is a membranous tube that passes from the anterior part of the urinary bladder to the outside of the body.
- The urethra contains two sphincters:
  1. internal sphincter
  2. external sphincter

Terms and Definitions That Are Related to the Urethra and Its Functions

- Stricture: closure of the urethra
- Urethritis: inflammation of the mucous membrane in the urethra
- Dysuria: difficult urination
- Cystitis: inflammation of the bladder
- Cystostomy: open-bladder surgery
- Cystectomy: removal of the bladder

Normal Renal Parenchyma

- A scan with the patient in the supine position will show three distinct segments of the kidney:
  1. poorly echoic medullary zone, which consists of numerous anechoic, triangle-shaped renal pyramids
  2. moderately echogenic renal cortex
  3. highly reflective central renal sinus
- The renal capsule and perinephric fat have a distinct layer of very reflective echoes that distinguish a normal right kidney from the liver, or the left kidney from the spleen.
- The thickness of this very reflective echogenic zone varies in relation to the amount of perinephric fat deposited around the kidney.

Renal Vessels

- The renal arteries are located posterolateral from the aorta, and are easiest to see when the patient is supine or in the LLD position.
- The right renal artery (RRA) extends from the posterolateral aorta to the central renal sinus. (On longitudinal scan, the RRA can be seen as a circular structure posterior to the IVC).
- The right renal vein (RRV) extends from the central renal sinus to the IVC.
- Both the RRA and the RRV appear as tubular structures in the transverse plane.
- Renal arteries have an echo-free central lumen with highly echogenic borders that consist of the vessel wall and surrounding retroperitoneal fat and connective tissue.
- Renal arteries lie posterior to the veins and can be seen with certainty if their junction with the aorta is seen.
- The left renal vein (LRV) flows from the central renal sinus, anterior to the aorta, posterior to the SMA to join the IVC. (The LRV is a tubular structure on transverse scan). "Nutcracker" phenomena is when the structure consists of the AO to LRV to SMA.
- The left renal artery (LRA) flows from the central renal sinus directly to the posterolateral border of the aorta.
- **Note:** The diaphragmatic crura run transversely in the paraaortic region.
- The diaphragmatic crura lie posterior to the renal arteries and should be identified by their lack of pulsations and no Doppler flow.
- The crura vary in echogenicity, depending on the amount of surrounding retroperitoneal fat. They may appear hypoechoic, like lymph nodes.

Renal Medulla

- The renal medulla consists of hypoechoic pyramids in a uniform distribution that are separated by bands of intervening parenchyma that extend toward the renal sinus.
- The pyramids are uniform in size, triangular shape, and distribution.
- The apex of the pyramid points toward the sinus, and the base lies adjacent to the renal cortex.
- The arcuate vessels lie at the base of the pyramids.
- The pyramids are located at the junction between the more-peripheral renal cortex and the central sinus.

Bertin's Columns

- Bertin's columns are prominent invaginations of the cortex located at varying depths within the medullary substance of the kidneys.
- These invaginated areas constitute normal cortex. The column may be the fusion of two septa into a single column that is twice the normal thickness.
- The columns are most exaggerated in patients with complete or partial duplication of renal sinus.
- Sonographic features of a renal mass effect produced by hypertrophied columns are as follows:
  - lateral indentation of the renal sinus
  - clear definition from the renal sinus
  - maximum dimension that does not exceed 3 cm
  - contiguity with the renal cortex
  - overall echogenicity similar to the renal parenchyma
  - "split-sinus" sign
  - lack of contour change on renal surface

CONGENITAL ANOMALIES
Dromedary Hump

- The dromedary hump is a cortical bulge that occurs on the lateral border of the kidney, typically more on the left. In some patients it may be so prominent that it looks like a neoplasm.
- The dromedary hump is likely the result of pressure by the spleen on the developing fetal kidney.
- Echogenicity is identical to the rest of the renal cortex.

Junctional Parenchymal Defect

- A junctional parenchymal defect is a triangular echogenic area in the upper pole of the renal parenchyma that can be seen during normal ultrasound scanning.
- The defect results from the normal extensions of the renal sinus in cases where there is distinct division between the upper and lower poles of the kidney.
- The kidneys develop from the fusion of two embryonic parenchymatous masses referred to as renunculi.
- In cases of partial fusion, parenchymal defects occur at the junction of the renunculi and are best demonstrated on sagittal scans.

Duplex Collecting System

- The duplex collecting system is a common normal variant that can be seen on ultrasound examination.
- It may be difficult for the sonographer to tell if the duplex collecting system is complete or incomplete because it is difficult to see the ureters well.
- The duplex kidney is usually enlarged and has smooth margins.
- The central renal sinus appears as two echogenic regions separated by a cleft of moderately echogenic tissue similar in appearance to the normal renal parenchyma.
- The pelvis of the lower pole is usually larger than the upper pole.

Sinus Lipomatosis

- Sinus lipomatosis is a condition that is characterized by the deposition of a moderate amount of fat in the renal sinus.
- The degree of proliferation of fibrofatty tissue varies.
- The renal sinus is composed of fibrous tissue, fat, lymphatic vessels, and renal vascular structures.
- On normal kidneys, this central zone appears as a bright area.
- In sinus lipomatosis, the abundant fibrous tissue may cause enlargement of the sinus region and increased echogenicity.

Extrarenal Pelvis

- The normal renal pelvis is a triangular-shaped structure.
- Its axis points inferiorly and medially.
- An intrarenal pelvis lies almost completely within the confines of the central renal sinus.
- This is usually small and foreshortened.
- The extrarenal pelvis tends to be larger, with long, major calices.
- On sonography the renal pelvis appears as a central cystic area that is either partially or entirely beyond the confines of the bulk of the renal substance.
- Transverse views are best to see continuity with the renal sinus.

RENAL ANOMALIES

- Renal anomalies are classified as abnormalities in number, size, position, structure, or form.
- Anomalies in number include agenesis or dysgenesis and supernumerary kidneys.
  - Agenesis: the absence or failure of formation
  - dysgenesis: defective embryonic development
  - supernumerary: exceeding the normal number

Solitary Kidney

- A solitary kidney is rare and results from unilateral renal agenesis.

- The sonographer must look for a small, nonfunctioning kidney before making a diagnosis of solitary kidney.
- Renal enlargement occurs with solitary kidney.

Pelvic Kidney

- If the kidney is not seen in the normal position in the renal fossa, the retroperitoneum and pelvis should be scanned.
- Most true ectopic kidneys are located in the bony pelvis and may be malrotated.
- A pelvic kidney may simulate a solid adnexal mass.
- A pelvic kidney may be associated with other abnormalities, such as vesicoureteral reflux and anomalous extrarenal pelvis.

Horseshoe Kidney

- Fusion anomalies of the kidneys include crossed renal ectopia, and a horseshoe kidney, which is the most common fusion anomaly.
- In a patient with a horseshoe kidney, there is fusion of the polar regions of the kidneys. Almost invariably, the lower poles are involved.
- This condition is usually associated with improper ascent and malrotation of the kidneys, usually in a lower retroperitoneal position. The renal pelves and ureters are more ventrally located.
- These kidneys usually lie closer to the spine than normal kidneys.
- The inferior poles lie more medially.
- The isthmus of the horseshoe kidney lies anterior to the spine and may simulate a solid pelvic mass.
- Pathologic conditions associated with this are pyelocaliectasis, anomalous extrarenal pelvis, and urinary calculi.

LABORATORY TESTS FOR RENAL DISEASE

Clinical Signs and Symptoms A patient with renal infection or disease process may experience any of the following symptoms: flank pain, hematuria, polyuria, oliguria, fever, urgency, or generalized edema.

Urinalysis

- A urinalysis is essential for the detection of urinary tract disorders in patients whose renal function is impaired or absent.
- The presence of an acute infection will cause hematuria, or red blood cells in the urine. Pyuria is pus in the urine.

Urine pH

- The abundance of hydrogen ions in a solution is called pH.
- pH refers to the strength of the urine as a partly acidic or alkaline solution.

- If urine contains an increased concentration of hydrogen ions, the urine is an acidic solution.
- pH is important in managing such diseases as bacteriuria and renal calculi.
- The formation of renal calculi partly depends on the pH of urine.
- Other conditions such as renal tubular acidosis and chronic renal failure are also associated with alkaline urine.

Specific Gravity

- The specific gravity is the measurement of the kidney's ability to concentrate urine.
- The concentration factor depends on the amount of dissolved waste products within it.
- An excessive intake of fluids or a decrease in perspiration may cause a large output of urine and a decrease in the specific gravity.
- A low fluid intake, excessive perspiration, or diarrhea will cause the output of urine to be low and the specific gravity to increase.
- The specific gravity is especially low in cases of renal failure, glomerular nephritis, and pyelonephritis.
- These diseases cause renal tubular damage, which affects the ability of the kidneys to concentrate urine.

Blood

- Hematuria is the appearance of red blood cells in the urine and may indicate early renal disease.
- An abundance of red blood cells in the urine may be suggestive of renal trauma, calculi, or pyelonephritis; or it may suggest glomerular or vascular inflammatory processes such as acute glomerulonephritis and renal infarction.
- Leukocytes may be present whenever there is inflammation, infection, or tissue necrosis originating from anywhere in the urinary tract.

Hematocrit

- Hematocrit refers to the relative ratio of plasma to packed cell volume in the blood.
- A decreased hematocrit level occurs with acute hemorrhagic processes secondary to disease or blunt trauma.

Hemoglobin

- The presence of hemoglobin in urine occurs whenever there is extensive damage or destruction of the functioning erythrocytes.
- This condition is injurious to the kidney and can cause acute renal failure.

Protein

- When glomerular damage is evident, albumin and other plasma proteins may be filtered in excess, thereby allowing the overflow to enter the urine. This condition then lowers the blood serum albumin concentration.

- Albuminuria is commonly found in patients with benign and malignant neoplasms, calculi, chronic infection, and pyelonephritis.

Creatinine Clearance

- The combination of specific measurements of creatinine concentrations in urine and blood serum levels is considered an accurate index for determining the glomerular filtration rate.
- Creatinine is a by-product of muscle energy metabolism. It is normally produced at a constant rate as long as the body muscle mass remains relatively constant.
- Creatinine goes through complete glomerular filtration without normally being reabsorbed by the renal tubules.
- A decreased urinary creatinine clearance indicates renal dysfunction because the decrease prevents the normal excretion of creatinine.

Blood Urea Nitrogen

- The blood urea nitrogen (BUN) is the concentration of urea nitrogen in blood, which is the end product of cellular metabolism.
- Urea is formed in the liver and carried to the kidneys through the blood, to be excreted in urine.
- Impairment of renal function and increased protein catabolism will result in BUN elevation in relation to the degree of renal impairment and rate of urea nitrogen excreted by the kidneys.

Serum Creatinine

- Renal dysfunction will also result in serum creatinine elevation.
- Blood serum creatinine levels are said to be more specific and more sensitive in determining renal impairment than BUN.

SPECIFIC CLINICAL SIGNS AND SYMPTOMS OF RENAL DISEASES

Renal Cystic Disease

Inflammatory or Necrotic Cysts

- Clinical symptoms include the following:
  - Flank pain
  - Hematuria
  - Proteinuria
  - White blood cells in urine
  - Elevated protein

Renal Subcapsular Hematoma

- Clinical symptoms include hematuria, and a decrease in hematocrit.

Renal Inflammatory Processes

Abscess

- Clinical symptoms include the acute onset of physical symptoms of fever, and the patient may have a palpable mass.
- Elevated WBC count
- Elevated pyuria

Acute Focal Bacterial Nephritis

- Clinical symptoms include fever, flank pain, and pyuria.
- An increase in BUN, albumin, and total plasma proteins are other symptoms.

Acute Tubular Necrosis

- Clinical symptoms (if caused by renal calculi) include: moderate to severe intermittent flank pain, vomiting, hematuria, infection, and leukocytosis with infection.

Chronic Renal Failure

- Increased concentration of urea in blood
- High urine protein excretion
- High BUN
- Increased creatinine
- Presence of granulocytes

Renal Cell Carcinoma

- Erythrocytosis may occur
- Leukocytosis
- Red blood cells in urine
- Pyuria
- Elevated LDH

RENAL NEOPLASM
Renal Cell Carcinoma

- Renal cell carcinoma comprises 85% of all kidney tumors.
- The frequency of occurrence in males is two times that of females, with peak incidence in the 70-year age range.
- With renal cell carcinoma, there is usually a solid parenchymal mass, frequently with areas of hemorrhage and necrosis.
- Occasionally, a renal cell tumor is predominately cystic.
- Irregular tumor calcification can be seen in 20% to 30% of these tumors.
- There is an increased frequency of dystrophic, irregular calcification inside the tumor. Ninety percent of all masses with nonperipheral calcification are carcinomas.
- There is an increased incidence of renal cell carcinoma in patients with von Hippel-Lindau disease and in those who are on chronic dialysis. Tumors tend to be multiple and bilateral, and there is an increased incidence of adenomas.
- The tumor appears bilateral in 0.1% to 1.5% of patients.

- Staging is as follows:
  Grade I confined to kidney
  Grade II spread to perinephric fat, but within Gerota's fascia
  Grade III spread to renal vein, IVC, regional lymph nodes
  Grade IV invasion of neighboring structures; distant metastases

Transitional Cell Carcinoma

- A transitional cell tumor is a tumor of the renal pelvis; however, these tumors are more frequently found in the bladder.
- Often there are multiple tumors.
- These tumors are three to four times more likely to occur in males than in females.
- The incidence of transitional cell carcinoma increases with age.

Ultrasound Findings

- On ultrasound examination, the sonographer will see a mass in the renal pelvis containing low level echoes, a widening of central sinus echoes, and a hypoechoic central area. Possibly the sonographer may be unable to detect any abnormalities.

Differential Diagnosis

- Other tumors of the renal pelvis such as squamous cell or adenoma
- Blood clot
- Fungus ball

Renal Lymphoma

- Sonographic findings of renal lymphoma are not specific.
- Lymphomatous involvement of the kidneys is usually a secondary process, either via the hematogenous spread or contiguous spread from the retroperitoneum.
  - Non-Hodgkin's lymphoma is more common than Hodgkin's.
  - Lymphoma is more common as a bilateral invasion, with multiple nodules.

Metastasis

- Common sites of metastases include the following:
  - Skin (melanoma)
  - Lymphoid tissue (lymphoma)
  - Cancer of lungs, breast, stomach, cervix, colon, pancreas

Wilms' Tumor, or Nephroblastoma

- Wilms' tumor, or nephroblastoma, is the most common solid renal mass found during childhood.
- Incidence of this tumor is as follows:

- Rare in newborn
- Peak incidence in second year of life
- 50% occur before third birthday
- 75% occur before fifth birthday
- Incidence extends into adulthood (i.e., there is poor prognosis of a cure)
- Associated with:
  - Beckswith-Wiedemann
  - Sporatic anoridia (no color in eye)
  - Omphalocele
  - Hemihypertrophy (one side of the body is larger than the other)
- 90% of patients with Wilms' tumor have a palpable abdominal mass.
- Other clinical findings include: abdominal pain, anorexia, nausea and vomiting, fever, and gross hematuria.
- Venous obstruction can result in leg edema, varicocele, or Budd-Chiari syndrome.
- These tumors tend to be large when detected.
- These tumors are multifocal in approximately 5% to 10% of patients.
- The sonographer must be able to separate these from adrenal masses (neuroblastoma).

Angiomyolipoma

- An angiomyolipoma is an uncommon benign renal tumor that is composed mainly of fat cells intermixed with smooth muscle cells and aggregates of thick-walled blood vessels.
- There may be hemorrhage in the tumor itself or in the subcapsular or perinephric spaces.

Ultrasound Findings

- Focal, solid hyperechoic mass
- There are two patterns of occurrence:
  1. (Accounts for 80% of cases) Tumor is solitary, nonhereditary, and found mostly in women who are between twenty and fifty years of age.
  2. Multiple tumors and bilateral renal involvement are seen in patients who are in their early teens who have tuberous sclerosis (20%).

Mesoplastic Nephroma

- Fetal renal hamartoma
- Mesenchymal hamartoma
- Mesoplastic nephroma is an uncommon benign neoplasm that represents the more common solid renal mass in children in the first few months of life.
- Most cases involve newborns or young infants.

Benign Renal Tumors

There are two common benign renal tumors: adenomas and oncocytomas.

- An adenoma can have calcifications.
- An oncocytoma resembles the spoke wheel patterns of enhancement with a central scar.
- To separate malignant from benign tumors, the sonographer should look at vessels and nodes, and look for metastasis, but should not rule out any possibilities of malignancy.

RENAL TRANSPLANT

On ultrasound examination, the sonographer should look for the following:

- Presence or absence of hydronephrosis
- Perirenal space (fluid collections)
- Doppler—diastolic flow
- Renal size
- Surgical results on ultrasound examination: perirenal collection (urinoma, lymphocele, hematoma, abscess)
- Medical:
  - obstruction, (dilation doesn't mean obstruction)
  - vascular to rule out thrombosis of vein or artery
  - rejection (increased renal size, prominent hypoechoic medullary pyramids, effacement of renal sinus fat, thickening of renal pelvis)
  - Acute tubular necrosis (ATN)
  - Cyclosporan toxicity (biopsy)
  - Diffuse infections

Doppler
- Increased resistive index (RI) (over 90%) means rejection or ATN
- Reversal of diastolic flow—renal vein thrombosis (Can see in rejection or ATN)

THE MALFUNCTIONING KIDNEY

- The excretory and regulatory functions of the kidneys are decreased in both acute and chronic renal failure.
- Acute renal failure is typically an abrupt, transient decrease in renal function and is often heralded by oliguria.
- The renal causes of acute azotemia include parenchymal disease (e.g., acute glomerulonephritis, acute interstitial nephritis, and acute tubular necrosis), renal vein thrombosis and, rarely, renal-artery occlusion.
- The etiologic basis of chronic renal failure includes obstructive nephropathies, parenchymal diseases, renovascular disorders, and any process that progressively destroys nephrons.
- The pathophysiologic states that cause varying degrees of renal malfunction have been categorized as prerenal, postrenal, and renal.
- Decreased perfusion of the kidneys causes prerenal failure that can be diagnosed by clinical and laboratory data alone.

- Prompt diagnosis and treatment are crucial for postrenal failure, which is potentially reversible.

Hydronephrosis

Hydronephrosis may be specific, with various sonographic findings.

- The dilated pyelocaliceal system appears as a separation of the renal sinus echoes by fluid-filled areas that conform anatomically to the infundibula, calices, and pelvis.
- The renal sinus and parenchyma become compressed with progressive obstruction, and in end-stage hydronephrosis, only multiple cystic spaces may be seen.
- It is possible to see the site of obstruction on scans under the following conditions:
  - Congenital obstruction of utero pelvic junction (UPJ) can be seen in utero.
  - Whenever hydronephrosis is seen, the ureters and bladder are scanned because dilation of these structures is indicative of obstruction of the ureterovesical junction or of the urethra.
- Localized hydronephrosis occurs as a result of strictures, calculi, focal masses, or a duplex collecting system.
- Possible sources of error when a mildly distended collecting system is seen include the following:
  - Overhydration
  - Underhydration
  - Extrarenal pelves
  - Previous urinary diversion procedures
- Post-void scanning techniques are helpful to avoid these errors.

Intrinsic Renal Disease
- Two classifications of disease processes of intrinsic renal disease have been described:
  1. One group produces a generalized increase in cortical echoes, which are believed to be caused by the deposition of collagen and fibrous tissue. This group includes:
     - Interstitial nephritis
     - Acute tubular necrosis
     - Amyloidosis
     - Diabetic nephropathy
     - Systemic lupus erythematosus
     - Myeloma
  2. A second group of diseases cause a predominant loss of normal anatomic detail, resulting in the inability to distinguish between the cortex and medullary regions of the kidneys. This group of diseases includes:
     - Chronic pyelonephritis
     - Renal tubular ectasia
     - Acute bacterial nephritis

- The end stage of many of these disease processes is renal atrophy, which can be seen on ultrasound examination by measuring renal length and cortical thickness.
- Some acute renal disorders can produce exactly the opposite findings; e.g., decreased parenchymal echogenicity and renal enlargement. Such disorders are:
  - Renal-vein thrombosis
  - Pyelonephritis
  - Renal-transplant rejection
- Interstitial edema is thought to be the most likely cause of these findings.

Acute Glomerulonephritis

- In acute glomerulonephritis, necrosis or proliferation of cellular elements (or both activities) occurs in the glomeruli.
- The vascular elements, tubules, and interstitium become secondarily affected, and the end result is enlarged, poorly functioning kidneys.
- Different forms of glomerulonephritis, including membranous, idiopathic, membranoproliferative, rapidly progressive and poststreptococcal, can be associated with abnormal echo patterns from the renal parenchyma on ultrasound examination.
- The increased cortical echoes probably result from changes within the glomerular, interstitial, tubular, and vascular structures.
- Clinical symptoms may include nephrotic syndrome, hypertension, anemia, and peripheral edema.

Acute Interstitial Nephritis

- Acute interstitial nephritis has been associated with infectious processes such as scarlet fever and diphtheria.
- It may be a manifestation of an allergic reaction to certain drugs.
- Clinical symptoms may include azotemia: uremia, proteinuria, hematuria, rash, fever, and eosinophilia.
- With this disease, the kidneys are enlarged and mottled.
- On ultrasound examination, the renal cortical echogenicity is increased.
- The greatest increase in echogenicity has been described in cases of diffuse active disease.
- There is a lesser increase in diffuse scarring.

Lupus Nephritis

- Systemic lupus erythematosus is a connective tissue disorder that is believed to be caused by an abnormal immune system.
- Females are affected more often than males; peak incidence is 20 to 40 years of age.
- The kidneys are involved in more than 50% of patients.
- Renal manifestations include hematuria, proteinuria, hypertension, renal vein thrombosis, and renal insufficiency.

- Sonography shows increased cortical echogenicity and renal atrophy.

Acquired Immune Deficiency Syndrome (AIDS)

- AIDS is a highly contagious disease.
- The AIDS virus destroys T cells and then replicates rapidly within the body.
- The virus affects many organs within the body.
- Unexplained uremia or azotemia may indicate renal dysfunction caused by the AIDS virus.
- It is not known if focal segmental glomerulosclerosis is primary or secondary.

Ultrasound Findings

- Echogenic parenchymal pattern
- Increase in cortical echogenicity
- Kidneys normal in size to enlarged

Sickle Cell Nephropathy

- Renal involvement is a common finding in patients with sickle cell disease.
- Abnormalities include the following:
  - Glomerulonephritis
  - Renal vein thrombosis
  - Papillary necrosis
  - Hematuria (common)
- The sonographic appearance of sickle cell nephropathy depends on the type of pathologic process that is involved.
  - With acute renal vein thrombosis, kidneys are enlarged, and there is decreased echogenicity secondary to edema.
  - Subacute cases show renal enlargement, with an increase of cortical echoes.
  - Diagnosis is specific if thrombosis is seen

Alport's Syndrome

- Alport's syndrome is a hereditary chronic nephritis associated with high-tone nerve deafness and ocular abnormalities.
- This disease affects males more often than females.
- Renal cortical echogenicity is increased because of cellular infiltration and fibrosis occurring in the interstitium.
- Glomerulosclerosis and tubular atrophy can also occur.
- The kidneys are commonly small, with compromised function.

Papillary Necrosis

- Many conditions may lead to papillary necrosis, such as sickle cell disease, diabetes, and others.
- Necrosis may develop within weeks or months after a kidney transplant.
- Patients previously treated for rejection and those with a kidney from a cadaver are at greatest risk for papillary necrosis.

- Ischemia has an important role in necrosis.
- Symptoms of necrosis suggest calculus or an inflammatory process.
- Patients may experience hematuria, flank pain, dysuria, hypertension, and acute renal failure.

Ultrasound Findings

- On ultrasound examination, the sonographer may see one or more fluid spaces at the corticomedullary junction that correspond to the distribution of the renal pyramids.
- Cystic spaces may be round or triangular.
- Sometimes arcuate vessels are seen.

Differential Diagnosis
- Congenital megacalices
- Hydronephrosis
- Post-obstructive atrophy

Renal Atrophy

- Renal atrophy results from numerous disease processes.
- The intrarenal anatomy is preserved, with uniform loss of renal tissue.
- Renal sinus lipomatosis occurs secondary to renal atrophy.
- More severe lipomatosis refers to a tremendous increase in renal sinus fat content in cases of marked renal atrophy as a result of hydronephrosis and chronic calculus disease.
- The kidneys appear enlarged, with a highly echogenic, enlarged renal sinus and a thin cortical rim.
- Renal sinus fat is easily seen on ultrasound examination.

RENAL FAILURE, INFARCTION, AND INFECTION
Acute Renal Failure

- Prerenal failure is secondary to hypoperfusion of the kidney.
- Renal failure may be caused by any of the following parenchymal diseases: acute glomerulonephritis, acute interstitial nephritis, acute tubular necrosis (ATN).
- Renal failure may also be caused by renal vein thrombosis or renal artery occlusion.
- Postrenal failure is usually caused by outflow obstruction and is potentially reversible.

Ultrasound Findings

- On ultrasound examination, the sonographer can differentiate between urinary outflow obstruction and parenchymal disease.
- Obstruction is responsible for approximately 5% of cases of acute renal failure.

Postrenal Failure

- Postrenal failure is often increased in patients with malignant neoplasm in any of the following locations:

- Bladder
- Prostate
- Uterus
- Ovaries
- Rectum
- Less common causes of postrenal failure include the following:
  - Retroperitoneal fibrosis
  - Paraortic lymph nodes
  - Retroperitoneal neoplasm
  - Renal calculi
  - Sloughed papilla
- The single most important issue with regard to diagnosis of acute renal failure is the presence or absence of urinary tract dilation.
- The degree of dilation doesn't necessarily reflect either the presence or severity of an obstruction.
- The sonographer should try to determine the level of obstruction.

Hydronephrosis

- Hydronephrosis is the separation of renal sinus echoes by fluid-filled areas.
- With progressive obstruction, renal parenchyma will be compressed.

Nonobstructive Hydronephrosis

Dilation of the renal pelvis does not always mean obstruction is present. Several other factors may cause the renal pelvis to be dilated:

- Reflux
- Infection
- High flow states (polyuria)
- Post-obstruction atrophy (once obstruction is relieved the obstruction can remain)
- Pregnancy dilation (the enlarged uterus can compress the ureter, usually more on the right side.)

False Positive Hydronephrosis

There are many conditions that may mimic hydronephrosis:

- Extrarenal pelvis
- Peripelvic cysts
- Reflux
- Transient diuresis
- Congenital megacalices
- Papillary necrosis
- Renal artery aneurysm (color can help distinguish between vascular enlargement and renal pelvis)
- Arterial-venous malformations (color can help distinguish these)

Localized Hydronephrosis

- Strictures
- Calculi
- Focal masses (transitional)
- Duplex system can be obstructed because of ectopic insertion of a ureter. In females it can insert below the external urinary sphincter and cause dribbling.

False Negative Hydronephrosis

- In patients with retroperitoneal fibrosis or necrosis, the sonographer should give a fluid challenge to see if the renal pelvis dilates.
- Distal calculi may cause no obstruction at the time of ultrasound examination; IVP is more sensitive to distal calculi.
- Staghorn calculus can mask associated dilation.

Major Hydronephrosis

- Dilated calices radiate from a larger central fluid collection, the renal pelvis.
- With major hydronephrosis, the affected kidney usually retains a normal shape.
- The sonographer will see fluid-filled sacs in a radiating pattern.

Acute Tubular Necrosis

- Acute tubular necrosis is the most common medical renal disease to produce acute renal failure.
- This condition can be reversible.

Ultrasound Findings

- Enlarged kidneys
- Hyperechoic pyramids that can revert to normal appearance

Differential Diagnosis

- Nephrocalcinosis

Chronic Renal Disease

- With chronic renal disease, there is a diffusely echogenic kidney, with a loss of normal anatomy.
- It is a nonspecific ultrasound finding. Chronic renal disease can be caused by multiple etiologies; i.e., AIDS can cause the kidneys to be echogenic.
- If chronic renal disease is bilateral, small kidneys are identified. This may be caused by hypertension, chronic inflammation, or chronic ischemia.

Infections

- Infections can progress from pyelonephritis to focal bacterial nephritis to abscess.

Pyonephrosis

- Pyonephrosis occurs when pus is found within the obstructed renal system.

- It is often associated with severe urosepsis.
- Pyonephrosis represents a true urologic emergency that requires urgent percutaneous drainage.
- Pyonephrosis usually occurs secondary to longstanding ureteral obstruction caused by calculus disease, stricture, or a congenital anomaly.

Ultrasound Findings

- Low-level echoes with fluid debris levels

Emphysematous Pyelonephritis

- Emphysematous pyelonephritis is air in the parenchyma; i.e., diffuse gas forming a parenchymal infection.
- This condition is commonly found in patients with diabetes.
- Emphysematous pyelonephritis is unilateral.
- The condition necessitates an emergency nephrectomy.

Xanthogranulomatous Pyelonephritis

- Xanthogranulomatous pyelonephritis is uncommon, but can result in chronic obstruction and infection.
- This condition also causes destruction of the renal parenchyma.
- Clinical symptoms include a nonfunctioning kidney, staghorn calculus; i.e., large kidneys, and multiple infections, such as proteus and *E. coli.*

Ultrasound Findings

- On ultrasound examination, staghorn calculus may be present. Peripelvic fibrosis can prevent staghorn from shadowing.
- Parenchyma is replaced by cystic spaces.
- The affected kidney is increased in size.
- Wave patterns can be diffuse or segmental.

Nephrocalcinosis

Ultrasound Findings

- Echogenic pyramids that may not have associated shadowing

Renal Cystic Disease

Simple Renal Cyst

- With a simple renal cyst, the exact pathogenesis is not known.
- A simple renal cyst is generally believed to represent retention cysts that occur secondary to tubular obstruction, vascular occlusion, or focal inflammation.
- These simple cysts affect 50% of adults over 50 years of age.

Ultrasound Findings

- No internal echoes
- Acoustic enhancement
- Clear demarcation of back wall
- Spherical or slightly ovoid shape

- Low-level echoes within a renal cyst may be caused by one of the following:
  - Artifact (sensitivity too high, or transducer frequency too low)
  - Infection
  - Hemorrhage
  - Necrotic cystic tumor
  - Technique: high gain of reverberation from wall

Atypical Cysts
- An atypical cyst with low-level echoes may represent a hemorrhagic cyst.

Ultrasound Findings
- Echoes within cyst
- Septae
- Mural nodules or calcifications (1% to 3% of cysts calcify with "rim-like" calcification, usually benign; now up to 20% are malignant)

Parapelvic Cyst
- A parapelvic cyst arises in the renal hilum but doesn't communicate with collecting system.

Ultrasound Findings
- No septations
- Can have irregular borders because they compress adjacent renal sinus structures
- Parapelvic cyst may obstruct; peripelvic cyst doesn't
- Symptoms are infrequent; however, the cyst can cause pain, hypertension, obstruction
- Sonographer should differentiate from hydronephrosis by connecting the dilated renal pelvis centrally.

Cysts Associated with Multiple Renal Neoplasms
- von Hippel-Lindau
- Tuberous sclerosis
- Acquired cystic disease of dialysis

von Hippel-Lindau
- "Cerebello retinal hemangioblastomatosis"
- Genetic disorder; autosomal dominant
- Retinal angiomas
- Cerebellar hemangioblastomas
- Abdominal cysts and tumors occur:
  - renal and pancreatic cysts
  - renal adenomas
  - frequent multiple and bilateral renal adenocarcinoma

Tubular Sclerosis
- "Bourneville's disease"
- Genetic disorder; autosomal dominant
- Multiple renal cysts
- Multiple and bilateral renal angiomyolipomas

- Cutaneous, retinal, and cerebral hamartomas
- Clinical triad: convulsive seizures, mental deficiency, adenoma sebaceum

Acquired Cystic Disease of Dialysis
- Patients undergoing dialysis have an increased incidence of having renal cysts.
- These patients also have an increased incidence (up to seven times that of the general population) of renal adenomas and cancer.
- Incidence increases, particularly after the first 3 years following a transplant.
- Cysts can suffer spontaneous bleeding.

Congenital Cystic Disease
Polycystic Renal Disease
There are two kinds of polycystic renal disease: infantile and adult.

- Infantile is an autosomal-recessive disease.
- Sometimes in utero, the fetus has large kidneys that are echogenic on ultrasound examination; the fetus develops renal failure and dies.
- In juvenile polycystic renal disease, there is bile duct proliferation, periportal fibrosis, portal hepatic varices, and nephromegaly.
- Adult polycystic disease is autosomal dominant.
- Adults are affected later in life. Renal failure is not as severe in onset as with younger patients. An adult patient usually has hypertension in the 30 to 40-year age range.
- The patient may have spontaneous bleeding in the cyst and therefore pain.
- Enlarged kidneys are eventually replaced by cysts.
  - The renal sinus is obliterated.
  - Associated abnormalities include Willis' circle aneurysm in 20% of patients; liver cysts in 50%, splenic cyst in 10%, and pancreatic cyst in 10%.

Multicystic Dysplastic Kidney
- Multicystic dysplastic kidney is a nonhereditary renal dysplasia.
- It is the most common palpable abdominal mass found in neonates.
- This condition is unilateral, with enlarged nonfunctioning kidneys. The kidneys can be small and calcified in adults.
- Multiple cysts of varying size with no normal parenchyma are often seen.
- The sonographer must be able to distinguish these cysts from hydronephrosis by connecting to the renal pelvis.
- Associated problems:
  - Ureteral atresia
  - Contralateral UPJ (in 33% of patients)
  - Nonfunctioning kidney
  - Atretic renal artery

Medullary Cystic Disease
- Medullary sponge kidney:
  - Benign
  - Rare in children
  - Tubular ectasia
  - Calcium found in 40% to 80% of affected patients (nephrocalcinosis)
  - Not hereditary
  - Associated with Carroli's disease of the liver
- Medullary cystic disease (nephronopthisis):
  - Small echodense kidneys
  - Autosomal recessive
  - Salt-wasting nephropathy present in young adults
  - Tubular atrophy; glomerulosclerosis
  - Multiple small cysts under 2 cm

Multilocular Cystic Nephroma
- Multiloculated cystic mass
- Multilocular cystic nephroma
  - Benign
  - Multiple cystic spaces
  - Does not communicate with renal pelvis
  - Peaks in infants and adults

Review Exercise A • Normal Renal Parenchyma

1. Define the three distinct segments of the kidney. _____

_____

_____

2. Where are the renal arteries located, and what is the best view to image them? _____

_____

_____

3. Where are the crura found and how can the sonographer define the crura from the vascular structures? _____

_____

_____

4. What is the sonographic appearance of the renal medulla? _____

_____

_____

_____

5. Describe Bertin's column. How can the sonographer confuse this variant with a renal mass? _____

_____

_____

6. What is a dromedary hump, and where is it commonly found? _____

_____

_____

7. Where is the junctional parenchymal defect most commonly found and what is its appearance on ultrasound examination? _____

_____

_____

8. Describe the duplex collecting system and its appearance on ultrasound examination. _____

_____

_____

9. Why does sinus lipomatosis produce such an echogenic renal image? _____

_____

_____

10. What is the ultrasound appearance of an extrarenal pelvis? _____

_____

_____

11. What should the sonographer look for in a patient with a pelvic kidney? _____

_____

_____

12. The horseshoe kidney has several distinguishing features on ultrasound examination. What are they? _____

_____

_____

Review Exercise B • Laboratory Tests for Renal Disease

1. Describe the clinical signs and symptoms that a patient with renal infection or disease process may have. _____

_____

_____

_____

2. Describe the urinalysis laboratory test and discuss when it is used. _____

_____

_____

_____

3. What does urine pH tell the clinician about renal disease? _____

_____

_____

_____

4. Describe the laboratory test for specific gravity. _____

_____

_____

_____

5. What is the significance of hematuria? _____

_____

_____

_____

6. What does a decreased hematocrit mean on a clinical basis? _____

_____

_____

_____

7. What does the presence of hemoglobin in the urine signify? _____

_____

_____

8. Describe the test for creatinine clearance. _____

_____

_____

_____

9. A common laboratory test used for renal disease is BUN. What does this abbreviation stand for and how does this test work? _____

_____

_____

_____

10. What are the clinical symptoms of renal cystic disease? _____

_____

_____

11. What are the clinical symptoms of a renal subcapsular hematoma? _____

_____

_____

_____

12. What are the clinical symptoms of a renal abscess? _____

_____

_____

_____

13. What are the clinical symptoms of acute focal bacterial nephritis? _____

_____

_____

14. What are the clinical symptoms of acute tubular necrosis? _____

_____

_____

15. What are the clinical symptoms of chronic renal failure? _____

_____

_____

16. What are the clinical symptoms of renal cell carcinoma? _____

_____

_____

Review Exercise C • Renal Cystic Disease

1. Describe the ultrasound appearance of a simple renal cyst. _____

_____

_____

2. What is the distinction between a simple renal cyst and an atypical cyst? _____

_____

_____

3. What is the definition of a parapelvic cyst? Describe the ultrasound appearance. _____

_____

_____

_____

4. What renal cysts are associated with multiple renal neoplasms? _____

_____

_____

_____

5. What is von Hippel-Lindau disease? _____

_____

_____

_____

6. What renal abnormalities are found in patients with tubular sclerosis? _____

_____

_____

_____

7. Discuss the formation of renal cystic disease in patients who are on long-term dialysis. _____

_____

_____

_____

8. Discuss polycystic renal disease. _____

_____

_____

_____

9. Describe the difference between medullary sponge kidney and medullary cystic disease. _____

_____

_____

_____

10. What is a multilocular cystic nephroma? _____

_____

_____

_____

11. Discuss the findings in a multicystic dysplastic kidney. _____

_____

_____

_____

12. What are other causes of a multiloculated renal mass? _____

_____

_____

_____

Review Exercise D • Renal Neoplasm

1. What is the most common of all renal tumors? _____

_____

_____

2. Describe the appearance of renal cell carcinoma as seen on ultrasound examination. _____

_____

_____

3. Describe the staging of renal cell carcinoma. _____

_____

_____

_____

4. What is the ultrasound appearance of transitional cell carcinoma? _____

_____

_____

5. Describe the ultrasound appearance of renal lymphoma. _____

_____

_____

6. Name the most common primary sites of tumor metastases to the kidney. _____

_____

_____

7. The most common tumor of childhood is Wilms' tumor. Describe the clinical findings the sonographer should consider in the evaluation of a Wilms' tumor. _____

_____

_____

8. Describe the composition of an angiomyolipoma of the kidney. _____

_____

_____

9. How can the sonographer attempt to separate a benign or malignant tumor of the kidney? _____

_____

_____

Review Exercise E • The Malfunctioning Kidney

1. What happens to the excretory and regulatory functions of the kidneys in acute and chronic renal failure? _____

_____

_____

_____

2. How can the sonographer be sure the diagnosis of hydronephrosis is correct? _____

_____

_____

3. Describe how intrinsic renal disease may be demonstrated by examining the renal parenchyma with ultrasound examination. _____

_____

_____

_____

4. Discuss acute glomerulonephritis in terms of ultrasound symptoms and clinical signs. _____

_____

_____

_____

5. Acute interstitial nephritis has been associated with infectious processes. What is the ultrasound appearance of this disease? _____

_____

_____

6. What is lupus nephritis? Describe the clinical and ultrasound findings. _____

_____

_____

_____

7. What is the effect of AIDS on the kidneys? How does it appear on ultrasound examination? _____

_____

_____

_____

8. What is the ultrasound appearance of sickle cell disease in the kidneys? _____

_____

_____

9. What is renal atrophy? _____

_____

_____

Review Exercise F • Renal Failure, Infarction, and Infection

1. What are the three stages of renal failure that may occur? _____

_____

_____

_____

2. How can the sonographer differentiate between urinary tract disease and obstruction? _____

_____

_____

3. What is the definition of hydronephrosis? _____

_____

_____

_____

4. What should the sonographer look for in determining hydronephrosis? _____

_____

_____

_____

5. What are the three grades of hydronephrosis? _____

_____

_____

_____

6. What is meant by the term "nonobstructive" hydronephrosis? _____

_____

_____

_____

7. What are the causes of false-positive hydronephrosis? _____

_____

_____

_____

8. How would a renal infarction appear on ultrasound examination? _____

_____

_____

_____

9. What is the most common medical renal disease that produces renal failure? _____

_____

_____

_____

_____

10. What is the cause of chronic renal disease and how is it seen on the ultrasound image? _____

_____

_____

_____

11. What is the natural course of a renal infection, and how do these infections affect the kidneys? _____

_____

_____

_____

_____

12. Describe the condition of pyonephrosis. What are its causes and ultrasound findings? _____

_____

_____

_____

13. Describe nephrocalcinosis and its ultrasound findings. _____

_____

_____

_____

14. Describe the sonographic technique and considerations that should be made before the evaluation of the renal

mass. _____

_____

_____

_____

_____

15. How are renal masses categorized, and what are their ultrasound characteristics? _____

_____

_____

_____

_____

16. What are the categories of renal cystic disease? _____

_____

_____

_____

17. Describe the characteristics of a simple renal cyst. _____

_____

_____

_____

18. What are the characteristics of a parapelvic cyst? _____

_____

_____

_____

19. Describe the difference between polycystic renal disease, juvenile disease, and infantile autosomal recessive renal disease. _____

_____

_____

_____

20. What are the findings in multicystic dysplasic kidney disease? _____

_____

_____

21. Describe the findings in medullary cystic disease. _____

_____

_____

_____

Self-Test • The Urinary System

1. The process of disposing of metabolic wastes is called:

   a. urea

   b. excretion

   c. deamination

   d. urination

2. Urea is produced mainly in the _____ , then transported to the _____ by the circulatory system.

   a. ureter; aorta

   b. kidney; liver

   c. liver; kidney

   d. pancreas; kidney

3. Urine is conducted from the renal pelvis to the urinary bladder by the:

   a. urethra

   b. uterua

   c. nephrons

   d. ureter

4. Urine in the major calices next passes into the:

   a. minor calices

   b. papilla

   c. renal capsule

   d. renal pelvis

5. The outer portion of the kidney is the:

   a. renal corpusle

   b. renal capsule

   c. renal sac

   d. perirenal space

6. The kidneys are located in the:

   a. peritoneal cavity

   b. retroperitoneal cavity

   c. perirenal cavity

   d. perirenal space

7. The renal corpuscle consists of a tuft of capillaries, the _____ , surrounded by _____ .

   a. glomerulus; Bowman's capsule

   b. afferent arteriole; efferent arteriole

   c. Henle's loop; convoluted tubule

   d. peritubular capillaries; Henle's loop

8. Blood flows into the glomerulus through a(n) _____ arteriole.

    a. efferent arteriole

    b. afferent arteriole

    c. peritubular

    d. glomerular

9. The process of returning most of the filtrate to the blood is known as:

    a. glomerular filtration

    b. tubular reabsorption

    c. tubular secretion

    d. refiltration

10. The urinary _____ is a temporary storage sac for urine.

    a. sac

    b. bladder

    c. pelvis

    d. system

Match the following (Note that one answer will be used twice):

excretion	renal capsule	pyramids
elimination	renal cortex	papilla
urea	renal medulla	glomerulus
uric acid	renal pelvis	Bowman's capsule
creatinine	major calices	Henle's loop
hilus	minor calices	urethra

11. _____ when urine leaves the bladder, it flows through this structure

12. _____ network of capillaries in the renal corpuscle

13. _____ surrounds the renal corpuscle

14. _____ removal of metabolic wasteswastes

15. _____ discharging undigested or unabsorbed food from the digestive tract

16. _____ amino group converted to ammonia

17. _____ formed from the breakdown of nucleic acids

18. _____ ureters and blood vessels connect the kidney at this point

19. _____ peripheral area of kidney

20. _____ formed from breakdown of nucleic acids

21. _____ urine flows into this hollow structure

22. _____ four to eight funnel-shaped calices

23. _____ several cone-shaped regions within the kidney

24. _____ middle area of the kidney

25. _____ means "nipple"

26. In a healthy individual, red blood cells may occasionally be found in the urine (true or false).

27. Blood in the urine is always related to a malignant invasive renal mass (true or false).

28. Three distinct segments seen within the kidney are:

    a. pyramids, cortex, pelvis

    b. medullary zone, cortex, renal sinus

    c. pyramids, medullary zone, renal sinus

    d. cortex, pelvis, capsule

29. What helps to distinguish the kidney from the liver?

    a. pyramids

    b. renal sinus

    c. capsule and perinephric fat

    d. pararenal sinus

30. Renal arteries arise from the:

    a. anterior aortic wall

    b. anterolateral aortic wall

    c. posterior aortic wall

    d. posterolateral aortic wall

31. Name the vessel that lies posterior to the IVC.

    a. left renal artery

    b. right renal vein

    c. left renal vein

    d. right renal artery

32. The course of the _____ flows _____ to aorta and _____ to the SMA.

    a. right renal vein; posterior; anterior

    b. left renal vein; anterior; posterior

    c. right renal artery; anterior; posterior

    d. left renal artery; posterior; anterior

33. What is the probable cause of a dromedary hump?

    a. congenital mass

    b. result of pressure on fetal kidney by spleen

    c. prominent Bertin's column

    d. engorged renal pyramid

Match the following variations in renal development:

34. _____ junctional parenchymal defect

35. _____ duplex collecting system

36. _____ sinus lipomatosis (use for 3 answers)

37. _____ extrarenal pelvis

38. _____ renal agenesis

39. _____ supernumerary kidney

40. _____ pelvic kidney (use for 3 answers)

41. _____ horseshoe kidney (use for 2 answers)

    a. may simulate a solid adnexal mass

    b. may simulate hydronephrosis

    c. accumulation of fat in the renal sinus

    d. failure of formation

    e. malrotation

    f. fusion of the lower poles

    g. central renal sinus duplicated

    h. lies within the confines of the central renal sinus

    i. triangular area in the upper pole of the renal parenchyma

    j. enlargement of the sinus area

    k. simulates lymphadenopathy

    l. exceeds normal number

    m. associated with vesicoureteral reflex

42. The retroperitoneal space is the area between the:

    a. anterior portion of parietal peritoneum and the posterior abdominal wall muscles

    b. posterior portion of parietal peritoneum and the posterior abdominal wall muscles

    c. anterior portion of parietal peritoneum and the anterior abdominal wall muscles

    d. posterior portion of visceral peritoneum

43. The retroperitoneal space encloses the aorta and inferior vena cava (true or false).

44. The kidneys lie on what group of muscles?

    a. iliacus, piriformis

    b. iliacus, psoas

    c. psoas, quadratus lumborum

    d. iliacus, quadratus lumborum

45. The left kidney is in contact with the:

    a. spleen, pancreas, and gallbladder

    b. spleen, gallbladder, and duodenum

    c. pancreas, colon, and portahepatis

    d. spleen, pancreas, colon, and jejunum

46. The right kidney is in contact with the:

    a. spleen, colon, and adrenal gland

    b. liver, colon, and adrenal gland

    c. liver, pancreas, and gallbladder

    d. liver, gallbladder, and splenic flexure

47. The renal hilum exits the kidney on the lateral surface (true or false).

48. The ureter runs inferior to the renal hilum to enter the anterior wall of the bladder (true or false).

49. The kidneys are _____ long, _____ thick, _____ wide.

    a. 9 cm to 12 cm; 3 cm; 4 cm

    b. 5 cm to 10 cm; 3 cm; 6 cm

    c. 5 cm to 12 cm; 6 cm; 4 cm

    d. 7 cm to 9 cm; 5 cm; 3 cm

50. The kidney is encased within the:

    a. paranephric space

    b. perinephric space

    c. renal capsule

    d. renal cortex

51. Outside the renal capsule is the:

    a. perinephric fat

    b. paranephric space

    c. renal fascia

    d. renal medulla

52. The _____ surrounds the answer in number 10.

    a. paranephric space

    b. anterior and posterior layers of renal fascia

    c. posterior perirenal space

    d. perinephric fat

53. The renal pyramids are also called the:

    a. renal cortex

    b. perirenal sinus

    c. medulla

    d. papilla

54. The area surrounding the renal pyramids is called:

    a. renal cortex

    b. perirenal fat

    c. medulla

    d. papilla

55. The renal artery is superior to the renal veins (true or false).

56. The adrenal glands are peritoneal structures (true or false).

57. The adrenal glands are surrounded by:

   a. perinephric fascia

   b. perinephric capsule

   c. crus

   d. paranephric fat

58. The term *Gerota's fascia* refers to the perirenal or renal fascia (true or false).

59. The blood supply to the adrenals is via the:

   a. suprarenal branch of the inferior phrenic artery

   b. suprarenal branch of the aorta

   c. suprarenal branch of renal artery

   d. inferior vena cava

60. The left adrenal vein drains into the:

   a. inferior vena cava

   b. adrenal vena recess

   c. left renal vein

   d. left gonadal vein

61. A triangular-shaped lesion on the peripheral border of the kidney would most likely represent a(n):

   a. renal tumor

   b. artifact from rib

   c. inferior vena cava compression

   d. junctional parenchymal defect

62. Hydration of the patient may result in:

   a. prominent renal pyramids

   b. prominent renal pelvis

   c. dilated ureter

   d. increased renal blood flow

63. In normal patients with a distended urinary bladder, the direction of ureteral jets would be posterior to anterior (true or false).

64. The left renal vein courses:

   a. posterior to the inferior vena cava

   b. anterior to the inferior vena cava

   c. anterior to the aorta

   d. anterior to the superior mesenteric artery

65. The vessel seen posterior to the inferior vena cava on the sagittal scan represents the:

   a. right adrenal artery

   b. right renal artery

   c. left renal artery

   d. left renal vein

66. The kidneys begin their development in the pelvis and migrate into the posterior retroperitoneal space (true or false).

67. The renal cortex is more echogenic than the renal pelvis (true or false).

68. The smallest arteries seen with color flow and Doppler in the kidneys are:

    a. interlobar

    b. arcuate

    c. pyramidal

    d. minute renal

69. Renal sonography is not helpful in evaluating:

    a. obstructive uropathy

    b. cyst formation

    c. renal function

    d. angiomyolipoma

70. Persistent fever, swelling, and tenderness are indicative of:

    a. malignancy

    b. infection

    c. hydronephrosis

    d. angiomyloma

71. A potential space located between the liver edge and right kidney is:

    a. Morison's pouch

    b. Douglas's pouch

    c. cul-de-sac

    d. Winhauer's space

72. Hypernephromas commonly invade the IVC via the:

    a. renal vein

    b. renal artery

    c. portal vein

    d. splenic vein

73. Pyonephrosis refers to the:

    a. presence of blood in a dilated collecting system

    b. presence of pus in a dilated collected system

    c. presence of urine in a dilated collecting system

    d. presence of a perinephric abscess

74. Acquired renal cystic disease often develops in patients who are undergoing hemodialysis. Of the following, which is the most common complication?

    a. lymphocele

    b. urinoma

    c. hemorrhage

    d. tumor

75. Which statement is not true of crossed renal ectopia?

   a. It is a common renal congenital anomaly

   b. It may be fused or unfused

   c. It produces no clinical symptoms

   d. It produces hematuria

76. An enlarged Bertin's column leads to a frequent misdiagnosis of:

   a. cyst formation

   b. hydronephrosis

   c. pseudotumor

   d. spontaneous hemorrhage

77. Which phrase is false regarding angiomyolipomas of the kidney?

   a. they contain adipose and smooth muscle tissue

   b. they are usually singular and unilateral

   c. they may be mistaken for a renal cell CA

   d. they are usually mistaken for hydronephrosis

78. The left renal vein:

   a. has a shorter course than the right

   b. has a longer course than the right

   c. passes anterior to the IVC

   d. passes posterior to the aorta

79. An extremely large echogenic renal sinus that appears to engulf the entire renal parenchymal outline would suggest the possibility of:

   a. hydronephrosis

   b. lipomatosis

   c. hypernephroma

   d. nephrocalcinosis

80. Adult polycystic renal disease appears on a sonogram as:

   a. a single unilateral cyst

   b. multiple cysts of varying sizes

   c. a complex mass

   d. dense echoes within the kidney

81. The early sonographic appearance of renal transplant rejection is:

   a. enlargement

   b. decrease in renal size

   c. increased echogenicity

   d. rupture

82. The differential diagnosis of pseudohydronephrosis can be made if the:

a. patient is obese

b. bladder is too full

c. patient has hematuria

d. kidney contains calculi

83. A dromedary hump would present itself sonographically as a:

a. fatty tumor of kidney

b. fluid-filled structure within the kidney

c. bulge on lateral border of left kidney

d. funnel-shaped tube at the hilus

84. A benign fatty tumor of the kidney is:

a. angiomyolipoma

b. hypernephroma

c. neuroblastoma

d. lymphoma

85. Gerota's fascia refers to:

a. the area around the gallbladder

b. the stomach muscles

c. the area around the esophagus

d. the area around the kidney

e. the area above the right kidney and below the liver edge

86. A triangular area in the upper pole of the renal parenchyma most likely represents:

a. extrarenal pelvis

b. sinus lipomatosis

c. renal agenesis

d. junctional parenchymal defect

87. A _____ may simulate mild hydronephrosis.

a. renal adenoma

b. hydroureter

c. hypernephroma

d. parapelvic cyst

88. Of the following renal tumors, which is not a benign lesion?

a. hamartoma

b. angiomyolipoma

c. hypernephroma

d. adenoma

89. Which of the following is not a function of the kidney?

    a. excretion of the by-products of metabolism

    b. regulation of red blood cell production

    c. regulation of vitamin D metabolism

    d. secretion of cholecystokinin

90. Another term for a renal abscess is a:

    a. carbuncle

    b. nephrius

    c. renalitis

    d. pus

91. Neuroblastomas are tumors that:

    a. metastasize to bone, lymph, and liver

    b. are benign

    c. exhibit a hypoechoic pattern with good through transmission

    d. contain hair, calcium, and skin tissue

92. Three distinct segments seen within the kidney are:

    a. pyramids, cortex, and pelvis

    b. medullary zone, cortex, and renal sinus

    c. pyramids, medullary zone, and renal sinus

    d. cortex, pelvis, and capsule

93. All of the following statements about the kidneys are true except:

    a. the kidneys are intraperitoneal in location

    b. the average adult kidneys measure approximately 9 cm to 12 cm in length

    c. the kidneys may move with respiration

    d. the anteroposterior thickness of the normal adult kidneys is approximately 4 cm to 5 cm

94. The renal sinus echoes are produced by:

    a. pelvis and calices, renal vessels, fat, and areolar tissue

    b. perinephric fat

    c. renal parenchyma

    d. all of the above

95. The renal parenchyma is separated into the cortex and medulla by the:

    a. glomeruli

    b. renal fat

    c. arcuate vessels

    d. renal pelvis

96. The best approach for the evaluation of the left kidney is:

   a. supine

   b. prone

   c. RAO

   d. coronal

97. To fulfill the criteria of a cyst, one must demonstrate sonographically:

   a. an anechoic structure

   b. distal acoustic enhancement

   c. smooth walls

   d. all of the above

98. Bertin's column may be confused with a pseudotumor. This may be found:

   a. in the cortex that is surrounding and separating the renal pyramids and is unusually large

   b. in the major calices as a rudimentary ureter

   c. in the minor calices as a rudimentary calix

   d. outside the renal capsule

99. In cases of renal trauma, sonography may be helpful in identifying a hematoma within the renal parenchyma. A hematoma typically presents as:

   a. a sonolucent mass

   b. an echogenic mass

   c. a semicystic, semisolid mass

   d. all of the above

100. Hydronephrosis may be best demonstrated sonographically by which of the following patterns?

   a. a distorted shape of the kidney outline

   b. multiple cystic masses throughout the renal parenchyma

   c. a fluid-filled pelvocaliceal collecting system

   d. a hyperechoic pelvocaliceal collecting system

101. Hydronephrosis may be caused by all except:

   a. angiomyolipoma

   b. calculi

   c. a congenital and/or inflammatory stricture

   d. pregnancy

102. Within the renal sinus, the following can be found except:

   a. renal pyramids

   b. minor calices

   c. major calices

   d. the renal pelvis

   e. vessels

   f. lymphatics

103. The renal cortex contains:

a. Bowman's capsule and convoluted tubules

b. renal pyramids

c. major calices

d. minor calices

e. all of the above

104. A congenital abnormality in which both kidneys are united at their lower poles is termed:

a. Bertin's column

b. dromedary hump

c. horseshoe kidney

d. polycystic kidney

105. Adult polycystic disease may be characterized by all of the following except:

a. it is a latent disease until the third or fourth decade of life

b. it is an autosomal-dominant disease

c. it may be associated with cysts in the liver, pancreas, and spleen

d. the involved kidneys are small and extremely echogenic

106. Horseshoe kidneys may be confused sonographically with which of the following entities?

a. carcinoma of the head of the pancreas

b. lymphadenopathy

c. hypernephroma

d. Wilms' tumor

107. In acute renal disease, kidney size is

a. generally enlarged

b. generally small

c. not affected

d. enlarged after one year

108. Which statement about the kidneys is false?

a. the kidneys are rigidly fixed on the abdominal wall

b. the kidneys consist of an internal medullary and external cortical substance

c. the kidneys rest on the psoas and quadratus lumborum muscles

d. renal pyramids are found within the medullary region

109. The left renal vein runs:

a. between the aorta and the superior mesenteric artery

b. posterior to the aorta

c. posterior to the inferior vena cava

d. parallel to the portal vein

110. On the medial border of each kidney is the renal hilum, which contains:

   a. the renal vein

   b. the renal artery

   c. the proximal ureter

   d. all of the above

111. The kidneys, the perinephric fat, and the adrenal glands are all covered by:

   a. the true capsule

   b. Gerota's fascia

   c. peritoneum

   d. Glisson's capsule

112. If a heavy deposition of fat (sinus lipomatosis) is found within the kidney on renal sonography, the renal sinus will appear:

   a. enlarged

   b. mostly echo free

   c. mostly echogenic

   d. all of the above

113. Which of the following is least likely to be confused with hydronephrosis?

   a. an angiomyolipoma

   b. a multicystic kidney

   c. sinus lipomatosis

   d. a central renal cyst

114. A hypertrophied Bertin's column is a:

   a. benign tumor of the kidney

   b. malignant tumor of the kidney

   c. normal renal variant

   d. benign tumor of adrenal origin

115. With any renal tumor one should also check for:

   a. paraaortic nodes

   b. liver metastases

   c. tumor invasion of the IVC

   d. all of the above

116. A pelvic kidney has a(n):

   a. abnormal appearance in a normal location

   b. normal appearance in an abnormal location

   c. normal appearance in a normal location

117. Which of the following statements is true?

    a. the right kidney lies slightly higher than the left

    b. the right kidney lies slightly lower than the left

    c. both kidneys always lie at the same level

118. Signs of renal disease include all of the following except:

    a. oliguria

    b. palpable flank mass

    c. generalized edema

    d. polyuria

    e. Murphy's sign

119. The term "supernumerary kidney" refers to:

    a. a pseudokidney in the renal fossa

    b. a double-collecting system

    c. the complete duplication of the renal system

    d. the pelvic kidney

120. To best evaluate the internal composition of a cyst, one should change:

    a. the TGC

    b. the overall gain

    c. the transducer to a higher frequency

    d. all of the above

121. Clinical symptoms associated with inflammatory renal masses include all of the following except:

    a. fever

    b. chills

    c. flank pain

    d. hypoglycemia

122. Which of the following disorders may not produce a complex sonographic pattern?

    a. an infected cyst

    b. a hemorrhagic cyst

    c. hematomas

    d. a congenital cyst

Case Reviews

1. Discuss the congenital anomalies shown in Figures 8-4 to 8-8.

a. (Figure 8-4)   b. (Figure 8-5)

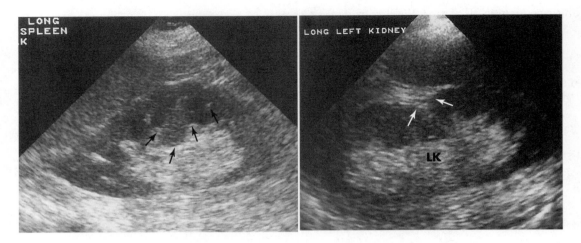

c. (Figure 8-6)   d. (Figure 8-7)

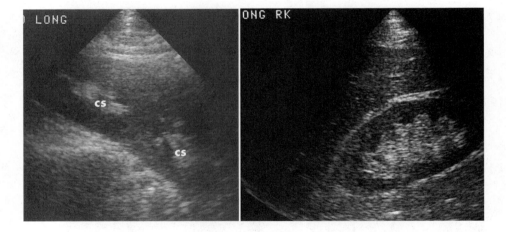

e. (Figure 8-8)

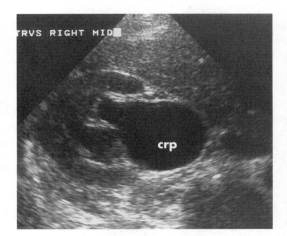

2. A 2-year-old male was brought to the hospital. He had a pulsatile abdominal mass. Laboratory values were within normal limits. What are your ultrasound findings (Figure 8-9)?

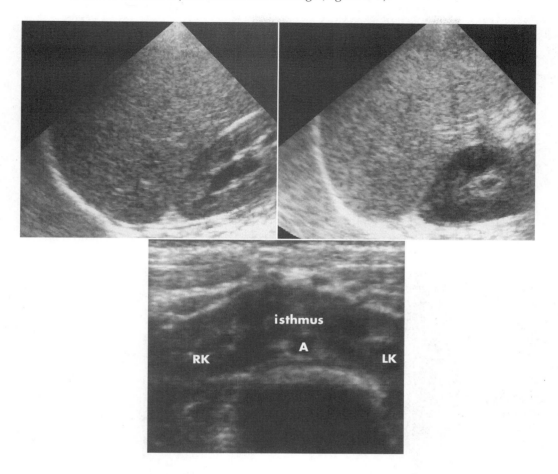

3. A 24-year-old female came to the hospital with localized, cramping pelvic pain. The kidneys were also evaluated during the ultrasound examination. What are your ultrasound findings (Figure 8-10)?

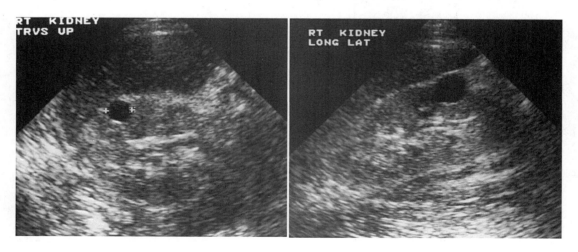

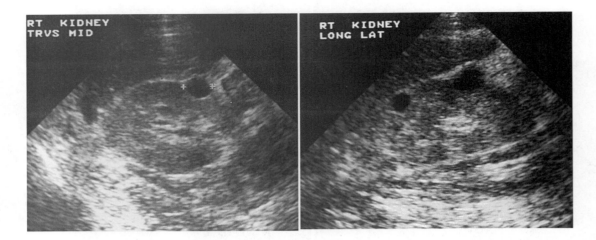

4. A 55-year-old patient had bilateral flank pain. He commented that his mother died from renal disease, but he didn't know the specifics of her disease. Scans were made of both kidneys. What are your ultrasound findings (Figure 8-11)?

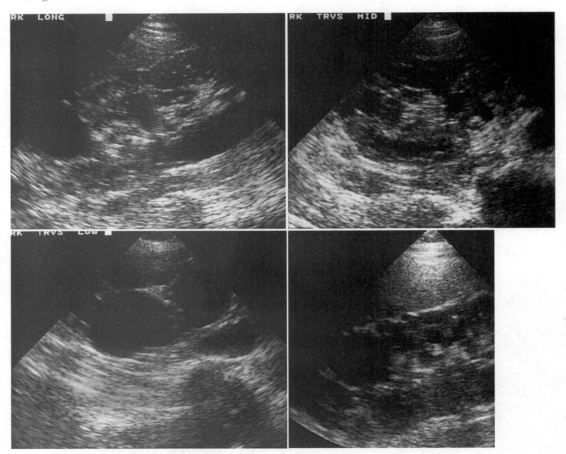

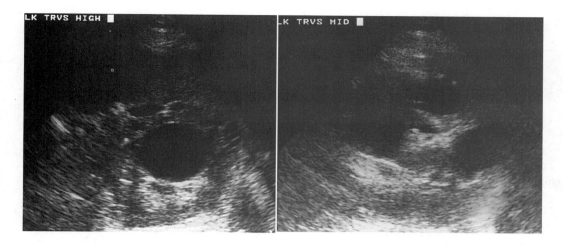

5. A 41-year-old male had bilateral flank pain extending into the right upper quadrant. Laboratory results showed hematuria and proteinuria. The man had been treated for hypertension for 4 years. What are your ultrasound findings (Figure 8-12)?

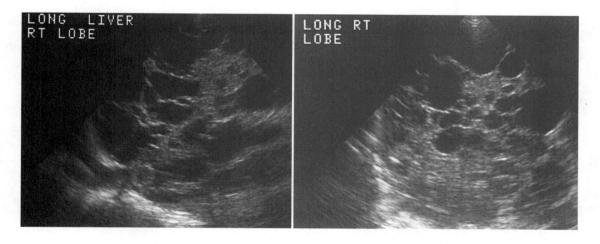

6. A young patient came to the hospital with bilateral flank pain and recurrent UTIs. What are your ultrasound findings (Figure 8-13)?

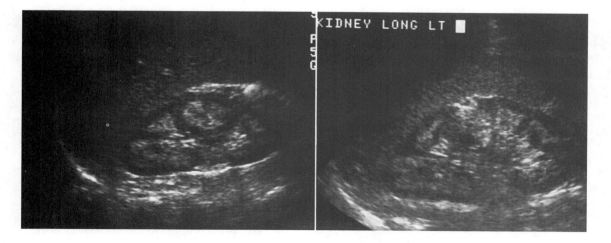

7. A 62-year-old male had hematuria and mild flank discomfort. What are your ultrasound findings (Figure 8-14)?

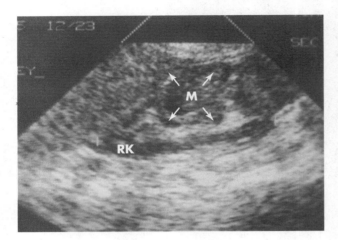

8. A 56-year-old male came to the hospital complaining that he had been experiencing gross hematuria and flank pain for the past 4 months. What are your ultrasound findings (Figure 8-15)?

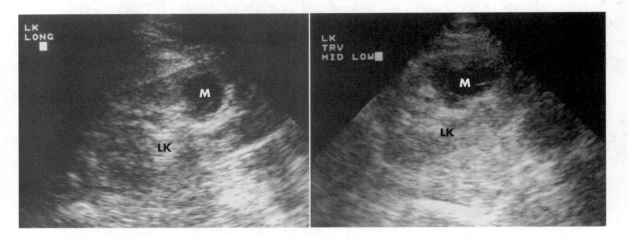

9. A 2-year-old has a large palpable abdominal mass and nausea and vomiting. What are your ultrasound findings (Figure 8-16)?

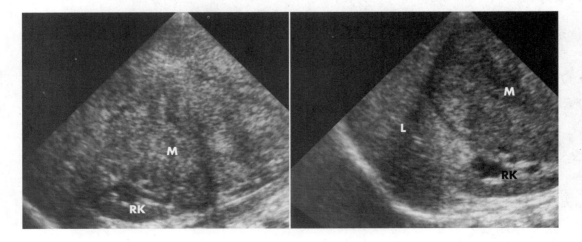

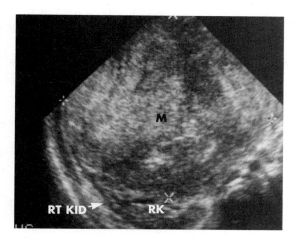

10. An 18-month-old child presented with nausea and vomiting and a palpable abdominal mass. What are your ultrasound findings (Figure 8-17)?

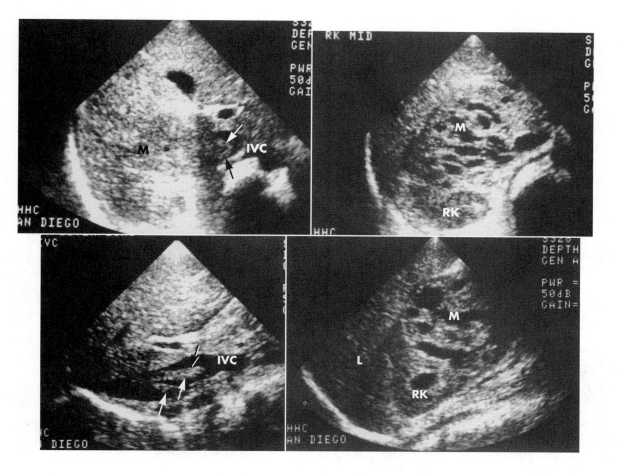

11. A 29-year-old female complained of RLQ fullness. No adenexal masses were found. What are your ultrasound findings (Figure 8-18)?

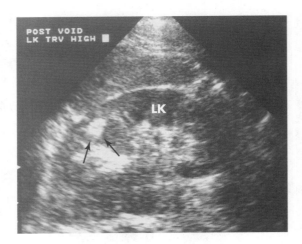

12. A 30-year-old female came to the hospital with pelvic pain. Evaluation of the kidneys was made after the normal pelvic ultrasound. What are your ultrasound findings (Figure 8-19)?

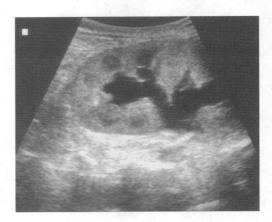

13. A middle-aged female was told to drink several glasses of water before her pelvic ultrasound. What are your ultrasound findings (Figure 8-20)?

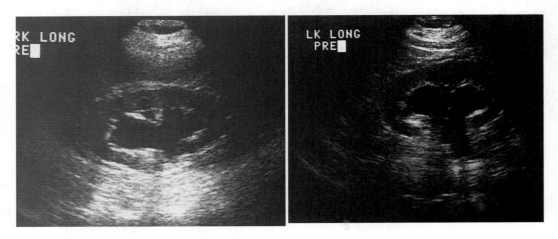

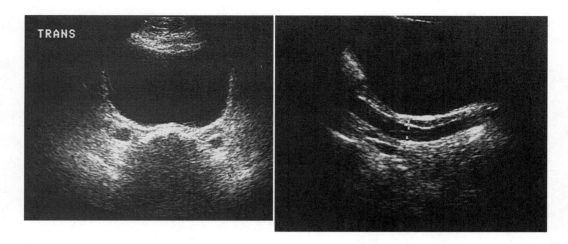

14. A young female with lupus erythematosus came to the hospital with flank pain. What are your ultrasound findings (Figure 8-21)?

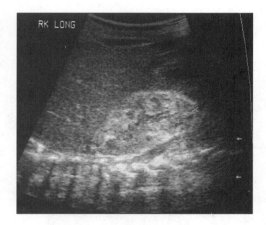

15. A 68-year-old diabetic male had flank pain. What are your ultrasound findings (Figure 8-22)?

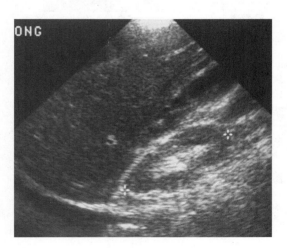

16. A young patient arrived at the ER with an elevated white count, and had experienced fever for the past 3 days. What are your ultrasound findings (Figure 8-23)?

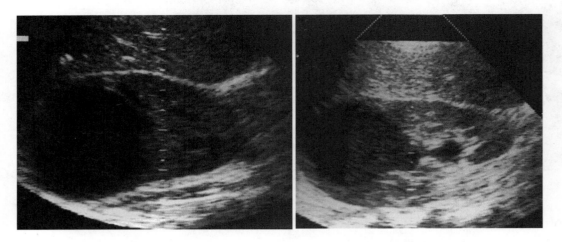

17. A 24-year-old male had a positive urine culture for *E. coli*. He had experienced repeated renal inflammatory processes. What are your ultrasound findings (Figure 8-24)?

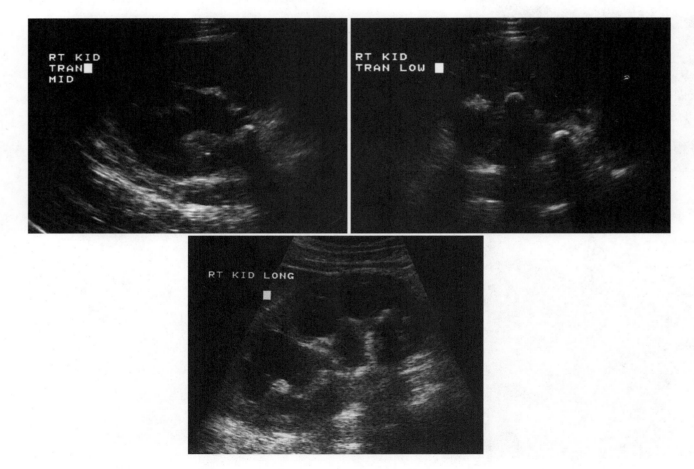

18. A 60-year-old female came to the hospital with burning, intense abdominal pain, and a feeling of fullness over the past 24 hours. What are your ultrasound findings (Figure 8-25)?

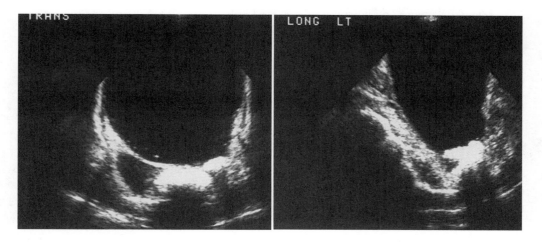

19. A 55-year-old male with a renal transplant came to the hospital with early signs of obstruction. What are your ultrasound findings (Figure 8-26)?

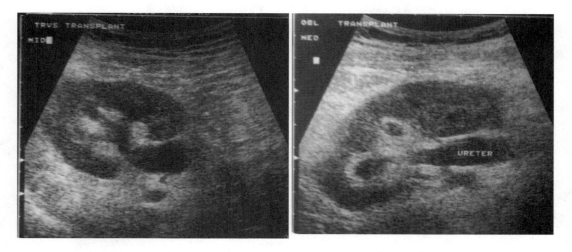

20. A 45-year-old diabetic female s/p renal transplant. What are your ultrasound findings (Figure 8-27)?

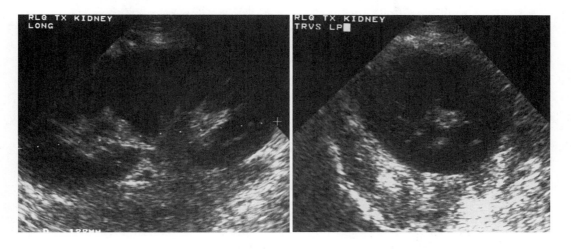

21. A 30-year-old female who had a renal transplant 14 years ago had right upper quadrant and midabdominal pain. She had rigors and chills, but was afebrile. What are your ultrasound findings (Figure 8-28)?

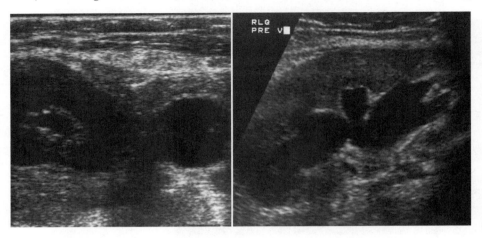

22. A 41-year-old male had abnormal renal function tests and an elevated BUN after renal transplantation. What are your ultrasound findings (Figure 8-29)?

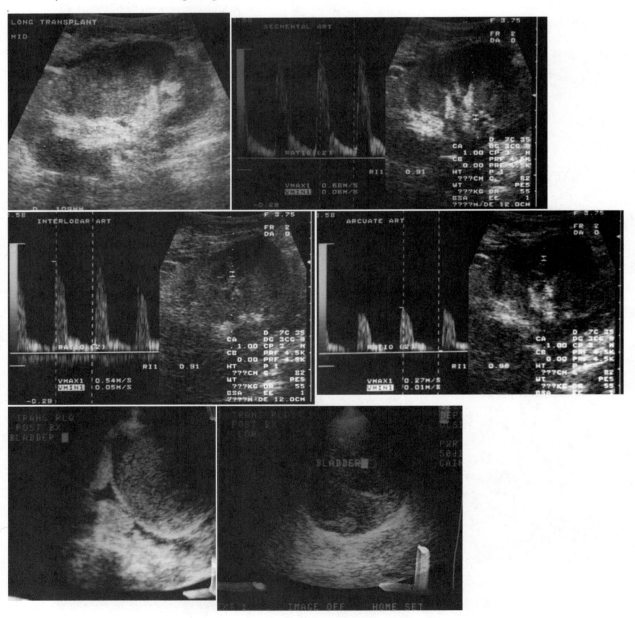

Answers to Review Exercise A

1. The supine scan shows three distinct segments of the kidney: a poorly echoic medullary zone that consists of numerous anechoic, triangle-shaped renal pyramids, a moderately echogenic renal cortex, and a highly reflective central renal sinus. The renal capsule and perinephric fat have a distinct layer of very reflective echoes that differentiate a normal right kidney from the liver (or left kidney from the spleen). The thickness of this very reflective echogenic zone varies in relation to the amount of perinephric fat deposited around the kidney.

2. The renal arteries are located on the posterolateral aortic wall. The arteries are best seen with the patient in the supine and left lateral decubitus positions. The right renal artery extends from the posterolateral wall of the aorta to enter the central renal sinus.

    On the longitudinal scan, the right renal artery can be seen as a circular structure posterior to the inferior vena cava. The right renal vein extends from the central renal sinus directly into the inferior vena cava. Both vessels appear as tubular structures in the transverse plane.

    The renal arteries have an echo-free central lumen with highly echogenic borders that consist of vessel wall and surrounding retroperitoneal fat and connective tissue. They lie posterior to the veins and can be demonstrated with certainty if their junction with the aorta is seen.

    The left renal artery flows from the central renal sinus directly to the posterolateral wall of the aorta. The left renal vein flows from the central renal sinus anterior to the aorta and posterior to the superior mesenteric vein to join the inferior vena cava. It is seen as a tubular structure on the transverse scan. It may be referred to as the "nutcracker" phenomena; i.e., "aorta-left renal vein-superior mesenteric artery."

3. The diaphragmatic crura run transversely in the paraaortic region. The crura lie posterior to the renal arteries and should be identified by their lack of pulsations and no Doppler flow.

    They vary in echogenicity, depending on the amount of surrounding retroperitoneal fat. They may appear hypoechoic, like lymph nodes.

4. The renal medulla consists of hypoechoic pyramids disbursed in a uniform distribution that are separated by bands of intervening parenchyma that extend toward the renal sinus. The pyramids are uniform in size, triangular shape, and distribution. The apex of the pyramid points toward the sinus, and the base lies adjacent to the renal cortex. The arcuate vessels lie at the base of the pyramids. The pyramids are located at the junction between the more-peripheral renal cortex and the central sinus.

5. Bertin's column is a prominent invagination of the cortex located at varying depths within the medullary substance of the kidneys. This area is normal cortex. The column may be the fusion of two septa into a single column that is twice the normal thickness. The column is most exaggerated in patients with complete or partial duplication.

    Sonographic features of a renal mass effect produced by a hypertrophied Bertin's column are as follows: a lateral indentation of the renal sinus, a clear definition from the renal sinus, or a maximum dimension that does not exceed 3 cm. In addition, there is contiguity with the renal cortex, and the overall echogenicity is similar to the renal parenchyma.

6. The dromedary hump is a cortical bulge that occurs on the lateral border of the kidney, typically more on the left. In some patients it may be so prominent that it looks like a neoplasm. It probably is the result of pressure on the developing fetal kidney by the spleen. The echogenicity is identical to the rest of the renal cortex.

7. A junctional parenchymal defect is a triangular echogenic area in the upper pole of the renal parenchyma that can be seen during normal ultrasound scanning. The defect results from the normal extensions of the renal sinus in cases where there is distinct division between the upper and lower poles of the kidney.

    The kidneys develop from the fusion of two embryonic parenchymatous masses referred to as renunculi. In cases of partial fusion, parenchymal defects occur at the junction of the renunculi and are best demonstrated on sagittal scans.

8. The duplex collecting system is a common normal variant that can be seen. Usually the sonographer cannot tell if it is complete or incomplete because it is difficult to see the ureters well. The duplex kidney is usually enlarged and has smooth margins. The central renal sinus appears as two echogenic regions separated by a cleft of moderately echogenic tissue similar in appearance to the normal renal parenchyma. The pelvis of the lower pole is usually larger than the upper pole.

9. Sinus lipomatosis is a condition that is characterized by the deposition of a moderate amount of fat in the renal sinus. The degree of proliferation of fibrofatty tissue varies.

    The renal sinus is composed of fibrous tissue, fat, lymphatic vessels, and renal vascular structures. On normal kidneys, this central zone appears as a bright area. In sinus lipomatosis, the abundant fibrous tissue may cause enlargement of the sinus region and increased echogenicity.

10. The normal renal pelvis is a triangular-shaped structure. Its axis points inferiorly and medially. An intrarenal pelvis lies almost completely within the confines of the central renal sinus. This is usually small and foreshortened. The extrarenal pelvis tends to be larger, with long, major calices. On sonography the renal pelvis appears as a central cystic area that is either partially or entirely beyond the confines of the bulk of the renal substance. Transverse views are best to see continuity with the renal sinus.

11. If the kidney is not seen in the normal position in the renal fossa, the retroperitoneum and pelvis should be scanned. Most true ectopic kidneys are located in the bony pelvis and may be malrotated. The pelvic kidney may simulate a solid adnexal mass. It may be associated with other abnormalities, such as vesicoureteral reflux and anomalous extrarenal pelvis.

12. Fusion anomalies of the kidneys include crossed renal ectopia, and a horseshoe kidney, which is the most common. In a patient with a horseshoe kidney, there is fusion of the polar regions of the kidneys during fetal development that almost invariably involves the lower poles. Usually this condition is associated with improper ascent and malrotation of the kidneys, usually in a lower retroperitoneal position. The renal pelves and ureters are more ventrally located. These kidneys usually lie closer to the spine than normal kidneys. The inferior poles lie more medially. The isthumus of the kidney lies anterior to the spine and may simulate a solid pelvic mass. Pathologic conditions associated with this are pyelocaliectasis, anomalous extrarenal pelvis, and urinary calculi.

Answers to Review Exercise B

1. A patient with renal infection or disease process may experience any of the following symptoms: flank pain, hematuria, polyuria, oliguria, fever, urgency, or generalized edema.

2. This test is essential for the detection of urinary tract disorders in patients whose renal function is impaired or absent. Most renal inflammatory processes will introduce a characteristic exudate for a specific type of inflammation into the urine. The presence of an acute infection will cause hematuria, or red blood cells in the urine. Pyuria will cause pus in the urine.

3. The abundance of hydrogen ions in a solution is called pH. The pH refers to the strength of the urine as a partly acidic or alkaline solution. The abundance of hydrogen ions in a solution is called pH. If urine contains an increased concentration of hydrogen ions, the urine is an acidic solution. Urine pH is very important in managing such diseases as bacteriuria and renal calculi. The formation of renal calculi partly depends on the pH of urine. Other conditions such as renal tubular acidosis and chronic renal failure are also associated with alkaline urine.

4. The specific gravity is the measurement of the kidney's ability to concentrate urine. The concentration factor depends on the amount of dissolved waste products within it. An excessive intake of fluids or a decrease in perspiration may cause a large output of urine and a decrease in the specific gravity. A low fluid intake, excessive perspiration, or diarrhea will cause the output of urine to be low and the specific gravity to increase.

   The specific gravity is especially low in cases of renal failure, glomerular nephritis, and pyelonephritis.

These diseases cause renal tubular damage, which affects the ability of the kidneys to concentrate urine.

5. Hematuria is the appearance of red blood cells in the urine and may indicate early renal disease. An abundance of red blood cells in the urine may be suggestive of renal trauma, calculi, or pyelonephritis; or it may suggest glomerular or vascular inflammatory processes such as acute glomerulonephritis and renal infarction.

   Leukocytes may be present whenever there is inflammation, infection, or tissue necrosis originating from anywhere in the urinary tract.

6. Hematocrit refers to the relative ratio of plasma to packed cell volume in the blood. A decreased hematocrit level occurs with acute hemorrhagic processes secondary to disease or blunt trauma.

7. The presence of hemoglobin in urine occurs whenever there is extensive damage or destruction of the functioning erythrocytes. This condition is injurious to the kidney and can cause acute renal failure.

8. The combination of specific measurements of creatinine concentrations in urine and blood serum levels is considered an accurate index for determining the glomerular filtration rate. Creatinine is a by-product of muscle energy metabolism. It is normally produced at a constant rate as long as the body muscle mass remains relatively constant.

   Creatinine goes through complete glomerular filtration without normally being reabsorbed by the renal tubules. A decreased urinary creatinine clearance indicates renal dysfunction because the decrease prevents the normal excretion of creatinine.

9. The blood urea nitrogen (BUN) is the concentration of urea nitrogen in blood, which is the end product of

cellular metabolism. Urea is formed in the liver and carried to the kidneys through the blood, to be excreted in urine. Impairment of renal function and increased protein catabolism will result in BUN elevation in relation to the degree of renal impairment and rate of urea nitrogen excreted by the kidneys.

10. Clinical symptoms include the following: flank pain, hematuria, proteinuria, white blood cells in urine, and elevated protein.

11. The clinical symptoms are hematuria and a decrease in hematocrit.

12. The clinical symptoms are acute onset of symptoms including fever, a palpable mass, elevated WBC count, and elevated pyuria.

13. The clinical symptoms are fever, flank pain, pyuria, increased BUN, increased albumin, and increased total plasma proteins.

14. The clinical symptoms (if caused by renal calculi) are moderate to severe intermittent flank pain, vomiting, hematuria, infection, and leukocytosis with infection.

15. The clinical symptoms are increased concentration of urea in blood, high urine protein excretion, high BUN, increased creatinine, and the presence of granulocytes.

16. The clinical symptoms are erythrocytosis, leukocytosis, red blood cells in urine, pyuria, and elevated LDH.

Answers to Review Exercise C

1. A simple renal cyst is generally believed to represent a retention cyst that occurs secondary to tubular obstruction, vascular occlusion, or focal inflammation. It may occur in as many as 50% of adults over 50 years of age. The sonographer should be careful not to confuse cysts with the renal pyramids.

   Ultrasound findings include no internal echoes, acoustic enhancement, clear demarcation of back wall, and a spherical or slightly ovoid shape. Low level echoes within real cysts are the result of one of the following: artifacts, infection, hemorrhage, or a necrotic cystic tumor. Technique used is high gain or reverberation from wall.

2. Atypical renal cyst ultrasound findings include echoes within, septae, and mural nodules or calcifications (1% to 3% of cysts calcify with "rim-like" calcification, usually benign; up to 20% are malignant). An atypical cyst with low-level echoes may represent hemorrhage. CT/MR may help define texture.

3. A parapelvic cyst arises in the renal hilum but doesn't communicate with collecting system.

   Ultrasound findings include no septations and irregular borders because of compression of adjacent renal sinus structures. The parapelvic cyst may obstruct; peripelvic cyst doesn't. Symptoms are infrequent and can cause pain, hypertension, and obstruction. The sonographer can differentiate from hydronephrosis by trying to connect them centrally.

4. Renal cysts that are associated with multiple renal neoplasms are von Hippel-Lindau, tuberous sclerosis, and acquired cystic disease of dialysis.

5. von Hippel-Lindau is an autosomal-dominant disease that is associated with the following neoplasms: "cerebello retinal hemangioblastomatosis," retinal angiomas, cerebellar hemangioblastomas, and abdominal cysts and tumors including renal and pancreatic cysts, renal adenomas, and frequent multiple and bilateral renal adenocarcinoma.

6. Tubular sclerosis is an autosomal-dominant lesion that is associated with multiple renal cysts and multiple and bilateral renal angiomyolipomas.

7. Patients on dialysis have an increased incidence of having renal cysts. These patients also have an increased incidence (up to seven times that of the general population) of renal adenomas and cancer. The incidence increases, particularly after the first 3 years following a transplant. The cysts can suffer spontaneous bleeding.

8. There are two kinds of polycystic renal disease: infantile and adult. Infantile is autosomal recessive. Sometimes in utero the fetus has large kidneys that are echogenic on ultrasound examination; the fetus develops renal failure and dies. In juvenile polycystic disease, there is bile duct proliferation, periportal fibrosis, portal hepatic varices, and nephromegaly. Adult polycystic disease is autosomal dominant. Adults are affected later in life. Renal failure is not as severe in onset. An adult patient usually has hypertension in the 30 to 40-year age range. Patients may have spontaneous bleeding in cysts and pain. Enlarged kidneys are replaced by cysts. The renal sinus is obliterated. Associated abnormalities include Willis' circle aneurysm in 20% of patients; liver cysts in 30% to 50%, and splenic or pancreatic cysts in 10%.

9. Two conditions in which the sonographer can see small cysts in the kidney are medullary sponge kidney and medullary cystic disease.

   Medullary sponge kidney is benign, and is rare in children. There is tubular ectasia; calcium is found in 40% to 80% of affected patients. This condition is also called *nephrocalcinosis*. Medullary sponge kidney is not hereditary.

Medullary cystic disease, or nephronopthisis, is a condition in which the kidneys are small and echodense. This disease is autosomal recessive. Salt-wasting nephropathy is present in young adults. There is tubular atrophy, which is glomerulosclerosis. Cysts are under 2 cm.

10. This is a multiloculated cystic mass or nephroma. The nephroma is benign. It presents with multiple cystic spaces and does not communicate with the renal pelvis.

11. This disease is a nonhereditary renal dysplasia. It is the most common palpable abdominal mass found in neonates. It is unilateral, with an enlarged nonfunctioning kidney. The kidney can be small and calcified in adults. Multiple cysts of varying size with no normal parenchyma are often seen. The sonographer must be able to separate it from renal hydronephrosis. Other findings include ureteral atresia, contralateral UPJ (33%), and atretic renal artery.

12. Causes of neoplasm include renal CA, cystic nephroma, and Wilms' tumor. Causes of cystic disease include localized renal cyst, a septated cyst, and segmental multicystic disease. Echinococcosis is an inflammatory cause. An organizing hematoma is a traumatic cause. A vascular lesion (AV fistula) can look cystic in the area of renal hilus; this can be ruled out with color.

Answers to Review Exercise D

1. Renal cell carcinoma is the most common of all renal tumors, comprising 85% of kidney tumors. The frequency of occurrence in males is two times that of females. The peak incidence usually does not occur until the sixth or seventh decade of life.

2. When found, it usually presents as a solid parenchymal mass, frequently with areas of hemorrhage and necrosis. Renal cell carcinoma is not usually echogenic unless calcification is present. Characteristically, the mass may be cystic or complex on ultrasound examination. Occasionally renal cell carcinoma may appear predominately as a cystic mass.

   Irregular tumor calcification can be seen in a small number of affected patients. Any calcified mass within the kidney will cause the sonographer to think of tumor; one should define the extent of involvement by scanning the renal veins, inferior vena cava, and right atrium of the heart. Color flow Doppler is useful to image the renal vein to observe flow rate; a low velocity may be seen if a lot of tumor obstruction is present.

   There is an increased incidence of renal cell carcinoma in patients with Von Hippel-Lindau disease or in patients on chronic dialysis. Tumors tend to be multiple and bilateral, and there is an increased incidence of adenomas. The tumor appears bilateral in 0.1% to 1.5% of patients.

3. Staging of renal cell carcinoma:
   Grade I confined to kidney
   Grade II spread to perinephric fat, but within Gerota's fascia
   Grade III spread to renal vein, IVC, regional lymph nodes
   Grade IV invasion of neighboring structures; distant metastases

4. This is the most common tumor of the renal collecting system. The tumor is often multiple, and is three to four times more likely to occur in males than in females. The incidence increases with age.

   On ultrasound examination, the mass is seen in the renal pelvis containing low-level echoes, widening of the central sinus echoes, and a hypoechoic central area. Clinically the patient may have a history of blood in the urine. The differential diagnosis would include other tumors of the renal pelvis such as squamous cell or adenoma, a blood clot, or a fungus ball.

5. The sonographic findings are not specific in patients with lymphoma involving the kidneys, although there is nonspecific enlargement of the kidney. The tumor is usually hypoechoic. The lymphomatous involvement of the kidneys is usually a secondary process, either via a hematogenous spread or contiguous spread from the retroperitoneum. Non-Hodgkin's lymphoma is more common than Hodgkin's. Lymphoma is more common as a bilateral invasion with multiple nodules.

6. Metastases to the kidneys is a relatively common finding at autopsy; however, it may also occur while the patient is alive. The most common primary sites of tumor spread are malignant melanoma, lymphoma, carcinoma of the lungs, breast, stomach, cervix, colon, or pancreas.

7. Nephroblastoma, or Wilms' tumor, is the most common solid renal mass found during childhood. Its incidence is rare in the newborn, with a peak incidence in the second year of life. Half of the tumors occur before the affected child's third birthday. The tumor may recur, so careful follow-up of the patient is important.

   Most of the cases present with a palpable abdominal mass. Other clinical findings may include abdominal pain, anorexia, nausea and vomiting, fever, or gross hematuria. Venous obstruction may result, with findings of leg edema, varicocele, or Budd-Chiari syndrome. The tumor may spread beyond the renal capsule and invade the venous channel, with tumor cells extending into the inferior vena cava and right atrium, with eventual metastases into the lungs. The tumor may be multifocal in a small percentage of patients.

8. This is an uncommon benign renal tumor composed mainly of fat cells. It is intermixed with smooth muscle cells and aggregates of thick-walled blood vessels. There may be hemorrhage in the tumor itself or in the subcapsular or perinephric spaces.

   On ultrasound examination, a focal, solid hyperechoic mass is typical of an angiomyolipoma. There are two primary patterns of occurrence, the most common being the tumor that is solitary, nonhereditary, and found in women who are between twenty and fifty

years of age. The other is one of multiple tumors with bilateral renal involvement found in teenagers who have tuberous sclerosis.

9. There are two common benign renal tumors: adenomas and oncocytomas. The adenoma can have calcifications. The oncocytoma resembles the spoke wheel patterns of enhancement with a central scar. To separate malignant from benign, the sonographer should look at the vascular flow patterns, the presence of nodes or metastasis surrounding the structure, or adjacent to the kidney. An ultrasound examination may distinguish the composition of a tumor, but it cannot give the histologic component of the mass.

Answers to Review Exercise E

1. The excretory and regulatory functions of the kidneys are decreased in both acute and chronic renal failure.

   Acute renal failure is typically an abrupt, transient decrease in renal function and is often heralded by oliguria. The renal causes of acute azotemia include parenchymal disease (e.g., acute glomerulonephritis, acute interstitial nephritis, and acute tubular necrosis), renal vein thrombosis and, rarely, renal-artery occlusion.

   The etiologic basis of chronic renal failure includes obstructive nephropathies, parenchymal diseases, renovascular disorders, and any process that progressively destroys nephrons.

2. Hydronephrosis may be specific, with many sonographic findings. The dilated pyelocaliceal system appears as a separation of the renal sinus echoes by fluid-filled areas that conform anatomically to the infundibula, calices, and pelvis. The renal sinus and parenchyma become compressed with progressive obstruction, and in end-stage hydronephrosis, only multiple cystic spaces may be seen.

   Whenever hydronephrosis is seen, the ureters and bladder are scanned because dilation of these structures is indicative of obstruction of the ureterovesical junction or of the urethra. A localized hydronephrosis occurs as a result of strictures, calculi, focal masses, or a duplex collecting system.

3. Intrinsic renal disease can be demonstrated by examining the renal parenchyma with ultrasound. Two classifications of disease processes have been described. One group produces a generalized increase in cortical echoes, believed to be caused by the deposition of collagen and fibrous tissue. This group includes interstitial nephritis, acute tubular necrosis, amyloidosis, diabetic nephropathy, systemic lupus erythematosus, and myeloma.

   A second group of diseases causes a predominant loss of normal anatomic detail, resulting in the inability to distinguish the cortex and medullary regions of the kidneys. This group of diseases includes chronic pyelonephritis, renal tubular ectasia, and acute bacterial nephritis.

   The end stage of many of these disease processes is renal atrophy, which can be seen on ultrasound examination by measuring renal length and cortical thickness.

   Some acute renal disorders can produce exactly the opposite findings; e.g., decreased parenchymal echogenicity and renal enlargement. Such disorders are renalvein thrombosis, pyelonephritis, and renal transplant rejection. Interstitial edema is thought to be the most likely cause of these findings.

4. Different forms of glomerulonephritis can be associated with abnormal echo patterns from the renal parenchyma on ultrasound examination. The increased cortical echoes probably result from changes within the glomerular, interstitial, tubular, and vascular structures.

   The patients have many symptoms, including the nephrotic syndrome, hypertension, anemia, and peripheral edema.

5. In acute interstitial nephritis, the kidneys are enlarged and mottled. On ultrasound examination, the renal cortical echogenicity is increased. The greatest increase in echogenicity has been described in cases of diffuse active disease.

6. Systemic lupus erythematosus is a connective tissue disorder believed to be caused by an abnormal immune system. Females are affected more often than males; peak incidence is at 20 to 40 years of age. The kidneys are involved in more than 50% of patients.

   The renal manifestations of lupus are hematuria, proteinuria, hypertension, renal vein thrombosis, and renal insufficiency. Sonography shows increased cortical echogenicity and renal atrophy.

7. AIDS is a highly contagious disease. The virus destroys T cells and then replicates rapidly within the

body. It affects many organs within the body. Patients experience with various symptoms. An echogenic parenchymal pattern is present on ultrasound examination. Cortical echogenicity is increased. Kidneys are normal in size to enlarged.

8. Renal involvement is a common finding in patients with sickle cell disease. Abnormalities include glomerulonephritis, renal vein thrombosis, papillary necrosis, and hematuria.

   The sonographic appearance of sickle cell nephropathy depends on the type of pathologic disorder. In acute renal vein thrombosis the kidneys are enlarged, with decreased echogenicity secondary to edema. In patients with subacute cases renal enlargement is present with increased cortical echoes.

9. Renal atrophy results from numerous disease processes. Intrarenal anatomy is preserved, with uniform loss of renal tissue. Renal sinus lipomatosis occurs secondary to renal atrophy. More severe lipomatosis refers to a tremendous increase in renal sinus fat content in cases of marked renal atrophy as a result of hydronephrosis and chronic calculus disease.

   The kidneys appear enlarged, with a highly echogenic, enlarged renal sinus and a thin cortical rim. Renal sinus fat is easily seen on ultrasound as very echogenic reflections.

Answers to Review Exercise F

1. Acute renal failure may occur in one of three stages: prerenal, renal, or postrenal failure. The prerenal stage is secondary to the hypoperfusion of the kidney.

   The renal stage may be caused by parenchymal diseases: acute glomerulonephritis, acute interstitial nephritis, or acute tubular necrosis. It may also be caused by renal vein thrombosis or renal artery occlusion.

   In postrenal failure, radiologic imaging plays a major role. This condition is usually caused by outflow obstruction and is potentially reversible. Postrenal failure is usually increased in patients with a malignancy of the bladder, prostate, uterus, ovaries, or rectum. Less frequent causes include retroperitoneal fibrosis and renal calculi.

2. On ultrasound examination, one can differentiate between urinary outflow obstruction and parenchymal disease. Obstruction is responsible for approximately 5% of acute renal failures. The most important issue is the presence or absence of urinary tract dilation. The degree of dilation doesn't necessarily reflect either the presence or severity of an obstruction. The sonographer should try to determine the level of obstruction. A normal ultrasound scan does not totally exclude urinary obstruction. In the clinical setting of acute obstruction secondary to calculi, a nondistended collecting system can be present.

3. Hydronephrosis is the separation of renal sinus echoes by interconnected fluid-filled areas. In patients with progressive obstruction, the renal parenchyma will be compressed.

4. If hydronephrosis is suspected, the sonographer should evaluate the bladder; if full, the sonographer should do a post-void longitudinal scan of each kidney to show the hydronephrosis has disappeared or remained the same. At the level of the obstruction, the sonographer should sweep the transducer back and forth in two planes to see if a mass can be distinguished.

5. There are three grades of hydronephrosis: Grade I refers to a small separation of the calyceal pattern, also known as *splaying*. The sonographer must be able to rule out a peripelvic cyst because the septations may be numerous, or renal vessels in the peripelvic area. (Color flow Doppler is extremely useful.) An extrarenal pelvis would protrude outside of the renal area, and the sonographer probably would not confuse this pattern with hydronephrosis. Grade II shows the "bear claw effect," with the fluid extending into the major and minor caliceal system. Grade III represents massive dilation of the renal pelvis with loss of renal parenchyma. In evaluating the patient for hydronephrosis, the sonographer should be careful to look for a dilated ureter, an enlarged prostate, which may cause the ureter to become obstructed, or an enlarged bladder, which may be secondary to an enlarged prostate. Bladder carcinoma may obstruct the pathway of the urethra, causing urine to back into the ureter and renal pelvis. A ureterocele may also block urine output. This condition occurs where the ureter inserts into the bladder wall. The ureter can turn inside out and obstruct the orifice.

6. Dilation of the renal pelvis does not always mean obstruction is present. Several other factors may cause the renal pelvis to be dilated, such as reflux, infection, high flow states (polyuria), postobstruction atrophy (once obstruction is relieved the obstruction can remain), or pregnancy dilation (the enlarged uterus can compress the ureter—usually occurs more on the right).

7. There are many conditions that may mimic hydronephrosis, such as extrarenal pelvis, parapelvic cysts, reflux, transient diuresis, congenital megacalices, papillary necrosis, renal artery aneurysm, which may be

distinguished by color Doppler, or an arterial-venous malformation, which also may be distinguished by color Doppler.

Localized hydronephrosis may be secondary to strictures, calculi, or focal masses (transitional). A duplex system can be obstructed because of an ectopic insertion of a ureter. In females it can insert below the external urinary sphincter and cause dribbling.

In patients with a false negative hydronephrosis, several techniques may be used to help distinguish the dilated renal pelvis from another condition. In patients with retroperitoneal fibrosis or necrosis, the sonographer should give a fluid challenge to see if the renal pelvis dilates. In patients with a distal calculi no obstruction may be seen unless the calculi has been there for several days. A staghorn calculus can mask an associated dilation.

The sonographer should be careful not to confuse adult polycystic disease and multicystic renal disease with severe hydronephrosis. In patients with severe hydronephrosis, the image would show dilated calices as they radiate from a larger central fluid collection in the renal pelvis. The kidney usually retains a normal shape. The sonographer would see fluid-filled sacs in a radiating pattern, or "cauliflower" configuration.

In patients with adult polycystic renal disease and multicystic renal disease, the renal cysts are randomly distributed, the contour is disturbed, and the cysts are variable in size.

Once the sonographer has shown that renal failure is not caused by obstruction, he/she should consider renal medical disease, which is the leading cause of acute renal failure.

8. Infarcts within the renal parenchyma appear as irregular masses somewhat triangular in shape along the periphery of the renal border. The renal contour may be somewhat lumpy in appearance. Remember that lobulations in the pediatric patient may be normal, except for the dromedary hump variant. In the adult patient, the renal contour should be smooth. The irregular area may appear to be slightly more echogenic than the renal parenchyma in the patient with a renal infarct.

9. This is the most common medical renal disease to produce acute renal failure, although it can be reversible. The ultrasound scan shows bilateral enlarged kidneys with hyperechoic pyramids; this can revert to normal appearance. The differential diagnosis would include nephrocalcinosis.

In pediatric patients the renal pyramids are very echogenic, without shadowing. The calculi may be too small to not cause dilation and shadowing. As renal function improves, the echogenicity decreases.

This can occur in the medulla or cortex. If this reverses, this is probably acute tubular necrosis.

10. This condition is characterized by a diffusely echogenic kidney with a loss of normal anatomy. It is a nonspecific ultrasound finding. Chronic renal disease can be caused by multiple etiologies. AIDS can cause the kidneys to be echogenic. If chronic renal disease is bilateral, small kidneys are identified. This may be caused by hypertension, chronic inflammation, or chronic ischemia.

11. There is a spectrum of severity. The disease can progress from pyelonephritis to focal bacterial nephritis to an abscess. An abscess can be transmitted through the parenchyma into the blood. Most renal infections stay in the kidney and are resolved with antibiotics. A perirenal abscess occurs from a direct extension.

12. This condition occurs when pus is found within the obstructed renal system. It is often associated with severe urosepsis and represents a true urologic emergency that requires urgent percutaneous drainage. It usually occurs secondary to longstanding ureteral obstruction from calculus disease, stricture, or a congenital anomaly.

The ultrasound findings include the presence of low-level echoes with a fluid debris level. The sonographer should be aware that an anechoic dilated system can occur; may have to do an ultrasound-guided aspiration or CT.

13. This disease process shows very echogenic pyramids with or without associated shadowing. Renal stones are very echogenic, with shadowing posterior. The patient may have a fever; this may indicate infection with hydronephrosis. When searching for renal stones, the sonographer should scan along the lines of the renal fat. Usually the stones are small and may not shadow.

14. Before the ultrasound examination for the evaluation of a renal mass, a complete review of the patient's chart and previous diagnostic examinations should be made by the sonographer. Many patients may have already had a previous imaging study, such as an intravenous pylogram, CT, or MR study. These films should be obtained before beginning the ultrasound study to tailor the examination to answer the clinical problem. The sonographer should evaluate the films for the shape and size of the kidney, determine the location of the mass lesion, look for distortion of the renal or ureter structure, and look for the presence of calcium stones or gas within the kidney.

15. Renal masses are categorized as cystic, solid, or complex by ultrasound evaluation. A cystic mass will appear sonographically with several characteristic features; i.e., a smooth, well-defined circular border, a

sharp interface between the cyst and renal parenchyma, no internal echoes (anechoic), and appear excellent through transmission beyond the posterior border.

A solid lesion would project as a nongeometric shape with irregular borders, poorly defined interface between the mass and the kidney, low-level internal echoes, weak posterior border as a result of the increased attenuation of the mass, and poor through transmission.

Areas of necrosis, hemorrhage, abscess, or calcification within the mass may alter the above classification and cause the lesion to fall into the complex category. This means the mass shows characteristics associated with both the cystic and solid lesions.

Real-time ultrasonography allows the sonographer to carefully evaluate the renal parenchyma in many stages of respiration. If the mass is very small, respiratory motion may cause it to move in and out of the field of view. With the combined use of careful evaluation of the best respiratory phase and the use of the cine-loop feature, most renal masses may be adequately imaged to determine their characteristic composition.

16. Renal cystic disease encompasses a wide range of disease processes that may be classified as simple renal cystic disease that may be typical, complicated, or atypical. The disease may be acquired or inherited, such as von Hippel-Lindau disease or tuberous sclerosis. More complex cystic disease includes adult polycystic, infantile polycystic, or multicystic disease. There may be cystic disease in the renal medulla or sinus.

17. Simple renal cysts are common, occurring in half of adults over 50 years of age. The renal cyst may be located anywhere in the kidney and is not of clinical significance unless it causes distortion of the adjacent calices or produces hydronephrosis or pain.

Sonographic features of a simple renal cyst include a well-defined mass lesion, smooth wall, and circular anechoic mass with good through transmission. The tadpole sign may be seen as narrow bands of acoustic shadowing posterior to the margins of the cyst along the lateral borders of enhancement.

A septum may be occasionally seen within the cyst as a well-defined linear line. This would mean the cyst was not a simple cyst, but a cyst with septations. Sometimes small sacculations or infoldings of the cystic wall may produce wall irregularity, and a cyst puncture or aspiration may be recommended to ascertain the pathology of the fluid within the mass.

Low-level echoes within a renal cyst may be caused by artifact (sensitivity too high, or transducer frequency too low); infection, hemorrhage, or a necrotic cystic tumor.

18. A parapelvic cyst is found in the renal hilum but doesn't communicate with the renal collecting system.

The ultrasound findings show a well-defined mass with no internal septations. It can have irregular borders because it may compress the adjacent renal sinus structures. The parapelvic cyst may obstruct the kidney; the peripelvic cyst does not. Clinical symptoms are infrequent, although the cyst can cause pain, hypertension, or obstruction.

The sonographer should be able to differentiate the parapelvic cyst from hydronephrosis by connecting the dilated renal pelvis centrally. The dilated renal pelvis may appear to look like a cauliflower, while the parapelvic cyst is more well-defined.

19. Polycystic renal disease may present in one of two forms: the infantile autosomal-recessive form, or the adult autosomal-dominant form.

The infantile form may occur in the fetus with large echogenic kidneys, which progresses to renal failure and eventually to intrauterine demise.

The juvenile form occurs with bile duct proliferation, periportal fibrosis, portal hepatic varices, and nephromegaly.

The adult form occurs later in life, with hypertension and renal failure not as severe in onset. The kidneys are enlarged as they are replaced bilaterally with multiple cysts. The cysts may grow so large as to obliterate the renal sinus. The cysts may have spontaneous bleeding, causing flank pain for the patient.

Associated abnormalities include a Willis' circle aneurysm in 20% of patients, liver cysts in 50%, splenic cysts in 10%, and pancreatic cysts in 10%.

20. This disease is a nonhereditary renal dysplasia that usually occurs unilaterally. Bilateral disease is incompatible with life. In neonates and children the kidneys are enlarged; in adulthood they may be small and calcified. The typical pattern is multiple cysts of varying size with no normal renal parenchyma.

Other findings may also be present, including ureteral atresia, which is failure of the ureter to develop from the caliceal system; contralateral uretoropelvic obstruction in 30% of patients (the development of the ureter from the bladder with retrograde filling); nonfunctioning kidney; or an atretic renal artery. This disease is the most common palpable abdominal mass in neonates.

21. This disease is autosomal recessive. It is caused by salt-wasting nephropathy occurring in young adults. The patient has small echodense kidneys, tubular atrophy, and glomerulosclerosis. There are multiple small cysts under 2 cm.

Answers to Self-Test

1. b	**42.** b	**83.** c
2. c	**43.** true	**84.** a
3. d	**44.** c	**85.** d
4. d	**45.** d	**86.** d
5. b	**46.** b	**87.** d
6. b	**47.** false	**88.** c
7. a	**48.** false	**89.** d
8. b	**49.** a	**90.** a
9. b	**50.** c	**91.** a
10. b	**51.** a	**92.** b
11. urethra	**52.** b	**93.** a
12. glomerulus	**53.** c	**94.** a
13. Bowman's capsule	**54.** a	**95.** c
14. excretion	**55.** true	**96.** d
15. elimination	**56.** false	**97.** d
16. urea	**57.** a	**98.** a
17. uric acid	**58.** true	**99.** d
18. hilus	**59.** d	**100.** c
19. cortex	**60.** c	**101.** a
20. uric acid	**61.** d	**102.** a
21. pelvis	**62.** b	**103.** a
22. major calyceal	**63.** true	**104.** c
23. pyramids	**64.** c	**105.** d
24. medulla	**65.** b	**106.** b
25. papilla	**66.** true	**107.** c
26. true	**67.** false	**108.** a
27. false	**68.** b	**109.** a
28. b	**69.** c	**110.** d
29. c	**70.** b	**111.** b
30. d	**71.** a	**112.** c
31. d	**72.** a	**113.** a
32. b	**73.** b	**114.** c
33. d	**74.** c	**115.** d
34. i	**75.** a	**116.** b
35. g	**76.** c	**117.** b
36. c, h, j	**77.** d	**118.** e
37. b	**78.** b	**119.** c
38. d	**79.** b	**120.** c
39. l	**80.** b	**121.** d
40. a, e, m	**81.** a	**122.** d
41. f, k	**82.** b	

Answers to Case Reviews

1. (Figure 8-4) The dromedary hump *(arrow)* is a cortical bulge that occurs on the lateral border of the kidney, typically more on the left than the right.
(Figure 8-5) A junctional parenchymal defect *(arrows)* is a triangular echogenic area in the upper pole of the renal parenchyma.
(Figure 8-6) This shows duplex collecting system. The central renal sinus *(cs)* appears as two echogenic regions separated by a cleft of moderately echogenic tissue similar in appearance to the normal renal parenchyma.
(Figure 8-7) This is a longitudinal scan of the right kidney, showing increased renal sinus fat consistent with renal sinus lipomatosis.
(Figure 8-8) This shows an extrarenal pelvis. It is a transverse scan of the right kidney showing the renal

pelvis appearing as a cystic area *(erp)* that extends beyond the confines of the bulk of the renal substance.

2. (Figure 8-9) *A* and *B,* Longitudinal scans of the right and left kidneys in a pediatric patient. It was very difficult to record the lower poles of both kidneys. *C,* Transverse scan of the renal area shows a hypoechoic tissue mass connected with both kidneys. This represented the isthmus of the horseshoe kidney.

3. (Figure 8-10) These are transverse and longitudinal scans of two small renal cysts along the lateral wall of the kidney. The borders are smooth and well defined. No internal echoes are seen.

4. (Figure 8-11) Patients with polycystic disease show enlargement of both kidneys, with multiple small cystic areas throughout. *A* to *C,* Longitudinal and transverse scans of the right kidney. *D* to *F,* Longitudinal and transverse scans of the left kidney. All of the cysts were distinct lesions and did not connect with the central renal sinus to indicate hydronephrosis.

5. (Figure 8-12) About one third of the patients with polycystic renal disease will also have polycystic liver disease. This severe case shows multiple cysts throughout the liver parenchyma. Often the cysts are so complex that it becomes difficult to distinguish the renal parenchyma from the liver.

6. (Figure 8-13) Longitudinal scans of a young patient with medullary sponge kidney show nephrocalcinosis and an echogenic medullary renal parenchyma.

7. (Figure 8-14) Renal cell carcinoma is seen in this 62-year-old male who presented with hematuria. The mass is complex *(arrows),* distorting the renal parenchyma. This shows a longitudinal scan of the mass as it distorts the central renal parenchyma.

8. (Figure 8-15) This shows longitudinal and transverse scans of a transitional cell carcinoma. The mass is hypoechoic and is located near the renal sinus.

9. (Figure 8-16) The tumor arises from the right kidney *(RK)* and compresses the renal sinus. It is clearly separate from the liver *(L).* This was a Wilms' tumor of the kidney.

10. (Figure 8-17) One of the complications of a Wilms' tumor is the spread beyond the renal capsule into the renal vein and inferior vena cava. This 18-month-old child had a huge complex tumor, with extension into the inferior vena cava *(arrows).* The longitudinal scan *(C)* shows the dilated IVC, with tumor echoes along the posterior border. The tumor may extend into the right atrium of the heart.

11. (Figure 8-18) An incidental finding of an angiomyolipoma is seen in the upper pole of the left kidney *(arrows).*

12. (Figure 8-19) This shows hydronephrosis of the kidney. The dilated pyelocaliceal system appears as a separation of the renal sinus echoes by fluid-filled areas that conform anatomically to the infundibula, calices, and pelvis.

13. (Figure 8-20) A distended urinary bladder may cause "pseudohydronephrosis" of both kidneys and ureters. The patient should be scanned after the bladder has been emptied. *C* and *D* show the distended ureters in transverse and longitudinal sections.

14. (Figure 8-21) Patients with lupus nephritis will show a very echogenic renal parenchymal pattern as compared with the liver. Renal atrophy is usually present.

15. (Figure 8-22) This shows atrophy of the right kidney in a patient with renal ischemia.

16. (Figure 8-23) Findings in a patient with pyonephrosis include a fluid/debris level within a well-defined mass lesion.

17. (Figure 8-24) A patient with xanthogranulomatous pyelonephritis shows a large, nonfunctioning right kidney secondary to a stone. Multiple areas of shadowing are seen within the renal parenchyma from the renal stones.

18. (Figure 8-25) These are transverse and longitudinal scans of a patient with a ureterovesical stone (echogenic area with shadowing) at the distal segment of the ureter.

19. (Figure 8-26) The hyperechogenic cortex appears as swollen sonolucent pyramids against the background of increased echogenicity of the outer and interpyramidal cortex. In addition, this patient had obstruction near the distal ureter, causing mild dilation of the renal pelvis and ureter.

20. (Figure 8-27) Distortion of the renal outline caused by localized areas of swelling involving both the cortex and the pyramids is secondary to early rejection. The renal sinus echoes may appear compressed.

21. (Figure 8-28) A tender cystic collection of fluid was located above and to the right of the umbilicus and anterior to the IVC represented an infected lymphocele. The patient also had mild to moderate hydronephrosis.

22. (Figure 8-29) These show abnormal flow patterns in a patient with rejection.
    A, Large hypoechoic area along the anterior border of the kidney, with compression of the calyceal system.
    B, Abnormal flow pattern in the segmental artery, with decreased diastolic flow and increased R.I. to .9.
    C, Abnormal flow in the interlobar artery.
    D, Abnormal flow in the acruate artery.
    E, Ther patient had a renal biopsy; status post-biopsy shows fine stippled echoes throughout the bladder, indicating hematoma within the bladder. Prebiopsy and postbiopsy scans should routinely be made to search for hematoma collections around the kidney or within the bladder.

CHAPTER
9
The Spleen

OBJECTIVES

At the completion of this chapter, students will show orally, in writing, or by demonstration that they will be able to:

1. Describe the location, size, and position of the spleen.
2. Describe the internal and surface anatomy of the spleen.
3. Illustrate the cross-sectional anatomy of the spleen and adjacent structures.
4. Describe the appearance and significance of splenic congenital anomalies.
5. Recall the functions of the spleen.
6. Select pertinent laboratory tests and radiologic procedures.
7. Explain the use of laboratory tests in the evaluation of the spleen.
8. Identify regressive and circulatory changes affecting the spleen.
9. Summarize the affect of systemic infections and anemia on the spleen.
10. Identify those conditions that cause splenomegaly by explaining their clinical significance.
11. Differentiate between sonographic appearances by explaining the clinical significance of primary tumors and cysts that involve the spleen.
12. State four diseases of the spleen seen in children and young adults.
13. Create high-quality diagnostic scans demonstrating the appropriate anatomy in all planes pertinent to the spleen.
14. Select the correct equipment settings appropriate to individual body habitus.
15. Distinguish between the normal and abnormal sonographic appearances of the spleen.

To further enhance learning, students should use marking pens to color the anatomic illustrations that follow.

SPLEEN

FIGURE 9-1

Relationship of Spleen to Adjacent Structures

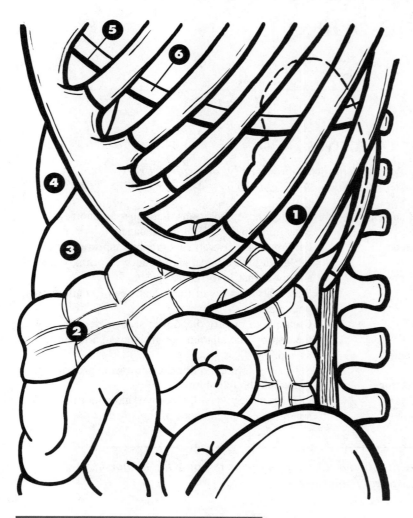

The spleen is an intraperitoneal organ that is almost completely covered with peritoneum except for a small area at the hilum. The spleen lies in the left hypochondrium, with its axis along the shaft of the tenth rib (Figure 9-1). Its lower pole extends forward as far as the midaxillary line. It is of variable size and shape but is generally considered to be ovoid, with a convex superior and a concave inferior surface. The ends of the spleen are posterior and anterior extremities, and its borders are superior and inferior.

1 spleen
2 transverse colon
3 stomach
4 liver
5 diaphragm
6 costodiaphragmatic recess

FIGURE 9-2
Spleen and Its Surrounding Structures

Relational Anatomy

Anterior to the spleen lies the stomach, the tail of the pancreas, and the left colic flexure (Figure 9-2). The left kidney lies along the medial border of the spleen. Posteriorly the diaphragm, left pleura, left lung, and ninth, tenth, and eleventh ribs are in contact with the spleen.

Blood is supplied by the splenic artery, which immediately divides into six branches after entering the splenic hilum.

The splenic vein leaves the splenic hilum and joins the superior mesenteric vein to form the portal vein.

The lymph vessels emerging from the hilum pass through a few lymph nodes along the course of the splenic artery and drain into the celiac nodes. The nerves to the spleen accompany the splenic artery and are derived from the celiac plexus.

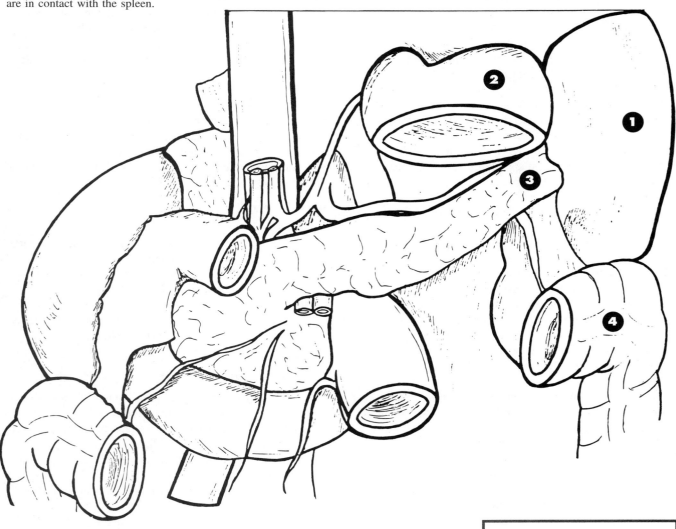

1	spleen
2	stomach
3	tail of the pancreas
4	descending colon

Spleen Review Notes

ANATOMY

- The spleen is the largest organ of the reticuloendothelial system.
- It plays an important role in the defense mechanism of the body.
- It is involved in pigment and lipid metabolism.
- Its architecture consists of white pulp (lymphoid tissue) and intervening red pulp (red blood cells and reticulum cells).
- It is normally devoid of hematopoietic activity.
- It is rarely the primary site of disease.
- It is often affected by a systemic disease process.
- It lies between the left hemidiaphragm and stomach, related to the 8th to 11th ribs but has poor contact with the diaphragm—big LLL, ascites, deformity of left hemidiaphragm, small horizontal spleen.
- The diaphragm is seen as a bright, curvilinear echogenic structure close to the proximal superolateral surface of the spleen.
- The medial surface is related to the stomach, tail of pancreas, left kidney, and splenic flexure of colon. Close proximity to these structures facilitates extention of inflammatory processes.
- The spleen is covered with peritoneum except for the hilum.
- It is held in place by lienorenal, gastrosplenic, and phrenicolic ligaments.
- The ligaments are derived from layers of peritoneum that form the greater and lesser sacs.
- An LUQ mass may displace the spleen inferiorly.
- Caudad displacement may be secondary to subclavian abscess, splenic cysts, and left pleural effusion.
- Cephalad displacement leads to left lung volume loss, left pneumothorax, paralysis of left hemidiaphragm, and large intraabdominal mass.
- Post-repair of congenital ventral hernia leads to an abnormally shaped spleen and liver, which will be more ventrally located.
- "Upside down spleen" involves rotation on the long AP axis, with the hilus directed cephalad or lateral. This may mimic a left suprarenal mass.
- A normal spleen with medial lobulation between the pancreas tail and left kidney may be confused with a cystic mass in the tail of the pancreas on ultrasound examination with the patient in the prone position.
- Anatomy varies in contour and orientation:
  - orange-segment—44%
  - tetrahedal—42%
  - triangular—14%
- The configuration also varies:
  - compact spleen; narrow hilus, even borders
  - disrupted spleen; widespread hilus

- notched anterior border
- thumblike lobe at inferior pole
- expanded portion or "tubercle" at upper medial pole
- "Wandering spleen"/splenic torsion is observed as ectopic, aberrant, floating, splenic ptosis. The name refers to migration of the spleen from its normal location in the LUQ. It is the result of an embryologic anomaly of the supporting ligaments of the spleen. (For splenomegaly and abdominal laxity, multiple pregnancies and too many hormones may be predisposing factors.) The patient initially shows an abdominal or a pelvic mass, with intermittant pain and volvulus (splenic torsion). Sonographers should use a color flow to map vascularity and note the typical splenic pattern to identify spleen tissue.

TECHNIQUE

- No patient preparation is needed.
- Various positions include supine and right lateral decubitus or prone in inspiration; transverse and sagittal.
- A normal pattern is homogeneous with internal echoes slightly less or equal to liver.

SPLENIC SIZE

- Volume index:
  Width > trans. at xyphoid in normal or at widest point
  Thickness (AP) > enlarged spleen
  Length > longitudinal—midaxillary line (splenomegaly-measure at longitudinal supine point)
  Multiply values:
  Width × Thickness × Length >>>> Splenic volume index (SVI) = 8 to 34 in 95% of normal spleens
- 27 (cube of three values)

ACCESSORY SPLEEN

- An accessory spleen results from failure of fusion of separate splenic masses forming on the dorsal mesogastrium.
- It is commonly located in the splenic hilum or along the splenic vessels of associated ligaments.
- It may occur from the diaphragm to the scrotum.
- It is usually small.
- There are usually no clinical problems such as torsion and infarction.
- It may simulate the surrounding structure and look like a "tumor" mass.
- Ultrasound can detect the splenic appearance, location, and blood supply.
- It is a round or an oval solid structure.
- It has similar echogenicity as splenic tissue.
- It is surrounded by high-amplitude interfaces that separate it from adjacent parenchymal organs.
- It may be near the splenic hilum—splenocolic ligament.

FOCAL DISEASE

- Focal disease may be single or multiple.
- It may be found in normal or enlarged spleens.
- Major nontraumatic causes for focal splenic defects include tumors (benign and malignant), infarction, abscesses, and cysts.
- Splenic defects may be incidental (seen on another imaging study) or specific (splenic infarct or abscess).

TUMORS OF THE SPLEEN
Benign Primary Neoplasms (rare)

- Hamartomas
- Cavernous hemangiomas
- Cystic lymphangiomas

Hamartomas

- Hamartomas have solid and cystic components.
- They are hyperechoic.
- They produce no symptoms.
- They may be solitary or multiple.
- They are well defined and not encapsulated.
- They are composed of lymphoid tissue or are a combination of sinuses and structures equivalent to pulp cords of normal splenic tissue.

Cavernous Hemangiomas

- This large, inhomogeneous echogenic mass has multiple, small hypoechoic areas.
- There are no symptoms; the incidence is 1 in 600.
- Patients show symptoms when the size of spleen increases, compressing other organs. This sometimes leads to anemia and a low-grade infection.
- Splenic rupture with peritoneal symptoms can occur in 25% of patients.
- There is a mixed ultrasound appearance, including infarction with coagulated blood or fibrin in cavities.
- Unspecific ultrasound features are also seen. (The differential includes hydatid cyst, abscess, dermoid, and mets.)

Cystic Lymphangiomas

- This benign malformation of the lymphatics is composed of endothelium-lined cystic spaces.
- It appears as a mass with extensive cystic replacement of splenic parenchyma.
- Lymphangiomatosis affects predominately the somatic soft tissue (found in neck, axilla, mediastinum, retroperitoneum, and soft tissues of extremities).
- Cystic lymphangioma may involve multiple organ systems or may be confined to solitary organs such as the liver, spleen, kidney, or colon.
- Splenic involvement is rare.
- A multicystic appearance is characteristic.

Malignant Primary Neoplasm (rare)

- Hemangiosarcoma is a rare malignant neoplasm arising from vascular endothelium of the spleen.
- It looks similar to cavernous hemangioma (mixed cystic pattern).
- It can also be hyperechoic.

Lymphoma (common)

- The spleen is commonly involved in lymphoma.
- It is difficult to detect splenic lymphoma.
- The pattern is typically hypoechoic.
- Focal areas are also seen.

Metastases (uncommon)

- Metastases are the result of hematogenous spread.
- The spleen is the tenth most common site (from breast, lung, ovary, stomach, melanoma, and prostate)
- It is usually associated with splenic involvement of other organs.
- Mets may be microscopic; patients rarely display symptoms.
- Splenic infarction with associated perisplenitis has been attributed to tumor emboli.
- Metastases may show as focal with a hypoechoic or hyperechoic pattern.
- Melanoma deposits appear hypoechoic but of higher echo amplitude than lymphoma; some are echodense.

Infarction (common)

- Infarction is caused by septic emboli and local thromboses in patients with pancreatitis, subacute bacterial endocarditis, leukemia, lymphomatous disorders, sickle cell anemia, sarcoidosis, and polyarteritis nodosa.
- Its appearance depends on the onset of the infarct.
- A fresh hemorrhagic infarct is hypoechoic.
- A healed infarct with scar tissue appears as an echogenic, wedge-shaped lesion with the base toward the subcapsular surface of the spleen.

Abscess (uncommon)

- Abscesses are uncommon probably because of phagocytic activity of the efficient reticuloendothelial system and leukocytes.
- The system may be breached from the following:
  - SBE
  - septicemia
  - decreased immunologic states
  - drug abuse
- An abscess may be spread from distant foci.
- There may be history of trauma.
- Invasion of extrinsic process may involve perinephric or subphrenic abscess, perforated gastric or colonic lesions, or pancreatic abscess.

- Direct extension of inflammatory processes from adjacent organs occurs in 10% of cases.
- Mortality is increased if the diagnosis is delayed.
- Clinical findings are subtle and include fever, LUQ tenderness, abdominal pain, left shoulder pain, flank pain, and a big spleen.
- One third of patients have an increased left hemidiaphragm or pleural effusion.

Ultrasound Findings

- Mixed echo patterns:
  - Hypoechoic often with hyperechoic foci that represent debris or gas
  - Thick or shaggy walls
  - Anechoic
  - Poor definition
  - Increased to decreased transmission (depending on presence of gas)

Cysts (uncommon)

- Cysts are classified as parasitic or nonparasitic in origin.
- Echinococcus is the only parasite that forms splenic cysts (uncommon in the United States).
- Parasitic cysts appear as anechoic lesions with possible daughter cysts and Ca^{++} or as solid masses with fine internal echoes and poor distal enhancement.
- Nonparasitic cysts of the spleen have been categorized as either true or "primary."
- Cysts (epidermoid cysts) contain an epithelial lining and are considered to be of congenital origin or are false or "secondary" cysts lacking a cellular lining, probably developing as a result of prior trauma to the spleen and accounting for 80% of nonparasitic splenic cysts.
- Epithelial-lined cysts (spidermoid cysts) are usually solitary and unilocal and rarely contain Ca^{++}.
- The internal surface of the cyst may be smooth or trabeculated.
- Fluid may be clear or turbid and may contain protein, iron, bilirubin, fat, and cholesterol crystals.
- Cysts occur more frequently in females (50% occur in patients under 15 years of age).
- Patients are initially seen with an asymptomatic LUQ mass.

Ultrasound Findings

- Hypoechoic or anechoic foci with well-defined walls and increased through transmission
- Internal echoes at increased gain
- Hemorrhage producing fluid level in some cases

DIFFUSE DISEASE

- Erythropoietic abnormalities:
  - Sickle cell
  - Hereditary spherocytosis
  - Hemolytic anemia
  - Chronic anemia
  - Polycythemia vera
  - Thalassemia
  - Myeloproliferative disorders
- Pathology: congestion of red pulp and RE cell hypertrophy
  - production of isoechoic pattern, same as liver
- Granulocytopoietic abnormalities:
  - Cases of reactive hyperplasia due to acute or chronic infection
  - Splenitis (e.g., sarcoid, TB)
  - Lymphoid hyperplasia of white pulp and lymphocytes, neutrophils, and/or phagocytic cells in the red pulp
  - Splenomegaly seen as diffusely hypoechoic (less dense than liver)
- Myeloproliferative disorders:
  - Acute and chronic myelogenous leukemias
  - Polycythemia vera
  - Myelofibrosis
  - Megakaryocytic leukemia
  - Erythroleukemia
- Isoechoic ultrasound pattern
- Hypoechoic compared with liver findings
- Lymphopoietic abnormalities:
  - Lymphoietic leukemias
  - Lymphoma
  - Hodgkin's disease

Ultrasound Findings

- Diffusely hypoechoic splenic pattern
  - Focal lesions possibly present
  - Non-Hodgkin's reported as having isoechoic echo-pattern
- The spleen is isoechoic in RE disorders and in congestion.

TRAUMA

- Blunt trauma is the most common cause.
- The tear may result in linear or stellate lacerations and capsular tears and may result from traction from adhesions or suspensary ligaments, puncture wounds from foreign bodies or rib fractures, subcapsular hematomas, avulsion of vascular pedicle, and laceration of short gastric vessels.
- Free blood can be seen immediately after trauma.
- Delayed ruptures may develop subcapsular hematoma, with subsequent rupture or small splenic laceration that was temporarily tamponaded.

Clinical Findings

- LUQ pain (100%)
- Left shoulder pain (50%)
- Left flank pain (36%)
- Dizziness (21%)

Signs
- LUQ tenderness
- Hypotension
- Decreased hemoglobin level

Ultrasound Findings
- Findings include splenomegaly with progressive enlargement and an irregular splenic border. Hematoma, contusion (splenic inhomogeneity), subcapsular and pericapsular fluid collections (subcapsular hematoma), free intraperitoneal blood, and left pleural effusion are also seen.
- Focal hematomas are represented by intrasplenic fluid collections.
- In subcapsular hematomas, perisplenic fluid is seen.
- Blood exhibits various echo patterns depending on the age of the trauma.
- After 24 hours, hemorrhage may appear hyperechoic (may be difficult to distinguish from normal splenic tissue; may see double contour).
- As protein and cells reabsorb, hematoma becomes organized and fluid becomes hyperechoic.
- Focal areas represent tiny splenic lacerations that give rise to small collections of blood interspersed with disrupted splenic pulp (contusion).

- With time, hematoma will become more fluid or lucent appearing.
- Echo free, intraperitoneal fluid probably represents blood intermixed with peritoneal transudate due to presence of blood within the cavity.
- Healing takes weeks to months.
- Free fluid disappears quicker because fluid is moved across the pleural and peritoneal membranes rapidly (2 to 4 weeks).
- Intrasplenic hematomas and contusions take longer because the fluid, protein, and necrotic debris must be resorbed from within a solid organ in which the blood supply has already been focally disrupted.
- When the spleen returns to normal, small, irregular foci may remain or parenchyma may be normal.

THE SPLEEN AND CONGENITAL HEART DISEASE
- Asplenia and polysplenia syndromes
- Complex cardiac malformations, bronchopulmonary abnormalities, and visceral hetoerotaxia (anomalous placement of organs or major blood vessels)
  - Horizontal liver
  - Malrotation of gut
  - Interruption of IVC with azygous continuation

Review Exercise • The Spleen

1. Describe the functions of the spleen. _____

_____

_____

_____

2. Discuss the location and shape of the spleen. _____

_____

3. What is an accessory spleen, and where is it usually found? _____

_____

_____

4. Describe the lymph vessels located near the spleen. _____

_____

_____

5. Name the ligaments attached to the spleen and their significance. _____

_____

_____

6. What is a wandering spleen? _____

_____

_____

7. What is the significance of splenic agenesis? _____

_____

_____

_____

8. What are the two types of splenic congestion and how do they affect the splenic size? _____

_____

_____

_____

9. Name the causes for nontraumatic focal defects in the spleen. _____

_____

_____

10. Name the common benign primary tumors of the spleen. _____

_____

_____

_____

11. Describe the ultrasound appearance of a hamartoma of the spleen. _____

_____

_____

_____

12. What is the ultrasound appearance of a cavernous hemangioma? _____

_____

_____

13. What is the ultrasound appearance of lymphoma? _____

_____

_____

14. Describe the course of metastases to the spleen. _____

_____

15. What is the cause for a splenic infarction? Describe the ultrasound appearance. _____

_____

_____

_____

_____

16. Discuss the occurrence of a splenic cyst and describe the difference between a true and false cyst. _____

_____

_____

_____

17. What are the ultrasound findings of a splenic cyst? _____

_____

_____

18. Give examples of erythropoietic abnormalities of the spleen and their ultrasound findings. _____

_____

_____

_____

19. What is an example of a granulocytopoietic abnormality of the spleen? Discuss the ultrasound findings. _____

_____

_____

_____

20. Discuss the ultrasound appearance of lymphopoietic abnormalities and give an example. _____

_____

_____

_____

21. Discuss the significance and findings in trauma to the spleen. _____

_____

_____

_____

Self-Test • The Spleen

1. Which of the following statements regarding the spleen are false?

   a. a prominent bulge along the medial surface of the spleen can be seen in normal patients

   b. the normal-sized spleen should not extend caudal to the midportion of the left kidney

   c. the spleen is a retroperitoneal organ

   d. the sonographic texture of the normal spleen is homogeneous

2. The best sonographic window to the left hemidiaphragm is the:

   a. spleen

   b. kidney

   c. stomach

   d. left lung

3. Splenomegaly may be the result of all of the following except:

   a. an inflammatory process

   b. a left subphrenic abscess

   c. metastatic disease to the spleen

   d. polycythemia vera

   e. chronic leukemia and lymphomas

4. An adrenal mass may displace the splenic vein:

   a. anteriorly

   b. posteriorly

   c. medially

   d. laterally

5. A fluid collection located between the diaphragm and the spleen may represent:

   a. a pleural effusion

   b. a subcapsular hematoma

   c. a subphrenic abscess

   d. a lesser sac abscess

6. Patients with right-side heart failure and elevated systemic venous pressure may develop:

   a. fatty liver

   b. portal-systemic anastomoses

   c. marked dilation of the intrahepatic veins

   d. nonfocal liver disease

7. The normal sonographic texture of the spleen is:

   a. homogeneous with internal echoes equal to those of the liver or less echogenic than the liver

   b. hypoechoic

   c. strongly echopenic but more echogenic than the liver

   d. hyperechoic

8. The spleen is:

    a. the center for hematopoietic activity

    b. the largest organ containing lymphoid tissue in the body

    c. not a part of the reticuloendothelial system

    d. a contributor to the production of alkaline phosphatase

9. Which statement describes the correct anatomic location of structures adjacent to the spleen?

    a. the diaphragm is anterior, lateral, and inferior to the spleen

    b. The fundus of the stomach and lesser sac are medial and posterior to the splenic hilum

    c. the left kidney lies inferior and medial to the spleen

10. Which of the following causes anterior displacement of the IVC?

    a. splenomegaly

    b. hydronephrosis

    c. enlarged lymph nodes

    d. pancreatitis

11. All of the following are functions of the spleen except:

    a. production of plasma cells

    b. production of lymphocytes

    c. destruction of red blood cells

    d. destruction of white blood cells

12. Cysts of the spleen are:

    a. infectious

    b. common

    c. of no clinical significance

    d. usually acquired

13. The spleen is variable in size, but it is considered to be which of the following?

    a. tetrahedral

    b. pentagonal

    c. triangular

    d. orange segment

14. When accessory spleens are present, they are usually located:

    a. at the inferior margin of the spleen

    b. on the posterior aspect of the spleen

    c. near the hilum of the spleen

    d. near the kidney

15. The splenic artery is located:

    a. posterior to the body of the pancreas

    b. medial to the pancreas

    c. on the superior margin of the pancreas

    d. lateral to the uncinate process

16. Anterior displacement of the splenic vein can be caused by:

    a. pancreatitis

    b. pseudocyst in the head of the pancreas

    c. left adrenal hyperplasia

    d. aneurysm of the hepatic artery

17. The major focal defects in the spleen may be caused by all of the following except:

    a. an accessory spleen

    b. tumors

    c. an infarction

    d. cysts

18. The most common benign neoplasms in the spleen include all of the following except:

    a. cavernous hemangiomas

    b. infarction

    c. cystic lymphangiomas

    d. hamartomas

19. A splenic rupture has been reported in patients with:

    a. leukemia

    b. lymphoma

    c. metastases

    d. hemangioma

20. Primary tumors that may metastasize to the spleen include all of the following except:

    a. melanoma

    b. ovary

    c. lung

    d. brain

21. What is the easiest patient position and sonographic technique used to demonstrate splenomegaly?

    a. The spleen normally measures less than 12 cm on a longitudinal decubitus scan.

    b. The spleen normally measures less than 10 cm on a longitudinal decubitus scan.

    c. The spleen measures less than 4 cm in a transverse scan.

    d. The spleen extends below the anterior aspect of the spine on a transverse scan.

22. With splenomegaly, the left kidney may be displaced:

    a. inferior

    b. cephalad

    c. medial

    d. anterior

23. Other areas that should be examined when ruling out a splenic rupture include all of the following except:

    a. liver and lesser sac

    b. pericardium

    c. pelvis

    d. renal gutter

24. What sonographic signs are present in a patient with histoplasmosis?

    a. calcifications

    b. cystic masses

    c. adenomas

    d. atrophy

25. What are the typical sonographic patterns of splenic infection?

    a. hyperechoic or hypoechoic mass

    b. calcifications

    c. atrophy

    d. enlargement

26. Which parasite is known to form splenic cysts?

    a. spherecyte

    b. splenocyte

    c. echinococcus

    d. ameobia

27. Which statement is not true in regards to portal hypertension?

    a. Ascites is rarely present.

    b. Splenomegaly is usually present.

    c. Portal vein size is not a reliable indicator of severity.

    d. Umbilical vein recanalization is virtually pathognomonic.

Which of the following statements are true concerning abdominal lymphoma?

28. _____ Retroperitoneal nodes appear as hypoechoic masses.

29. _____ It is considered retroperitoneal when located between the aorta and inferior vena cava.

30. _____ Mesenteric masses usually represent non-Hodgkin's lymphoma.

31. _____ Splenomegaly indicates intrinsic involvement of the spleen.

32. _____ Diffuse intrahepatic lesions can be differentiated from hepatic metastatic disease.

Case Reviews

1. A middle-aged man is scheduled for an abdominal ultrasound for right upper quadrant pain. Longitudinal decubitus **(A)** and transverse scans **(B)** of the left upper quadrant were also made. What are your findings (Figure 9-3)?

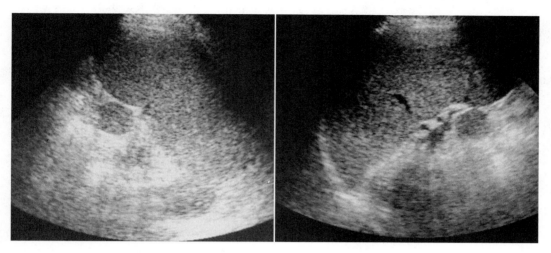

2. A 54-year-old man with rheumatoid arthritis is scheduled for an abdominal ultrasound to rule out medication-induced gallstones. What are your findings (Figure 9-4)?

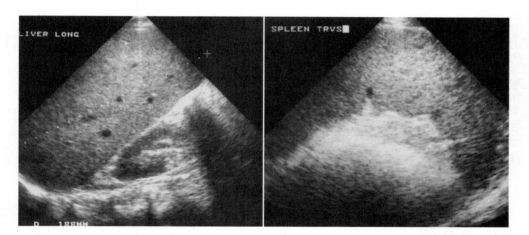

3. A young male is seen with anemia, fatigue, fever, dyspnea, and repeated infections. He was sent for an abdominal ultrasound to rule out the source of infection. What are your findings (Figure 9-5)?

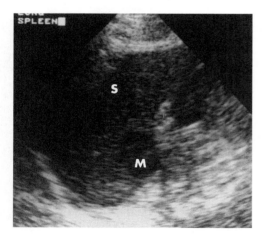

4. An asymptomatic farmer is scheduled for an abdominal ultrasound after calcifications were found on his routine upper gastrointestinal series. What are your findings (Figure 9-6)?

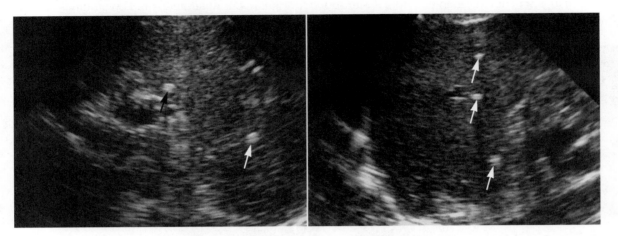

5. A young Mexican female is seen with chronic cough and vague upper abdominal pain. What are your findings (Figure 9-7)?

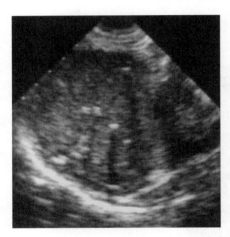

6. A young HIV-positive patient is seen with tenderness in the upper abdomen. What are your findings (Figure 9-8)?

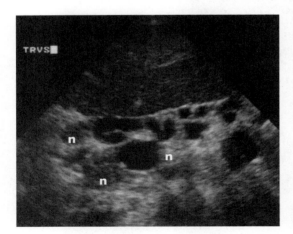

7. A 19-year-old woman presents with RUQ pain. What are your findings (Figure 9-9)?

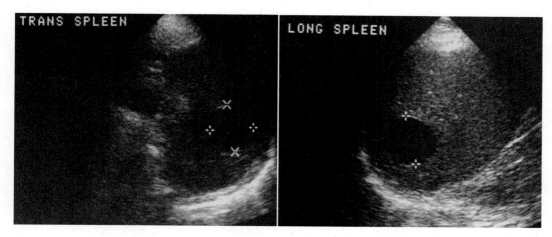

8. A 43-year-old, HIV-positive man with alcoholic pancreatitis and a pseudocyst in the tail of the pancreas comes to the ER with abdominal pain and fever. What are your findings (Figure 9-10)?

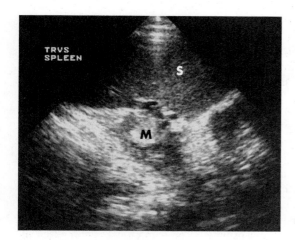

Answers to Review Exercise

1. The spleen is the largest single mass of lymphoid tissue in the body. It is active in blood formation during the initial part of fetal life. This function decreases gradually by the fifth or sixth month when the spleen assumes its adult characteristics and discontinues its hematopoietic activities. The spleen plays an important role in the defense mechanism of the body. The spleen is rarely the primary site of disease, although it is often affected by systemic disease processes.

2. The spleen lies in the left hypochrondrium, with its axis along the shaft of the tenth rib. Its lower pole extends forward as far as the midaxillary line.

   The spleen is of variable size and shape, (orange-segment, tetrahedral, triangular) but generally is considered to be ovoid with even borders and a convex superior and concave inferior surface.

3. Accessory spleens occasionally may be found near the hilum of the spleen. An accessory spleen results from the failure of fusion of separate splenic masses forming on the dorsal mesogastrium, most commonly located in the splenic hilum or along the splenic vessels or associated ligaments. They have been reported from the diaphragm to the scrotum and are usually solitary. They usually remain small and do not present as a clinical problem. The accessory spleen may simulate pancreatic, suprarenal, and retroperitoneal tumors.

4. The lymph vessels emerge from the splenic hilum, pass through other lymph nodes along the course of the splenic artery, and drain into the celiac nodes.

5. The ligaments are the lienorenal, gastrosplenic, and phrenicolic ligaments. These ligaments are derived from the layers of peritoneum that form the greater and lesser sacs. A mass in the left upper quadrant may displace the spleen inferiorly. Caudad displacement may be secondary to a subclavian abscess, splenic cyst, or left pleural effusion. A cephalic displacement may be the result of volume loss in the left lung, left pneumonia, paralysis of the left hemidiaphragm, or a large intraabdominal mass.

6. Wandering spleen refers to the migration of the spleen from its normal location in the left upper quadrant. It is the result of an embryologic anomaly of the supporting ligaments of the spleen. The patient is seen with an abdominal or a pelvic mass, intermittent pain, and volvulus (splenic torsion). The sonographer should use color Doppler to map the vascularity within the spleen. Complete torsion would show a decrease in the vascular pattern.

7. Complete absence of the spleen (asplenia or agenesis of the spleen) is rare and by itself causes no difficulties. However, it may occur as part of a asplenic or polysplenia syndrome in association with complex cardiac malformations, bronchopulmonary abnormalities, or visceral heterotaxis (anomalous placement of organs or major blood vessels) and includes a horizontal liver, malrotation of the gut, and interruption of the inferior vena cava with azygous continuation.

   Splenic agenesis may be ruled out by the demonstration of a spleen on ultrasound. The sonographer should be careful not to misidentify the bowel, which may lie in the same area normally occupied by the spleen. Color Doppler will help determine the splenic vascular pattern and thus differentiate it from the colon.

8. There are two types of splenic congestion, acute and chronic. In acute congestion, active hyperemia accompanies the reaction in the moderately enlarged spleen. In chronic venous congestion, diffuse enlargement of the spleen occurs.

9. The major nontraumatic causes for focal splenic defects include tumors (benign and malignant), infarction, abscesses, and cysts. Splenic defects may be incidental as seen on another imaging study or specific (e.g., splenic infarct, abscess).

10. Common benign primary tumors are the hamartoma, cavernous hemangioma, and cystic lymphangioma. Most of these tumors appear isoechoic as compared with normal splenic parenchyma. Splenomegaly is the first indicator of an abnormality.

11. The hamartoma has both solid and cystic components and is generally hyperechoic on ultrasound. The patient does not have symptoms. The tumor may be solitary or multiple and is considered well defined but not encapsulated. The hamartoma is composed of lymphoid tissue or a combination of sinuses and structures equivalent to pulp cords of normal splenic tissue.

12. The cavernous hemangioma represents a large, inhomogeneous echogenic mass with multiple small hypoechoic areas. The patient has no symptoms and only becomes symptomatic when the size of the spleen increases and compresses other organs. Complications occur when the tumor enlarges and causes a splenic rupture with peritoneal symptoms.

    The ultrasound appearance is a complex pattern; infarction with coagulated blood or fibrin in the cavities may be seen but is unspecific. The differential diagnosis includes a hydatid cyst, abscess, dermoid, or metastases.

13. The spleen is commonly involved in lymphoma. It may be difficult to detect splenic lymphoma by ultrasound. However, when seen, it appears as typically hypoechoic with some focal areas also seen.

14. Metastases are the result of a hematogenous spread from another primary site. The spleen is the tenth most common site (from breast, lung, ovary, stomach, melanoma, and prostate). The metastatic tumors may be microscopic, causing no symptoms for the patient. Careful evaluation of the splenic parenchyma should be made by the sonographer to detect the abnormalities of the splenic parenchyma.

15. An infarction is caused by septic emboli and local thrombosis in patients with pancreatitis, subacute bacterial endocarditis, leukemia, lymphocyte disorders, sickle cell anemia, sarcoidosis, or polyarteritis nodosa.

    The appearance of an infarct depends on its onset. A fresh hemorrhagic infarct is hypoechoic, whereas a healed infarct with scar tissue appears as an echogenic, wedge-shaped lesion, with the base toward the subcapsular surface of spleen.

16. Primary or epidermoid cysts contain an epithelial lining and are considered to be of congenital origin. False or "secondary" cysts lack a cellular lining, probably developing as a result of prior trauma to the spleen, and account for 80% of nonparasitic splenic cysts.

    True cysts are usually solitary and unilocular and rarely contain calcification. The internal surface of the cyst may be smooth or trabeculated. The fluid may be clear or turbid and may contain protein, iron, bilirubin, fat, and cholesterol crystals.

    Epidermoid cysts occur more frequently in females (50% in patients under 15 years of age). Clinically, patients are seen with an asymptomatic LUQ mass.

17. Ultrasound shows a hypoechoic or an anechoic foci with well-defined walls and increased through transmission. Epidermoid cysts can have internal echoes at increased gain. Hemorrhage within the cyst may produce a fluid level.

18. Erythropoietic abnormalities include sickle cell, hereditary spherocytosis, hemolytic anemia, chronic anemia, polycythemia vera, thalassemia, and myeloproliferative disorders. On ultrasound, they tend to produce an isoechoic pattern.

19. Granulocytopoietic abnormalities include cases of reactive hyperplasia resulting from acute or chronic infection (e.g., splenitis sarcoid, tuberculousis). On ultrasound, splenomegaly is seen with a diffusely hypoechoic pattern (less dense than the pattern of the liver).

    Patients who have had a previous granulomatous infection will be seen with bright echogenic lesions on ultrasound, with or without shadowing. Histoplasmosis and tuberculosis are the most common; sarcoidosis is rare. The sonographer may also find calcium in the splenic artery.

20. Lymphopoietic abnormalities include lymphoietic leukemias, lymphoma, and Hodgkin's disease. Ultrasound shows a diffusely hypoechoic splenic pattern with focal lesions. Patients with non-Hodgkin's lymphoma have been reported as having an isoechoic echopattern.

    Chronic myelogenous leukemia may be responsible for more extreme splenomegaly than any other disease. Chronic lymphatic leukemia produces a less severe degree of splenomegaly.

21. The spleen is most commonly injured as the result of blunt abdominal trauma. If the patient has severe left upper quadrant pain secondary to trauma, a splenic hematoma or subcapsular hematoma should be considered. The tear may result in linear or stellate lacerations and capsular tears and may result from traction from adhesions or suspensory ligaments, puncture wounds from foreign bodies or rib fractures, subcapsular hematomas, avulsion of vascular pedicle, and laceration of short gastric vessels.

    There are two outcomes from blunt trauma. If the capsule is intact, the outcome may be intraparenchymal or subcapsular hematoma; if the capsule ruptures, a focal or free intraperitoneal hematoma may form. Free intraperitoneal blood can be seen immediately after trauma. Delayed ruptures may develop a subcapsular hematoma with subsequent rupture or a small splenic laceration that was temporarily tamponaded.

    The patient typically is seen with left upper quadrant pain, left shoulder pain, left flank pain, or dizziness. On clinical evaluation, the patient may be tender over the LUQ and hypotensive and show a decreased hemoglobin level, indicating a bleed.

    The most prominent finding is splenomegaly, with progressive enlargement as the bleed continues. In addition, an irregular splenic border, hematoma, contusion (splenic inhomogeneity), subcapsular and pericapsular fluid collections, free intraperitoneal blood, or left pleural effusion may be present. Fresh hemorrhage may appear hypoechoic. (This may be difficult to distinguish from normal splenic tissue—look for "double contour" sign depicting the hematoma as separate from the spleen.) As the protein and cells reabsorb, the hematoma becomes organized and the fluid becomes hyperechoic and similar to splenic tissue. Focal areas represent tiny splenic lacerations that give rise to small collections of blood interspersed with a disrupted splenic pulp (contusion). With time the hematoma will become more fluid or lucent appearing.

    The echo-free, intraperitoneal fluid probably represents blood intermixed with peritoneal transudate resulting from the presence of blood within the cavity. Healing of the lesion takes time, often extending into months. The free fluid disappears quicker because the fluid is moved across the pleural and peritoneal membranes rapidly (2 to 4 weeks). Intrasplenic hematomas and contusions take longer because the fluid, protein, and necrotic debris must be resorbed from

within a solid organ in which the blood supply is already focally disrupted. When the spleen returns to normal, small irregular foci may remain or the parenchyma may be normal.

Answers to Self-Test

1. c	**12.** c	**23.** b
2. a	**13.** b	**24.** a
3. b	**14.** c	**25.** a
4. a	**15.** c	**26.** c
5. c	**16.** c	**27.** a
6. c	**17.** a	**28.** true
7. a	**18.** b	**29.** true
8. a	**19.** d	**30.** false
9. c	**20.** d	**31.** false
10. c	**21.** a	**32.** false
11. c	**22.** a	

Answers to Case Reviews

1. (Figure 9-3) Accessory spleen. These extra splenic tissue masses are usually found near the hilum or inferior border of the spleen (arrows). It may be confused with the tail of the pancreas or nodes in the splenic hilum.

2. (Figure 9-4) Amyloidosis of the spleen. Patients with secondary amyloidosis usually suffer from another chronic infectious or inflammatory disease, such as tuberculosis, osteomyelitis, rheumatoid arthritis, and Crohn's disease. The cause of amyloidosis is unknown. In systemic diseases leading to amyloidosis the spleen is the organ most frequently involved, although almost all organs are affected, most often the kidneys, liver, and spleen. This patient showed hepatosplenomegaly with increased congestion in the liver and splenic parenchyma.

3. (Figure 9-5) Longitudinal scan in a patient with acute myelogenous leukemia. An isoechoic pattern is seen as the splenic parenchyma is hypoechoic as compared with the pattern of the liver. *S,* Spleen; *M,* mass.

4. (Figure 9-6) **A,** Transverse and **B,** longitudinal scans of a patients with granulomatous infection. The bright echogenic lesions are seen within the splenic parenchyma, (arrows).

5. (Figure 9-7) Splenic calcifications are seen in this young female with tuberculosis.

6. (Figure 9-8) Multiple nodes are seen along the splenic hilum, with prominent splenic vascular structures. Color Doppler should be used to make sure the hypoechoic structures are not vascular channels.

7. (Figure 9-9) This young patient with RUQ pain had an incidental finding of a splenic cyst. The borders are well defined, and the mass is anechoic.

8. (Figure 9-10) Ultrasound findings revealed a complex mass in the area of the previous pseudocyst. This may represent an infected pseudocyst with purulent fluid, hemorrhage within the pseudocyst, or fatty deposition. This patient had multiple nodes along the head of the pancreas (not shown).

CHAPTER

10
Retroperitoneal Structures

OBJECTIVES

At the completion of this chapter, students will show orally, in writing, or by demonstration that they will be able to:

1. Describe the location, size, and position of the retroperitoneal area.
2. Illustrate the cross-sectional anatomy of the retroperitoneum and adjacent structures.
3. Know the signs of retroperitoneal disease.
4. Differentiate between sonographic appearances by explaining the clinical significance of masses that affect the retroperitoneum of the following diseases:
   a. lymphadenopathy
   b. primary neoplasms
   c. fluid collections

d. retroperitoneal fibrosis
e. metastasis
5. Know the pitfalls in the diagnosis of retroperitoneal disease.
6. Create high-quality diagnostic scans demonstrating the appropriate anatomy in all planes pertinent to the liver.
7. Select the correct equipment settings appropriate to individual body habitus.
8. Distinguish between the normal and abnormal appearances of the retroperitoneal structures.

To further enhance learning, students should use marking pens to color the anatomic illustrations that follow.

RETROPERITONEAL SPACE

FIGURE 10-1

Transverse Section of the Abdomen through the Epiploic Foramen

The retroperitoneal space is the area between the posterior portion of the parietal peritoneum and the posterior abdominal wall muscles (Figures 10-1 and 10-2). It extends from the diaphragm to the pelvis. Laterally the boundaries extend to the extraperitoneal fat planes within the confines of the transversalis fascia, and medially the space encloses the great vessels.

The retroperitoneal space is subdivided into three areas: the perinephric space (or fascia of Gerota), the anterior paranephric space, and the posterior paranephric space. The perinephric space surrounds the kidney and the perinephric fat. The anterior paranephric space includes the extraperitoneal surfaces of the gut and pancreas. The iliopsoas muscle, fat, and other soft tissues are within the posterior paranephric space.

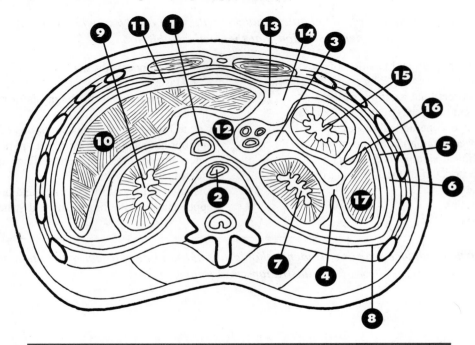

1	inferior vena cava	10	liver
2	aorta	11	falciform ligament
3	lesser sac	12	epiploic foramen
4	lienorenal ligament	13	greater sac
5	peritoneum	14	lesser omentum
6	subserous fascia	15	stomach
7	left kidney	16	gastrolienal ligament
8	diaphragm	17	spleen
9	right kidney		

FIGURE 10-2

Transverse Section of the Abdominal Cavity Showing the Reflections of the Peritoneum

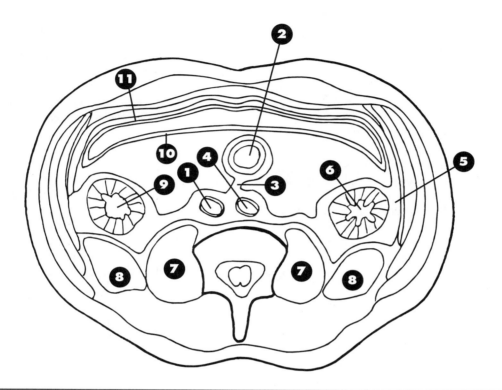

1	inferior vena cava	7	psoas major muscle
2	small intestine	8	quadratus lumborum muscle
3	mesentery of the small intestine	9	ascending colon
4	aorta	10	posterior layers of the greater omentum*
5	peritoneum	11	anterior layers of the greater omentum*
6	descending colon		

*There is generally no space between the anterior and posterior layers of the greater omentum; they are usually fused together.

Retroperitoneum Review Notes

ANATOMY

The retroperitoneum is delineated by the following:

- Anteriorly by the posterior peritoneum
- Posteriorly by the transversalis fascia
- Laterally by the lateral borders of the quadratus lumborum muscles and peritoneal leaves of the mesentery
- Superior to inferior, with the retroperitoneum extending from the diaphragm to the pelvic brim
- Superior to the pelvic brim, with the retroperitoneum partitioned into the lumbar and iliac fossae

- The pararenal and perirenal spaces are included in the lumbar fossa.
- Pathologic processes can stretch from the anterior abdominal wall to the subdiaphragmatic space, mediastinum, and subcutaneous tissues of the back and flank.
- The retrofascial space, which includes the psoas, quadratus lumborum, and iliacus muscles (muscles posterior to the transversalis fascia), is often the site of extension of retroperitoneal pathologic processes.

Anterior Pararenal Space

- The anterior pararenal space is bound anteriorly by the posterior parietal peritoneum and posteriorly by the anterior renal fascia.
- It is bound laterally by the lateroconal fascia formed by the fusion of the anterior and posterior leaves of the renal fascia.
- This space merges with the bare area of the liver by the coronary ligament.
- The pancreas, duodenal sweep, and ascending and transverse colon are the organs included in the anterior pararenal space.

Perirenal Space

- The perirenal space is surrounded by the anterior and posterior layers of the renal fascia (Gerota's fascia).
- These layers join and attach to the diaphragm superiorly, but they are united only loosely inferiorly at the level of the iliac crest, or superior border of the "false" pelvis.
- Collections in the perinephric space can communicate within the iliac fossa of the retroperitoneum.
- The lateroconal fascia, the lateral fusion of the renal fascia, proceeds anteriorly as the posterior peritoneum.
- The posterior renal fascia fuses medially with the psoas or quadratus lumborum fascia.
- The anterior renal fascia fuses medially with connective tissue surrounding the great vessels.
- This space contains the adrenal, kidney, and ureter; the great vessels, which also lie within this space, are largely isolated within their connective tissue sheaths.

- The perirenal space contains the adrenal and kidney (enclosed in a variable amount of echogenic perinephric fat, the thickest portion being posterior and lateral to the lower pole of the kidney).
- The kidney is anterolateral to the psoas muscle, anterior to the quadratus lumborum muscle, and posteromedial to the ascending and descending colon.
- The second portion of the duodenum is anterior to the kidney hilum on the right.
- On the left, the kidney is bounded by the stomach anterosuperiorly, the pancreas anteriorly, and the spleen anterolaterally.

Adrenal

Adult Adrenal

- Adrenal glands are anterior, medial, and superior to kidneys.
- The right adrenal is more superior to the kidney.
- The left adrenal is more medial.
- The medial portion of the right gland is immediately posterior to the IVC (above the level of the portal vein and lateral to the crus).
- The lateral portion of the gland is posterior and medial to the right lobe of the liver and posterior to the duodenum.
- The left is lateral or slightly posterolateral to the aorta and lateral to the crus.
- The superior portion is posterior to the lesser omental space, posterior to the stomach.
- The inferior portion is posterior to the pancreas.
- The splenic vein and artery pass between the pancreas and the left adrenal.
- The right is posterior to the IVC and the left is to the left of the aorta.
- Glands vary in size, shape, and configuration:
  - Right—triangular
  - Left—semilunar
- Internal texture is medium in consistency; cortex and medulla are not distinguished.
- Adrenal is a distinct hypoechoic structure; highly echogenic fat is sometimes seen.
- The adrenal is usually smaller than 3 cm (3 to 6 cm long, 3 to 6 mm thick, 2 to 4 cm wide).

Neonatal Adrenal

- The neonatal adrenal is characterized by a thin echogenic core surrounded by a thick transonic zone.
- A thick rim of transonicity represents the hypertrophied adrenal cortex; the echogenic core is the adrenal medulla.
- The infant adrenal is proportionally larger than the adult (one-third the size of the kidney; in adults, it is one-thirteenth the size).

Aorta

- The aorta enters the abdomen posterior to the diaphragm at L1 and passes posterior to the left lobe of liver.
- It has a straight course to L4, where it bifurcates.
- The slight anterior curve results from lumbar lordosis.

Inferior Vena Cava

- The inferior vena cava extends from the junction of the two common iliac veins to the right of L5 and travels cephalad.
- It curves anteriorly toward its termination in the right atrium.

Diaphragmatic Crura

- The diaphragmatic crura begin as tendinous fibers from lumar vertebral bodies, disks, and transverse processes of L3 on the right and L1 on the left.
- The right crus is longer, larger, and more lobular; it is associated with the anterior aspect of the lumbar vertebral ligament.
- The right renal artery crosses anterior to the crus and posterior to the IVC at the level of the right kidney.
- The right crus is bounded by the IVC anterolaterally and the right adrenal and right lobe of the liver posterolaterally.
- The left crus courses along the anterior lumbar vertebral bodies in a superior direction and inserts into the central tendon of the diaphragm.

Nodes

- Nodes surround the aorta and IVC and are sometimes located anterior to the spine.
- They are up to 1 cm in size.
- Common sites are paraaortic, paracaval, peripancreatic, renal hilar, and mesenteric.

Ultrasound Findings

- Rounded, focal, echopoor lesions 1 to 3 cm
- Larger, confluent echopoor masses often displacing the kidney laterally
- Mantle of nodes in paraspinal location
- "Floating" or anterior displaced aorta
- Mesenteric "sandwich" sign representing anterior and posterior node masses surrounding mesenteric vessels

Posterior Pararenal Space and Iliac Fossa

- The posterior pararenal space and iliac fossa are located between the posterior renal fascia and the transversalis fascia.
- They communicate with properitoneal fat, lateral to the lateroconal fascia.
- The space merges inferiorly with the anterior pararenal space and retroperitoneal tissues of the iliac fossa.
- The psoas muscle, the fascia of which merges with the posterior transversalis fascia, makes up the medial border of this posterior space.
- The space is open laterally and inferiorly.
- Blood and lymph nodes embedded in fat are found in the posterior pararenal space.

Iliac Fossa

- The region extends between the internal surface of the iliac wings from the crest to the iliopectineal line.
- Known as the *false* pelvis, it contains the ureter and major branches of distal great vessels and their lymphatics.
- The transversalis fascia extends into the iliac fossa as the iliac fascia.
- The renal fascia terminates at the level of the superior margin of the iliac fossa and mixes loosely with the iliac fascia.

Retrofascial Space

- The retrofascial space comprises the posterior abdominal wall, muscles, nerves, lymphatics, and areolar tissue behind the transversalis fascia.
- It is divided into three compartments:
  1. Psoas
  2. Lumbar (quadratus lumborum)
  3. Iliac by the leaves of the transversalis fascia
- The quadratus lumborum originates from the iliolumbar ligament, the adjacent iliac crest, and the superior borders of the transverse process of L3, L4 and inserts into the margin of the twelfth rib. It is adjoining and posterior to the colon, kidney, and psoas.
- The psoas spans from the mediastinum to the thigh, with the fascia attaching to the pelvic brim.
- The iliacus makes up the iliac space and extends the length of the iliac fossa. The psoas passes through the iliac fossa medial to the iliacus muscle and posterior to the iliac fascia. The two muscles merge as they extend into the true pelvis. The iliopsoas takes on a more anterior location caudally to lie along the lateral pelvic sidewall.

Pelvic Retroperitoneum

- The pelvic portion lies between the sacrum and pubis from back to front, pelvic peritoneal reflection above and the pelvic diaphragm (coccygeus and levator ani muscles) below, and the fascial investment of the lateral pelvic wall musculature (obturator internus and piriformis).
  - It has four subdivisions:
    1. Prevesical
    2. Rectovesical
    3. Presacral
    4. Bilateral pararectal (and paravesical) spaces

Prevesical

- The prevesical is also known as the *Retropubic space of Retzius'*.

- It spans from the pubis to the anterior margin of the bladder.
- It is bordered laterally by the obturator fascia.
- Connective tissue covering the bladder, seminal vesicles, and prostate is continuous with the fascial lamina within this space.
- The space is an extension of the retroperitoneal space of the anterior abdominal wall deep to the rectus sheath, which is continuous with the transversalis fascia.
- The space between the bladder and rectum is the rectovesical space.

Presacral Space

- The presacral space is located between the rectum and fascia covering the sacrum and posterior pelvic floor musculature.

Bilateral Pararectal Space

- The bilateral pararectal space is bounded laterally by the piriformis and levator ani fascia and medially by the rectum.
- It extends anteriorly from the bladder, medially to the obturator internus, and laterally to the external iliac vessels.
- Paravesical and pararectal spaces are traversed by ureters.
- Pelvic wall muscles, iliac vessels, ureter, bladder, prostate, seminal vesicles, and cervix are retroperitoneal structures within the true pelvis.
- The obturator internus muscle lines the lateral aspect of the pelvis.
- Posteriorly, the piriformis muscle is seen extending anterolaterally from the region of the sacrum.

Retroperitoneal Fat

- Lesions in the liver or Morison's pouch displace the echoes posterior and inferior.
- Renal and adrenal lesions cause anterior displacement.
- Extrahepatic masses shift the IVC anteromedially (anterior displacement of right kidney).

Review Exercise • The Retroperitoneum

1. Why are the adrenal glands so difficult to image with ultrasound? _____

_____

_____

_____

2. How should the sonographer position the patient to image the adrenal glands, what landmarks are used, and what is the texture of the glands? _____

_____

_____

3. What is the technique used to image the paraortic nodes? _____

_____

_____

_____

4. Define the boundaries of the retroperitoneal space. _____

_____

_____

_____

5. Describe the perirenal, anterior pararenal, and posterior pararenal space and its surrounding structures. _____

_____

_____

6. Define the boundaries the sonographer should search for in identifying the adrenal glands. _____

_____

_____

_____

7. What is the appearance of the neonatal adrenal gland? _____

_____

_____

_____

8. What are the two major node-bearing areas in the retroperitoneal cavity? _____

_____

_____

9. What is the best ultrasound approach to image the lymph nodes? _____

_____

_____

_____

10. What other organ should be evaluated in patients with lymphadenopathy? _____

_____

_____

_____

11. Describe where the posterior pararenal space is located and describe the landmarks associated with this space.

_____

_____

_____

_____

12. What is the iliacus and where is it found? _____

_____

_____

13. Describe the pelvic retroperitoneum and name the four subdivisions of the pelvic retroperitoneum. _____

_____

_____

_____

14. What structures are contained in the pelvic retroperitoneum? _____

_____

_____

15. What is the definition of a primary retroperitoneal tumor? _____

_____

_____

_____

Self-Test • Retroperitoneal Space

1. The retroperitoneal space is the area between the:

a. anterior portion of the parietal peritoneum and the posterior abdominal wall muscles

b. posterior portion of the parietal peritoneum and the posterior abdominal wall muscles

c. anterior portion of the parietal peritoneum and the anterior abdominal wall muscles

d. posterior portion of the visceral peritoneum

2. The retroperitoneal space encloses the aorta and inferior vena cava (true or false).

3. The kidneys lie on what group of muscles?

a. iliacus, piriformis

b. iliacus, psoas

c. psoas, quadratus lumborum

d. iliacus, quadratus lumborum

4. The left kidney is in contact with the:

a. spleen, pancreas, and gallbladder

b. spleen, gallbladder, and duodenum

c. pancreas, colon, and portahepatis

d. spleen, pancreas, colon, and jejunum

5. The right kidney is in contact with the:

a. spleen, colon, and adrenal

b. liver, colon, and adrenal

c. liver, pancreas, and spleen

d. liver, gallbladder, and splenic flexure

6. The ureter runs inferior to the renal hilum to enter the anterior wall of the bladder (true or false).

7. The kidney is surrounded by the:

a. paranephric space

b. perinephric space

c. renal capsule

d. renal cortex

8. Outside the renal capsule is the:

a. perinephric space

b. paranephric space

c. renal capsule

d. renal medulla

9. The adrenal glands are peritoneal structures (true or false).

10. The adrenal glands are demonstrated more easily in neonates than in the adult (true or false).

11. The adrenal glands are separated from the kidneys by the:

    a. perinephric fascia

    b. perinephric capsule

    c. crus

    d. perinephric fat

12. A triangular-shaped lesion on the peripheral border of the kidney would most likely represent a:

    a. renal tumor

    b. artifact from rib

    c. inferior vena cava compression

    d. junctional parenchymal defect

13. The vessel seen posterior to the inferior vena cava on the sagittal scan represents the:

    a. right adrenal artery

    b. right renal artery

    c. left renal artery

    d. left renal vein

14. The kidneys begin their development in the pelvis and migrate into the posterior retroperitoneal space (true or false).

15. Paraortic nodes are not visualized on ultrasound examination unless they are enlarged (true or false).

16. Name the structures that surround the tail of the pancreas:

    a. stomach, gallbladder, and duodenum

    b. common duct, gallbladder, and duodenum

    c. hepatic artery, stomach, and splenic artery

    d. stomach, splenic artery, and hilum of the spleen

17. Which of the following is not retroperitoneal?

    a. kidney

    b. aorta

    c. psoas muscle

    d. spleen

18. A retroperitoneal abscess may not be found within:

    a. the rectus abdominus muscle

    b. the psoas muscle

    c. the iliacus muscle

    d. the quadratus lumborum muscle

    e. none of the above

19. An adrenal mass may displace the splenic vein:

    a. anteriorly

    b. posteriorly

    c. medially

    d. laterally

20. The mass in the normal adult adrenal should measure more than _____ to be detected by ultrasound examination:

    a. 2 cm

    b. 2 mm

    c. 3 cm

    d. 3 mm

21. Which of the following causes anterior displacement of the IVC?

    a. splenomegaly

    b. hydronephrosis

    c. enlarged lymph nodes

    d. pancreatitis

22. Which of the following can be confused with the normal right adrenal gland?

    a. crus of the diaphragm

    b. bowel gas

    c. renal cyst

    d. aorta

23. Which of the following disorders may not produce a complex sonographic pattern?

    a. infected cyst

    b. hemorrhagic cyst

    c. hematomas

    d. congenital cyst

24. Horseshoe kidneys may be confused sonographically with which of the following diseases?

    a. carcinoma of the head of the pancreas

    b. lymphadenopathy

    c. hypernephroma

    d. Wilms' tumor

25. Which statement is false about adrenal carcinoma?

    a. These tumors usually produce steroids and are associated with one of the hyperadrenal syndromes.

    b. It is a nonsteroid-producing tumor.

    c. There is a strong tendency for invasion into the adrenal vein, inferior vena cava, and lymph glands.

    d. Metastases to regional and periaortic nodes are common.

26. What adrenal tumor is occasionally found in patients with hypertension?

    a. neuroblastoma

    b. adenoma

    c. myeliopoma

    d. pheochromocytoma

27. One of the most common childhood tumors is:

   a. adenoma

   b. pheochromocytoma

   c. neuroblastoma

   d. liposarcoma

28. On ultrasound a retroperitoneal hemorrhage may be recognized as:

   a. asymmetry of the psoas muscles

   b. concavity of the abdominal wall

   c. solid-appearing mass with shadowing

   d. anechoic mass with irregular boarders

29. A lymphocele may be defined as a:

   a. ragged, homogeneous irregular mass

   b. lymph-filled space without a distinct epithelial lining

   c. heterogenous irregular mass

   d. cystic space anterior to the aorta

30. Metastatic lymphopathy disease can occur by lymphatic or hematogeneous spread. It may be secondary to carcinoma of the:

   a. breast, lung, or testis

   b. pancreas, lung, or liver

   c. breast, gallbladder, or lung

   d. lung, ovary, or pancreas

Use the following terms to define the statements that follow.

anterior pararenal space	nodes	pelvic retroperitoneum
perirenal space	posterior pararenal space	retroperitoneal fat
diaphragmatic crura	retrofascial space	

31. _____ Lies between the sacrum and pubis from back to front, pelvic peritoneal reflection above and pelvic diaphragm below, and the fascial investment of the lateral pelvic wall musculature.

32. _____ Bounded anteriorly by the posterior parietal peritoneum and posteriorly by the anterior renal fascia.

33. _____ By knowing the displacement of this, the sonographer can diagnose the anatomic origin of the mass in the right upper quadrant.

34. _____ Surrounded by the anterior and posterior layers of the renal fascia.

35. _____ Made up of the posterior abdominal wall components, muscles, nerves, lymphatics, and areolar tissue behind the transversalis fascia.

36. _____ Begins as tendinous fibers from the lumbar vertebral bodies.

37. _____ Located between the posterior renal fascia and the transversalis fascia.

38. _____ Surround the aorta and inferior vena cava.

Case Reviews

1. A premature infant was delivered as a crash C-section. A mass was noted along the right flank. What are your findings (Figure 10-3)?

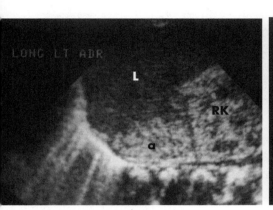 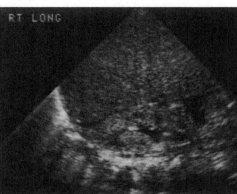 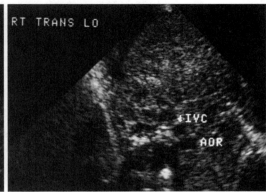

2. A 48-year-old man is seen with intermittent hypertensive episodes accompanied by palpitations, tachycardia, malaise, and sweating. What are your findings (Figure 10-4)?

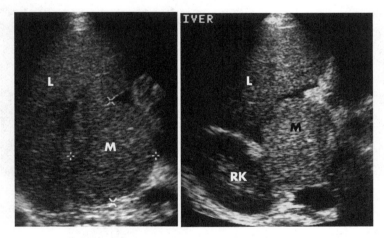

3. A 54-year-old woman with a history of breast cancer is seen with vague left upper quadrant pain. What are your findings (Figure 10-5)?

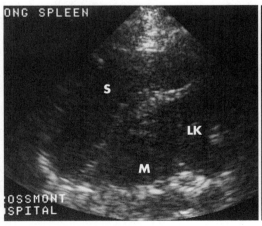 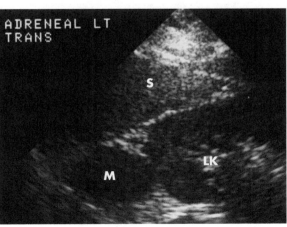

4. A 24-year-old man is seen with abdominal pain. What are your findings (Figure 10-6)?

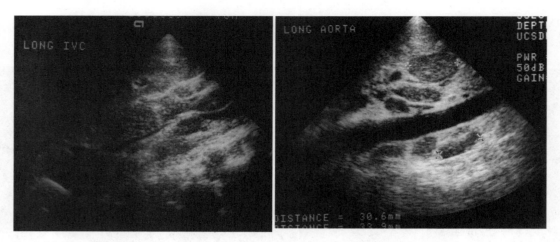

5. A 32-year-old woman is seen with right upper quadrant pain and fever. What are your findings (Figure 10-7)?

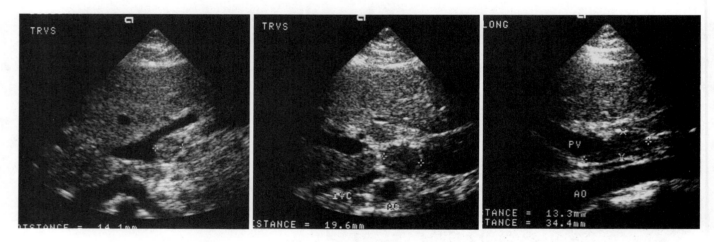

6. A 32-year-old man with AIDS is seen with abdominal pain and fever. What are your findings (Figure 10-8)?

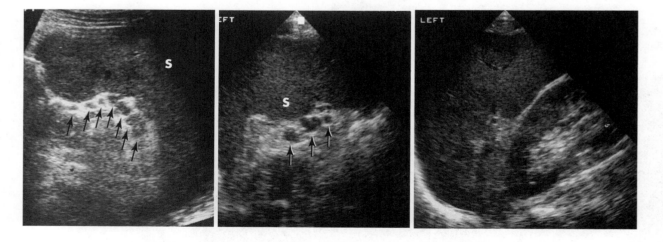

Answers to Review Exercise

1. Visualization of the adrenal glands has been difficult because of its small size, medial location, and surrounding perirenal fat. If the adrenal gland becomes enlarged secondary to disease, it becomes easier to image and separate from the upper pole of the kidney.

   Visualization of the adrenal area depends on several factors: the size of the patient and the amount of perirenal fat surrounding the adrenal area, the presence of bowel gas, and the ability to change the patient into multiple positions.

2. With the patient in the decubitus position the sonographer should attempt to align the kidney and ipsilateral paravertebral vessels (inferior vena cava or aorta). The right adrenal gland has a "comma" or triangular shape in the transaxial plane.

   The best visualization is obtained by a transverse scan with the patient in a left lateral decubitus position. As the patient assumes this position, the inferior vena cava moves forward and the aorta rolls over the crus of the diaphragm to offer a good window to image the upper pole of the right kidney and adrenal.

   If the patient is obese, it may be difficult to recognize the triangular or crescent-shaped adrenal gland. The adrenal should not appear rounded; this would be suggestive of a pathologic process.

   The longitudinal scan is made through the right lobe of the liver, perpendicular to the linear right crus of the diaphragm. The retroperitoneal fat must be recognized as separate from the liver, crus of the diaphragm, adrenal gland, and great vessel.

   The left adrenal gland is closely related to the left crus of the diaphragm and the anterior-superior-medial aspect of the upper pole of the left kidney. It may be more difficult to image the left adrenal because of stomach gas interference. The patient should be placed in a right lateral decubitus position and transverse scans made in an attempt to align the left kidney and the aorta. The left adrenal is seen by scanning along the posterior axillary line. The patient should be in deep inspiration in an effort to bring the adrenal and renal area into better view.

3. Paraortic nodes are normally not seen with ultrasound because they are beyond the limits of resolution. The nodes are only seen when they are enlarged secondary to metastasis, lymphoma, or inflammatory process.

   The nodes are generally located anterior to the inferior vena cava and aorta and along the origin of major vessels throughout the body. In some cases the enlarged nodes may be so prominent that they are seen posterior to the major vessels. Enlarged nodes may be found in the porta hepatis, renal, and the splenic hilum.

4. The retroperitoneal space is the area between the posterior portion of the parietal peritoneum and the posterior abdominal wall muscles. It extends from the diaphragm to the pelvis. Laterally the boundaries extend to the extraperitoneal fat planes within the confines of the transversalis fascia, and medially the space encloses the great vessels. It is subdivided into three categories: anterior pararenal space, perirenal space, and posterior pararenal space.

5. The perirenal space surrounds the kidney, adrenal, and perirenal fat. The anterior pararenal space includes the duodenum, pancreas, and ascending and transverse colon. The posterior pararenal space includes the iliopsoas muscle, ureter, branches of the inferior vena cava and aorta, and their lymphatics.

   The anterior pararenal space is bound anteriorly by the posterior parietal peritoneum and posteriorly by the anterior renal fascia. It is bound laterally by the lateroconal fascia formed by the fusion of the anterior and posterior leaves of the renal fascia. (This space merges with the bare area of the liver by the coronary ligament.) The pancreas, duodenal sweep, and ascending and transverse colon are the organs included in the anterior pararenal space.

   The perirenal space is surrounded by the anterior and posterior layers of the renal fascia (Gerota's fascia). These layers join and attach to the diaphragm superiorly, but they are united only loosely at their inferior margin at the level of the iliac crest or superior border of the "false" pelvis. Collections in the perinephric space can communicate within the iliac fossa of the retroperitoneum.

   The lateroconal fascia (the lateral fusion of the renal fascia) proceeds anterior as the posterior peritoneum. The posterior renal fascia fuses medially with the psoas or quadratus lumborum fascia. The anterior renal fascia fuses medially with connective tissue surrounding the great vessels. (This space contains the adrenal gland, kidney, and ureter; the great vessels, which also lie within this space, are largely isolated within their connective tissue sheaths.)

   The perirenal space contains the adrenal and kidney (enclosed in a variable amount of echogenic perinephric fat, the thickest portion being posterior and lateral to the lower pole of the kidney). The kidney is anterolateral to the psoas muscle, anterior to the quadratus lumborum muscle, and posteromedial to the ascending and descending colon.

   The second portion of the duodenum is anterior to the kidney hilum on the right. On the left the kidney is bounded by the stomach anterosuperiorly, the pancreas anteriorly, and the spleen anterolaterally.

6. In the adult patient, the adrenal glands are anterior, medial, and superior to the kidneys. The right adrenal is more superior to the kidney, whereas the left

adrenal is more medial to the kidney. The medial portion of the right adrenal gland is immediately posterior to the inferior vena cava (above the level of the portal vein and lateral to the crus). The lateral portion of the gland is posterior and medial to the right lobe of the liver and posterior to the duodenum.

The left adrenal gland is lateral or slightly posterolateral to the aorta and lateral to the crus of the diaphragm. The superior portion is posterior to the lesser omental space and posterior to the stomach. The inferior portion is posterior to the pancreas. The splenic vein and artery pass between the pancreas and the left adrenal gland.

7. The neonatal adrenal glands are characterized by a thin echogenic core surrounded by a thick transonic zone. This thick rim of transonicity represents the hypertrophied adrenal cortex; the echogenic core is the adrenal medulla. The infant adrenal is proportionally larger than the adult (one-third the size of the kidney; in adults it is one-thirteenth the size).

8. There are two major node-bearing areas in the retroperitoneal cavity: the iliac and hypogastric nodes within the pelvis and the paraortic group in the upper retroperitoneum. The lymphatic chain follows the course of the thoracic aorta, abdominal aorta, and iliac arteries. Common sites are the paraortic, paracaval, peripancreatic, renal hilar area, and mesenteric.

9. The lymph nodes lie along the lateral and anterior margins of the aorta and inferior vena cava, so the best scanning is done with the patient in the supine or decubitus position. It is always important to examine the patient in two planes, since the enlarged nodes seen in one plane may mimic an aortic aneurysm or tumor in only one plane.

Longitudinal scans may be made first to outline the aorta and search for enlarged lymph nodes. The aorta provides an excellent background for the hypoechoic nodes. Scans should begin at the midline and the transducer angled both to the left and right at small angles to image the anterior and lateral borders of the aorta and inferior vena cava.

Transverse scans are made from the level of the xyphoid to the symphysis. Careful identification of the great vessels, organ structures, and muscles is important. Patterns of a fluid-filled duodenum or bowel may make it difficult to outline the great vessels or may cause confusion in diagnosing lymphadenopathy.

Scans below the umbilicus are more difficult because of interference from the small bowel. Careful attention should be given to the psoas and iliacus muscles within the pelvis because the iliac arteries run along their medial border. Both muscles serve as a hypoechoic marker along the pelvic sidewall.

Enlarged lymph nodes can be identified anterior and medial to these margins. A smooth, sharp border of the muscle indicates no nodal involvement. The bladder should be filled to help push the small bowel out the pelvis and to serve as an acoustic window to better image the vascular structures. Color Doppler may also be used to help delineate the vascular structures.

10. Splenomegaly should also be evaluated in patients with lymphadenopathy. As the sonographer moves caudally from the xyphoid, attention should be on the splenic size and great vessel area to detect nodal involvement near the hilus of the spleen.

11. The posterior pararenal space is located between the posterior renal fascia and the transversalis fascia. It communicates with the peritoneal fat, lateral to the lateroconal fascia. The posterior pararenal space merges inferiorly with the anterior pararenal space and retroperitoneal tissues of the iliac fossa.

The psoas muscle, the fascia of which merges with the posterior transversalis fascia, makes up the medial border of this posterior space. This space is open laterally and inferiorly. The blood and lymph nodes embedded in fat may be found in the posterior pararenal space.

12. The iliacus makes up the iliac space and extends the length of the iliac fossa. The psoas passes through the iliac fossa medially to the iliacus. The iliacus and psoas muscles merge as they extend into the true pelvis. The iliopsoas takes on a more anterior location caudally to lie along the lateral pelvic sidewall.

13. The pelvic portion lies between the sacrum and pubis from back to front, pelvic peritoneal reflection above and pelvic diaphragm (coccygeus and levator ani muscles) below, and between the fascial investment of the lateral pelvic wall musculature (obturator internus and piriformis). There are four subdivisions: the prevesical, the rectovesical, the presacral, and the bilateral pararectal (and paravesical) spaces.

The prevesical space spans from the pubis to the anterior margin of the bladder. The space between the bladder and rectum is the rectovesical space. The presacral space lies between the rectum and fascia covering the sacrum and the posterior pelvic floor musculature. The bilateral pararectal space is bounded laterally by the piriformis and levator ani fascia and medially by the rectum.

The paravesical and pararectal spaces are traversed by the two ureters.

14. The pelvic wall muscles, iliac vessels, ureter, bladder, prostate, seminal vesicles, and cervix are retroperitoneal structures within the true pelvis. The obturator internus muscle lines the lateral aspect of the pelvis. Posteriorly, the piriformis muscle is seen extending anterolaterally from the region of the sacrum.

15. A primary retroperitoneal tumor is one that originates independently within the retroperitoneal space. The tumor can arise anywhere and is most likely malignant. As with other tumors, it may exhibit a variety of sonography patterns, from homogeneous to solid to a mixture of complex tissue mass.

Answers to Self-Test

1. b	**14.** true	**27.** c
2. true	**15.** true	**28.** a
3. c	**16.** d	**29.** b
4. d	**17.** d	**30.** a
5. b	**18.** a	**31.** pelvic retroperitoneum
6. false	**19.** a	**32.** anterior pararenal space
7. c	**20.** c	**33.** retroperitoneal fat
8. a	**21.** c	**34.** perirenal space
9. false	**22.** a	**35.** retrofascial space
10. true	**23.** d	**36.** diaphragmatic space
11. d	**24.** b	**37.** posterior pararenal space
12. d	**25.** b	**38.** nodes
13. b	**26.** d	

Answers to Case Reviews

1. (Figure 10-3) Adrenal hemorrhage in a 1-month-old neonate. The mass appears superior to the kidney as a complex lesion with multiple internal echoes and generalized enlargement of the gland. This hemorrhage should decrease in size over the next several weeks.

2. (Figure 10-4) This benign mass arises from the excess pheochromocytes of the medulla. The pheochromocytoma is a homogeneous solid tumor that has a weak posterior wall and decreased through transmission. This tumor can grow quite large, usually over 2 cm, but may grow as large as 5 to 6 cm. It can be unilateral or bilateral. The mass will displace the inferior vena cava anteriorly. *(A)* Longitudinal. *L,* Liver; *M,* mass. *(B)* Transverse. *L,* Liver; *RK,* right kidney; *IVC,* inferior vena cava; *M,* mass.

3. (Figure 10-5) Metastasis to the adrenal gland may result from primary cancer of the lung, breast or kidneys or melanoma. The mass may be difficult to differentiate from adenoma. This shows a patient with a large mass in the left adrenal gland representing metastases secondary to breast carcinoma. The mass is solid, well encapsulated, and within the adrenal gland. *S,* Spleen; *LK,* left kidney; *M,* adrenal mass.

4. (Figure 10-6) Paraortic nodes over 1 cm can be identified on ultrasound because they surround the aortic, inferior vena cava, mesenteric, and celiac vessels. The nodes usually appear as hypoechoic to low-level echogenicity, homogeneous, and with smooth borders. Longitudinal scans over the inferior vena cava *(A)* and aorta *(B)* show multiple nodes elevating the inferior vena cava and surrounding the aorta.

5. (Figure 10-7) Careful attention should be made over the paraortic area and celiac axis to evaluate for the enlarged nodes. As the nodes enlarge, they will create a mantle appearance surrounding the vessels. They may simulate an aortic aneurysm. On this patient, two paracaval nodes (cross-bars) were seen anterior to the aorta and inferior to the portal vein.

6. (Figure 10-8) Splenomegaly should be evaluated in patients with lymphadenopathy. Enlarged nodes *(arrows)* are seen in the area of the hilus of the spleen *(S).* This patient also has a metastatic lesion near the periphery of the spleen.

CHAPTER
11

The Peritoneal Cavity and Abdominal Wall

OBJECTIVES

At the completion of this chapter, students will show orally, in writing, or by demonstration that they will be able to:

1. Describe the various landmarks of the peritoneal cavity.
2. Define the internal, surface, and relational anatomy of the peritoneum.
3. Illustrate the cross-sectional anatomy of the peritoneum and adjacent structures.
4. Select the pertinent laboratory tests and other diagnostic procedures.
5. Differentiate between sonographic appearances by explaining the clinical significance of the pathologic processes as related to the peritoneum in the following diseases or conditions:
   a. ascites
   b. abscess
   c. hematomas
   d. biloma

   e. cystic lesions of the mesentery, omentum, and peritoneum
   f. lymphocele
   g. urinoma
   h. urachal cyst
   i. peritoneal metastases
   j. lymphoma
   k. hernia
6. Create high-quality diagnostic scans demonstrating the appropriate anatomy in all planes pertinent to the peritoneum.
7. Select the correct equipment settings appropriate to individual body habitus.
8. Distinguish between the normal and abnormal sonographic appearances of the peritoneal cavity.

To further enhance learning, students should use marking pens to color the anatomic illustrations that follow.

FIGURE 11-1

Transverse Section of the Abdominal Cavity Showing the Reflections of the Peritoneum

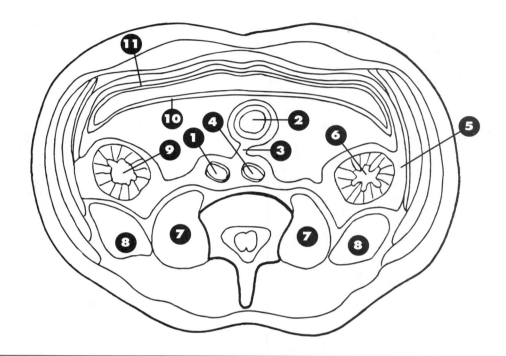

1   inferior vena cava

2   small intestine

3   mesentery of the small intestine

4   aorta

5   peritoneum

6   descending colon

7   psoas major muscle

8   quadratus lumborum muscle

9   ascending colon

10   posterior layers of the greater omentum*

11   anterior layers of the greater omentum*

There is usually no space between the anterior and posterior layers of the greater omentum; they are usually fused together.

FIGURE 11-2
Anterior View of the Abdominal Viscera
(Liver Pulled Upward)

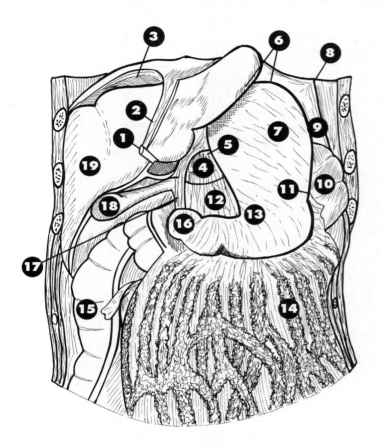

Lesser Omentum (Figure 11-2)

The visceral peritoneum covers the anterior surface of the stomach, and the lesser curvature forms the anterior layer of the lesser omentum. The lesser omentum has a free border on the right where it folds around the common bile duct, hepatic artery, and portal vein. This free border forms the anterior margin of the opening into the lesser sac. The peritoneum forms the posterior layer of the lesser omentum to become continuous with the visceral layer of peritoneum covering the posterior stomach wall.

The peritoneum leaves the greater curvature of the stomach to form the gastrosplenic omentum. At this point it reflects backward toward the abdominal wall to form the anterior layer of the lienorenal ligament. The peritoneum now covers the anterior surface of the pancreas, the aorta, and the inferior vena cava.

The peritoneum passes anteriorly over the right kidney to the lateral abdominal wall to reach the anterior abdominal wall, where it forms a continuous layer around the abdomen.

1	ligamentum teres	11	gastrosplenic ligament
2	falciform ligament	12	lesser omentum
3	hepatic coronary ligament	13	lesser curvature of the stomach
4	caudate lobe of the liver	14	greater omentum
5	hepatogastric ligament	15	ascending colon
6	cardiac ligament	16	pylorus
7	fundus of the stomach	17	epiploic foramen
8	diaphragm	18	gallbladder
9	parietal peritoneum	19	liver
10	spleen		

FIGURE 11-3
Sagittal Section Through the Abdomen and Pelvis

Sagittal View of the Peritoneum (Figure 11-3)

The parietal peritoneum along the anterior abdominal wall may be traced from the falciform ligament to the diaphragm. The visceral peritoneum covers the anterior and inferior surfaces of the liver to the porta hepatis. At this point it passes to the lesser curvature of the stomach as the anterior layer of the lesser omentum. It covers the anterior surface of the stomach to form the greater omentum. The apron fold of the greater omentum hangs anterior to the intestine and contains part of the lesser sac within it. The peritoneum then folds upward and forms the posterior layer of the greater omentum. At the transverse colon the peritoneum forms the posterior layer of the transverse mesocolon. The peritoneum passes over the anterior border of the pancreas and runs downward anterior to the third part of the duodenum.

The peritoneum leaves the posterior abdominal wall as the anterior layer of the mesentery of the small intestine. The visceral peritoneum covers the jejunum and forms the posterior layer of the mesentery. The peritoneum returns to the posterior abdominal wall into the pelvis to cover the anterior rectum. Here, in the female, it reflects onto the posterior vagina to form the rectouterine pouch, or Douglas' pouch. In the female the peritoneum passes over the vagina to its anterior surface to the upper surface of the bladder to the anterior abdominal wall. In the male it reflects off the bladder and seminal vesicles to form the rectovesical pouch.

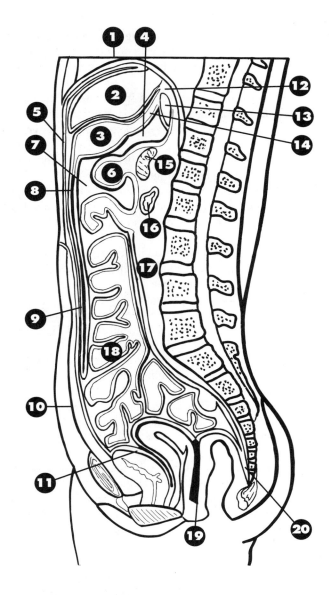

1	diaphragm	8	greater omentum	15	pancreas
2	liver	9	parietal peritoneum	16	duodenum
3	stomach	10	linea alba	17	retroperitoneum
4	omental bursa	11	vesicouterine pouch	18	intestine
5	gastric ligament	12	subphrenic space	19	rectouterine pouch
6	transverse colon	13	lesser omentum	20	anococcygeus ligament
7	peritoneal cavity	14	caudate lobe of the liver		

Peritoneal Cavity Review Notes

DETERMINATION OF INTRAPERITONEAL LOCATION

- Pleural versus subdiaphragmatic:
  - Because of the coronary ligament attachments, collections in the right posterior subphrenic space cannot extend between the bare area of the liver and the diaphragm.
  - Because the right pleural space extends medially to the attachment of the right superior coronary ligament, pleural collections may appear apposed to the bare area.
  - Pleural fluid will tend to distribute posteromedially.
- Subcapsular versus intraperitoneal:
  - Subcapsular liver and spleen collections are seen when inferior to the diaphragmatic echocomplex unilaterally and conforming to the shape of the organ capsule.
  - Subcapsular will be confined to the falciform ligament.
  - It may extend medially to the attachment of the superior coronary ligament.
- Retroperitoneal versus intraperitoneal:
  - The mass is confirmed when anterior renal displacement or anterior displacement of dilated ureters can be documented.
  - The mass interposed anteriorly or superiorly to kidneys can be located either intraperitoneally or retroperitoneally.
  - Fatty and collagenous connective tissues in the perirenal or anterior pararenal space produce echoes that are best demonstrated on sagittal scans.
  - Retroperitoneal lesions displace the echo ventrally and cranially; hepatic and subhepatic lesions produce inferior and posterior displacement.
  - Anterior displacement of SMA and SMV, splenic vein, renal vein, and IVC excludes an intraperitoneal location.
  - Large right-sided retroperitoneal masses rotate the intrahepatic portal veins to the left.
  - The left portal vein may flow from right to left rather than the umbilical portion entering the liver in a posteroanterior direction.
  - Right posterior hepatic masses of similar dimension produce minor displacement of the intrahepatic portal vein.
  - Primary liver masses should move simultaneously with the liver.
- Extraperitoneal versus intraperitoneal:
  - Delineation of the undisrupted peritoneal line demarcates extraperitoneal from intraperitoneal locations.
  - Demonstration of posterior or lateral bladder displacement suggests an extraperitoneal or retroperitoneal location.

SONOGRAPHIC IDENTIFICATION OF INTRAPERITONEAL COMPARTMENTS

- Perihepatic and upper abdominal compartments:
  - Ligaments on the right side of the liver form the subphrenic and subhepatic spaces.
  - The falciform ligament divides the subphrenic space into right and left components.
  - The ligamentum teres hepatis ascends from the umbilicus to the umbilical notch of the liver within the free margin of the falciform ligament before coursing within the liver.
  - The bare area is delineated by the right superior and inferior coronary ligaments, which separate the posterior subphrenic space from the right superior subhepatic space (Morison's pouch).
  - Lateral to the bare area and right triangular ligament, the posterior subphrenic and subhepatic spaces are continuous.
  - A single large and irregular perihepatic space surrounds the superior and lateral aspects of the left lobe of the liver, with the left coronary ligaments anatomically separating the subphrenic space into anterior and posterior compartments.
  - The left subhepatic space is divided into an anterior compartment (gastrohepatic recess) and a posterior compartment (lesser sac) by the lesser omentum and stomach.
  - The lesser sac lies anterior to the pancreas and posterior to the stomach.
  - With fluid in the lesser and greater omental cavities, the lesser omentum may be seen as a linear, undulating echodensity extending from the stomach to the porta hepatis.
  - Gastrosplenic ligament—The left lateral extension of the greater omentum connects the gastric greater curvature to the superior splenic hilum and forms a portion of the left lateral border of the lesser sac.
  - Splenorenal ligament—This ligament is formed by the posterior reflection of the peritoneum off the spleen and, passing inferiorly to overlie the left kidney, forms the posterior portion of the left lateral border of the lesser sac and separates the lesser sac from the renosplenic recess.
- The lesser omental bursa:
  - The lesser sac itself is subdivided into a larger lateroinferior and a smaller mediosuperior recess by the gastropancreatic folds, which are produced by the left gastric and hepatic arteries.
  - The lesser sac extends to the diaphragm.
  - The superior recess of the bursa surrounds the anterior, medial, and posterior surfaces of the caudate lobe, making the caudate a lesser sac structure.

- Lesser sac collections may extend a considerable distance below the plane of the pancreas by inferiorly displacing the transverse mesocolon or extending into the inferior recess of the greater omentum.
- Lower abdominal and pelvic compartments:
  - The supravesical space and medial and lateral inguinal fossae represent intraperitoneal paravesical spaces formed by indentation of the anterior parietal peritoneum by the bladder, obliterated umbilical arteries, and inferior epigastric vessels.
  - The retrovesical space is divided by the uterus into the anterior vesicouterine recess and posterior rectouterine sac (Douglas' pouch).
  - Peritoneal reflection over the dome of the bladder may have an inferior recess extending anterior to the bladder.
  - Ascites displaces the distended urinary bladder inferiorly but not posteriorly.
  - Intraperitoneal fluid will compress the bladder from its lateral-aspect in cases of loculation.
  - Fluid in the extraperitoneal prevesical space has a "yoke over Bell" configuration, displacing the bladder posteriorly and compressing it from the sides along its entire length.

ASCITES

- Serous ascites appears as echofree fluid regions indented and shaped by the organs and viscera it surrounds or between which it is interposed.
- The amount of intraperitoneal fluid depends on the location and volume.
- Peritoneal pressure, patient position, the area from which fluid originates, rapidity of accumulation, presence or absence of adhesions, density of fluid with respect to other abdominal organs, and degree of bladder fullness affect the ultrasonographic appearance.
- The fluid first fills Douglas' pouch, then the lateral paravesical recesses; it then ascends to both paracolic gutters.
- The major flow of fluid from the pelvis is via the right paracolic gutter.
- Ascites may involve the chest, and continue from the abdomen into the posterior mediastinum through the esophageal hiatus in patients with concomitant hiatal hernia.
- In a patient who is supine, small volumes of fluid first appear around the inferior tip of the right lobe in the superior portion of the right flank and in the pelvic cul-de-sac, followed by collection in paracolic gutters, lateral and anterior to the liver.
- Small bowel loops will sink or float in surrounding ascitic fluid, depending on the relative gas content and the amount of fat in the mesentery.
- The middle portion of the transverse colon usually floats on top of the fluid because of gas content, whereas the ascending portions of colon, which are

fixed retroperitoneally, remain in normal location with or without gas.
- Floating loops of small bowel, anchored posteriorly by the mesentery and with fluid between the mesenteric folds, have a characteristic anterior convex fan shape or arcuate appearance.
- An overdistended bladder may mask small quantities of fluid.
- Inflammatory or malignant ascites appears as fine or coarse internal echoes, loculation, or unusual distribution, matting or clumping of bowel loops, and thickening of interfaces between the fluid and neighboring structures.
- Hepatorenal recess occurs with generalized ascites, inflammatory fluid from acute cholecystitis, fluid caused by pancreatic autolysis, or blood from a ruptured hepatic neoplasm or ectopic gestation.
- Abdominal fluid collections do not persist as a normal part of the healing process 1 week after abdominal surgery.
- Loculated ascites tends to be more irregular in outline, shows less mass effect, and may change shape slightly with positional variation.

ABSCESS

- An abscess has a cystlike, fluid appearance to a solid composition.
- The sonographer may see well-defined debris, septa, gas (scattered air reflectors), and acoustic shadowing.
- The configuration depends on the anatomic compartment involved.
- Abscesses tend to hold their shape and displace or indent neighboring structures unless they meet with resistant boundaries such as the liver capsule or sacral promontory.
- The walls of the affected organ are typically fine and irregular.

HEMATOMA

- The echo characteristics of hematomas are highly variable and are dependent on the age of the collection and on the transducer frequency.
- In the acute phase a hematoma may be echofree with increased through transmission.
- The organization of a laminated clot or fragmentation of a hemolyzed clot within hematomas results in the generation of internal echoes.
- Coarse clumps of echogenic material may be a striking feature of chronic hematoma.
- The shape of a hematoma is determined by its location.
  - An intraperitoneal collection is ovoid or spherical and tends to displace rather than conform to adjacent structures.
  - A lenticular configuration is more likely to be encoun-

tered in instances when hemorrhage dissects along well-defined tissue planes.

- Intramural intestinal hemorrhage in hemophilia is seen as a tubular anechoic mass containing a core of strong echoes (bowel lumen), an appearance not unlike that of neoplastic or inflammatory diseases or other causes of bowel wall thickening.

BILOMA

- Extrahepatic loculated collections of bile may develop because of iatrogenic, traumatic, or spontaneous rupture of the biliary tree.
- Bilomas are cystic in nature.
- The sonographer may see weak, internal echoes, or a fluid-fluid level if clots or debris are not present.
- Bilomas are also characterized by sharp margins.
- Extrahepatic: usually crescentic, surrounding and compressing structures with which they come in contact
- The patient with a biloma may experience pain in the RUQ, or in the mid or LUQ areas.

INFLAMMATORY FLUID OF PANCREATIC ORIGIN

- Pancreatic pseudocysts are unilocular, multilocular, and ovoid or irregular.
- They are also characterized by smooth or ragged walls, anechoic echo patterns, debris, septations, and nondependent internal echoes caused by contained and adherent inflammatory masses.

CYSTIC LESIONS OF THE MESENTERY, OMENTUM, AND PERITONEUM

- Abdominal cysts may be embryologic, traumatic or acquired, neoplastic, or infective and degenerative.
- Mesenteric and omental cysts are uniloculated or multiloculated, with smooth walls and thin internal septations.
- Internal echoes are correlated with fat globules, debris, superimposed hemorrhage, or infection.
- A cystic lesion may follow the contour of the underlying bowel and conform to the anterior abdominal wall rather than produce distention.
- A hemorrhage into the omental or mesenteric cysts may cause rapid distension and may clinically mimic ascites.
- Peritoneal inclusion cysts are considered in the differential diagnosis when large adnexal cystic structures are identified in a young woman.
- Fungal infections may appear as peritoneal cystic lesions.

CEREBROSPINAL FLUID ASCITES

- Cerebrospinal fluid ascites is a rare complication of ventricular peritoneal (VP) shunting.
- This condition is characterized by a diffuse, nonloculated collection of cerebral spinal fluid (CSF) that occurs secondary to a primary failure of the peritoneal cavity to absorb spinal fluid.
- Cerebrospinal fluid ascites is indistinguishable from transudative ascites.

LYMPHOCELE

- A lymphocele is a lymph-filled space resulting from surgery.
- Lymphoceles are unilocular and usually retroperitoneal.
- Lymphoceles are elliptical with sharp margins and no internal echoes, but may have thin septations.

URINOMA

- A urinoma is an encapsulated collection of urine that may result from closed renal injury or surgical intervention, or may arise spontaneously secondary to an obstructing lesion.
- The extraperitoneal extravasation may be subcapsular or perirenal; the latter collections are sometimes termed *uriniferous pseudocysts.*
- They may leak around the ureter, where perinephric fascia is weakest, or into the adjoining fascial planes and peritoneal cavity.
- Cystic masses are most often oriented inferomedially, with upward and lateral displacement of the lower pole of the kidney and medial displacement of the ureter.

On ultrasound examination, the sonographer may see:

- Anechoic or low-level echoes
- Sharp margins
- Elliptical shape
- Indentation by adjacent solid organs
- Thin septa

URACHAL CYST

- A urachal cyst is caused by incomplete regression of the urachus during fetal development. Variations include:
  - patent urachus
  - urachal diverticulum
  - urachal sinus
  - urachal cyst

On ultrasound examination, a urachal cyst appears:

- As a mass between the umbilicus and the bladder
- Cystic
- There may be small or giant multiseptations extending into the upper abdomen.
- With mixed echogenicity
- As a bladder distention

PERITONEAL METASTASES

- Peritoneal metastases develop from cellular implantation across the peritoneal cavity.
- The most common primary sites are the ovaries, stomach, and colon.
- Other sites are the pancreas, biliary tract, kidneys, testicles, uterus sarcomas, melanomas, teratomas, and embryonic tumors.

The sonographer may see the following:

- Nodular, sheet-like, irregular configuration
- Small nodules along the peritoneal line

- Larger masses obliterate the line
- Adhesion to bowel loops

LYMPHOMA OF OMENTUM AND MESENTERY

- The omental band is a uniformly thick, hypoechoic band-shaped structure that follows the convexity of the anterior and lateral abdominal wall.
- This lymphoma is a lobulated confluent hypoechoic mass surrounding a centrally positioned echogenic area.
- The sandwich sign is a mass infiltrating the mesenteric leaves and encasing the SMA.

PRIMARY TUMORS OF THE PERITONEUM, OMENTUM, AND MESENTERY

- Secondary tumors and lymphoma are neoplasms that most commonly involve the peritoneum and mesentery.

- These are characterized by fibromatoses and fibrosing mesenteritis.
- They may also be lipomatous.
- Peritoneal and omental mesothelioma occur in middle-aged men.
- They are often caused by asbestos exposure.
- The patient experiences abdominal pain, weight loss, and ascites.
- This appears as a large mass with discrete smaller nodes scattered over large areas of visceral and parietal paritoneum.
- Or, it may appear as diffuse nodes and plaques that coat the abdominal cavity and envelope and mat together the abdominal viscera.

Abdominal Wall Review Notes

NORMAL ANATOMY

- Paired rectus abdominis muscles are delineated medially in the midline of the body by linea alba.
- Laterally the aponeuroses of external oblique, internal oblique, and transversus abdominis muscles unite to form a band-like, vertical fibrous groove called the linea semilunaris, or spigelian fascia.
- The sheath of three anterolateral abdominal muscles invests the rectus muscle both anteriorly and posteriorly.
- Midway between the umbilicus and symphysis pubis, the aponeurotic sheath passes anteriorly to the rectus muscle only.
- Below the line, the rectus muscle is separated from the intraabdominal contents only by the transversalis fascia and the peritoneum.
- The rectus muscles are a biconvex muscle group delineated by the linea alba and linea semilunaris.
- The peritoneal line is seen as discrete linear echogenicity in the deepest layer of the abdominal wall.

PATHOLOGY

Extraperitoneal Hematomas

- Rectus sheath hematomas are acute or chronic collections of blood lying either within the rectus muscle or between the muscle and its sheath.
- A rectus sheath hematoma may be the result of direct trauma, pregnancy, cardiovascular and degenerative muscle diseases, surgical injury, anticoagulation therapy, steroids, or extreme exercise.
- Clinically, the patient has acute, sharp, persistent nonradiating pain.
- An ultrasound study shows a mass that is anechoic, with scattered internal echoes.
- A bladder-flap hematoma is a collection of blood between the bladder and lower uterine segment, result-

ing from lower uterine transverse CS and bleeding from uterine vessels.
- A subfascial hematoma is blood in the prevesical space caused by disruption of inferior epigastric vessels or branches during CS.

Inflammatory Lesions

- Abdominal wall abscesses appear on ultrasound examination with anechoic or internal echoes, gas bubbles, and irregular margins.
- These lesions may be flat, spindle-shaped, or ovoid.

Neoplasms

- Neoplasms may be lipomas, desmoid tumors, or metastases.
- Neoplasms are hypoechoic to cystic, except for lipomas.
- A desmoid tumor is a benign fibrous neoplasm of the aponeurotic structures.
  - It most commonly arises in relation to the rectus abdominus muscle and its sheath.
  - Echo patterns of desmoid tumors are anechoic and hypoechoic.
  - These tumors are characterized by smooth and sharply defined walls.

Hernia

- A hernia may appear as a peristalsing bowel and may mimic other masses.
- It may be absent with incarceration.
- A hernia may involve the omentum only.
- It commonly originates near the junction of the linea semilunaris and the arcuate line.
- A spigelian hernia sac itself may dissect between the muscle layers or subcutaneous tissues to move elsewhere.

- A hernia penetrates both the transversus abdominus muscle and internal oblique muscle, expanding laterally in the space between two oblique muscles.
- The sonographer should scan obliquely between the anterior superior iliac spine and pubic crest and along the course of the inguinal ligament.
- The femoral artery and vein are seen anterior to the iliopubic junction.
- The psoas muscle and lymphatic channels occupy space between the anterior superior iliac spine and the iliopubic junction.
- Masses arising in relation to femoral vessels and beneath the inguinal ligament include the femoral hernias, lipomas, soft tissue sarcomas, and lymph node masses.
- Abdominals arising superior to femoral vessels and the inguinal ligament include direct and indirect inguinal hernias, ectopic testicles, and extension of femoral hernias.

ABSCESS FORMATION AND POCKETS IN THE ABDOMEN AND PELVIS

An abscess is a cavity formed by necrosis within solid tissue or a circumscribed collection of purulent material.

Clinical Symptoms and Lab Values

- Fever
- Chills
- Weakness
- Malaise
- Pain at the localized site of infection
- Normal liver function values
- Increased white blood cell
- Generalized sepsis
- Bacterial cultures (if superficial)

General Sonographic Appearance

Abscess collections can appear quite varied in their texture because of the length of time the abscess has to form, or the available space the abscess has to localize. Therefore many collections may appear predominantly fluid-filled with irregular borders; they can also be complex with debris floating within the cystic mass; or they may appear as more of a solid pattern. If the collection is in the pelvis, careful analysis of bowel patterns and peristalsis should be made in an attempt to separate the bowel from the abscess collection.

Classically an abscess appears on ultrasound examination as an elliptical sonolucent mass with thick and irregular margins. It tends to be under tension and displaces surrounding structures. A septated appearance may result from previous or developing adhesions. Necrotic debris produces low-level, internal echoes, which may be seen to float within the abscess. Fluid levels are secondary to layering, probably because of the setting of debris.

Liver

There are five major pathways through which bacteria can enter the liver and cause abscess formation:

1. Through the portal system
2. By way of ascending cholangitis of the CBD, which is the most common cause of liver bacteria in the US.
3. Via the hepatic artery (HA) secondary to bacteremia
4. By direct extension from an infection
5. By implantation of bacteria after trauma to the abdominal wall.

Renal

Renal abscesses are classified according to their locations.

A renal carbuncle is an abscess that forms within the renal parenchyma. Symptoms vary from none to fever, leukocytosis, and flank pain. Sonographic appearance is a discrete mass within the kidney—may be cystic or cystic with debris, or may be solid.

A perinephric abscess is usually the result of a perforated renal abscess that leaks purulent material into the tissues adjacent to the kidney. Sonographic appearance shows fluid collection around the kidney, or an adjacent mass that can vary from a cystic to more solid appearance.

Abdominal Abscess

85% of abdominal pelvic abscesses appear after surgery or trauma. The hepatic recesses and perihepatic spaces are the most common sites for abscess. The pelvic area is a common site also; free fluid below the transverse mesocolon often flows into Douglas' pouch and perivesical spaces.

Gas Containing Abscess. An abscess that contains gas appears with varying echo patterns. Generally the patterns appear as a densely echogenic mass with or without acoustic shadowing and otherwise increased through transmission. A teratoma may mimic the pattern of a gas-containing abscess, but the clinical history and x-ray examination will exclude abscess from the diagnosis. An abscess may be confused with a solid lesion because it may be difficult to determine the presence of through transmission.

Peritonitis and resultant abscess formation may be a generalized or localized process. Multiloculated abscesses or multiple collections should be documented and their size determined as accurately as possible to aid in planning drainage and for improved accuracy in follow-up studies.

Lesser-Sac Abscess. The small "slitlike" epiploic foramen usually seals off the lesser sac from inflammatory processes extrinsic to it. If the process begins within the lesser sac, such as with a pancreatic abscess, the sac may be involved in addition to other secondarily affected peritoneal and retroperitoneal spaces.

The differential diagnoses should include the following:

- Pseudocyst
- Pancreatic abscess

- Gastric outlet obstruction
- Fluid-filled stomach

Subphrenic Abscess. The LUQ is difficult to examine. The sonographer may alter the patient's position to right lateral decubitus to scan along the coronal plane of the body, or to the prone position to use the spleen as a window. The sonographer should be careful of pleural effusions. Another alternative is to scan the patient upright so the pleural area and subdiaphragmatic area may be better demonstrated.

Subcapsular collections of fluid within the liver may mimic loculated subphrenic fluid. Intraabdominal fluid may be differentiated by its smooth border and its tendency to conform to the contour of the liver. It displaces the liver medially, rather than indents the border locally, as subcapsular fluid might. A tense subphrenic abscess can displace the liver.

It may be difficult to distinguish a subphrenic abscess from ascites. The sonographer can look at the margins of the fluid collection to differentiate or can look for other fluid collections, such as in the pelvis, to distinguish ascites from fluid. Preperitoneal fat anterior to the liver may mimic a localized fluid collection.

An abscess will collect in the most dependent area of the body; therefore, all the gutters, pockets, and pouches should be evaluated, in addition to the spaces above and around various organs.

If an abscess is suspected; i.e., if the patient has a fever of unknown origin, the sonographer should evaluate these areas:

- Subdiaphragmatic (liver and spleen)
- Splenic recess and borders
- Hepatic recess and borders
- Liver and right kidney
- Pericolic gutters
- Lesser omentum
- Transverse mesocolon
- Morison's pouch
- Gastrocolic ligament
- Phrenicosplenic ligament
- Recesses between the intestinal loops and colon
- Extrahepatic falciform ligament
- Douglas' pouch
- Broad ligaments (female)
- Anterior to the urinary bladder
- Right subhepatic space (fluid ascends up right pericoloic gutter into Morison's pouch; when fluid fills Morison's pouch it spreads past coronary ligament and up over the dome of the liver.) The presence of a right subhepatic abscess generally implies previous contamination of the right subhepatic space.

Appendiceal Abscess

Acute appendicitis is the most common abdominal pathologic process that requires immediate surgery. Colicky pain at onset may be caused by obstruction of the appendix, which itself is caused by a fecalith at its origin at the cecum. The appendix becomes distended rapidly after obstruction.

- Symptoms of appendicitis are fever and severe pain near McBurney's point in the RLQ. (Draw straight line between the umbilicus and the anterior superior iliac spine and then move 2″ along the line from the iliac spine.)
- Laboratory values show an increase in white blood cells.
- Differential diagnoses may include:
  - PID
  - Twisted or ruptured ovarian cyst
  - Acute gastroenteritis
  - Mesenteric lymphadenitis
- A sonogram study will show a complex RLQ mass. The sonographer should examine other gutters to rule out differentials.

Abdominal Wall Masses

An abdominal wall collection usually occurs postoperatively. A sonogram may show cystic, complex, or solid characteristics. Generally an abdominal wall mass is very superficial and easy to locate.

Hematoma

Hematomas are caused by surgical injury to tissue and blunt or sharp trauma to the abdomen. Laboratory values may show a decrease in hematocrit and red blood cells, and the patient may go into shock. The sonographic appearance depends on the stage of the bleeding. New bleeds are primarily cystic with some debris (blood clots); as the blood begins to organize, the mass becomes more solid in appearance. New clots may be very homogeneous.

Hematomas may become infected and at any stage may be sonographically indistinguishable from abscess. They may mimic subphrenic fluid.

Lymphoceles

These collections generally look like loculated, simple fluid collections, although they may have a more complex, usually septated morphology. Differentiation from loculated ascites is usually possible because the mass effect of a lymphocele that is under tension will displace the surrounding organs. Differentiation from other fluid collections is mainly made by aspiration.

Peritoneum

The peritoneal lining is not seen as a distinct structure during sonography unless it is thickened. This is usually secondary to metastatic implants or to direct extension of a tumor from the viscera or mesentery. Primary mesotheliomas occur rarely.

Review Exercise A • Peritoneal Cavity and Abdominal Wall

1. Describe the technique used to image the peritoneal cavity and abdominal wall. _____

_____

_____

2. How does the sonographer differentiate between pleural and subdiaphragmatic fluid collections? _____

_____

_____

3. How does the sonographer differentiate between subcapsular and intraperitoneal fluid collections in the abdomen?

_____

_____

_____

4. How does the sonographer differentiate between retroperitoneal and intraperitoneal fluid collections? _____

_____

_____

_____

5. How does the sonographer differentiate between extraperitoneal and intraperitoneal fluid collections? _____

_____

_____

6. Use these terms to complete the following statements:

right triangular ligament   subphrenic and subhepatic spaces   lesser sac (use twice)
falciform ligament   bare area   gastrosplenic ligament
lesser omentum   gastrohepatic ligament   splenorenal ligament
ligamentum teres

a. Ligaments on the right side of the liver form the _____ and _____ .

b. The _____ divides the subphrenic space into right and left components.

c. The _____ ascends from the umbilicus to the umbilical notch of the liver within the free

margin of the falciform ligament before coursing within the liver.

d. The _____ is delineated by right superior and inferior coronary ligaments, which separate

the posterior subphrenic space from the right superior subhepatic space (Morison's pouch).

e. The left subhepatic space is divided into an anterior compartment (_____) and a posterior

compartment (_____) by the lesser omentum and stomach.

f. The _____ sac lies anterior to the pancreas and posterior to the stomach.

g. With fluid in the lesser and greater omental cavities, the _____ may be seen as a linear,

undulating echodensity extending from the stomach to the porta hepatis.

h. The _____ ligament is the left lateral extension of the greater omentum that connects the

gastric greater curvature to the superior splenic hilum and forms a portion of the left lateral border of the lesser sac.

i. The _____ ligament is formed by the posterior reflection of the peritoneum off the spleen

and passes inferiorly to overlie the left kidney, forms the posterior portion of the left lateral border of the lesser
sac and separates the lesser sac from the renosplenic recess.

7. What is another name for Douglas' pouch? _____

_____

_____

8. How does ascites displace the urinary bladder? _____

_____

_____

9. How does serous ascites appear on ultrasound examination? _____

_____

_____

10. How does inflammatory or malignant ascites appear on ultrasound examination? _____

_____

_____

11. Describe the sonographic appearance of an abdominal abscess. _____

_____

_____

_____

12. Describe the sonographic appearance of a hematoma. _____

_____

_____

_____

13. What is a biloma? Describe the sonographic appearance. _____

_____

_____

14. Discuss the sonographic appearance of cystic lesions of the mesentery, omentum, and peritoneum. _____

_____

_____

15. What is the sonographic appearance of a urinoma, and how does it form? _____

_____

_____

_____

16. Describe the sonographic appearance of lymphoma of the omentum and mesentery. _____

_____

_____

_____

17. What is the sonographic technique of examining a rectus sheath hematoma? What is the sonographic appearance? _____

_____

_____

18. How can the sonographer determine a hernia from a cystic mass? _____

_____

_____

Review Exercise B • Fluid Collections in the Abdomen and Pelvis

1. List the five areas in the abdominopelvic cavity where ascites or fluid collections may be found.

    a. _____

    b. _____

    c. _____

    d. _____

    e. _____

2. List two of the most common causes of abscess formation.

    a. _____

    b. _____

3. List the differential diagnoses for fluid collections.

    a. _____

    b. _____

    c. _____

    d. _____

    e. _____

    f. _____

4. How does the sonographer find McBurney's point and what disease is it associated with most often? _____

_____

5. What other areas should be scanned when searching for an appendiceal abscess?

    a. _____

    b. _____

    c. _____

    d. _____

6. A postsurgical patient has an ultrasound examination that demonstrates a primarily cystic mass with some solid components. No peristalsis is seen on real time. The differential diagnoses would include:

    a. _____

    b. _____

7. Where is Morison's pouch? _____

_____

_____

8. Where is Douglas' pouch? _____

_____

9. How can one distinguish among ascites and malignant ascites? _____

_____

_____

10. What are three fluid collections associated with renal transplants?

a. _____

b. _____

c. _____

11. What is the classic ultrasound appearance of a tuboovarian abscess? _____

_____

_____

12. What is the most common cause of secondary localized peritonitis in children? _____

13. What are the reasons for hematomas in children?

a. _____

b. _____

c. _____

14. What is iatrogenic? _____

15. What direction is the bowel pushed in a patient with ascites? _____

_____

_____

16. What position should the patient be placed in for a thoracentesis guidance? What care should the sonographer take in marking the location? _____

_____

_____

17. In what position should the patient be placed to show the fluid in Morison's pouch? _____

18. Describe how to localize the needle tip with ultrasonography during an interventional procedure. _____

_____

_____

_____

19. If a mass is shown in the LUQ, how could the sonographer prove that the fluid mass was in the stomach if the patient has a nasogastric tube and was restricted from fluid intake? _____

_____

_____

_____

20. Discuss the role of water in an ultrasound examination of the pancreas. _____

_____

_____

_____

Self-Test • Peritoneal Cavity and Abdominal Wall

1. Collections in the right posterior subphrenic space cannot extend between the bare area of the liver and the:

    a. right kidney

    b. diaphragm

    c. right pleural space

    d. coronary ligament

2. Primary liver masses should move simultaneously with the liver (true or false).

3. Posterior or lateral displacement of the bladder suggests a mass to be:

    a. intraperitoneal

    b. supraperitoneal

    c. retroperitoneal

    d. infraperitoneal

4. _____ on the right side of the liver form the subphrenic and subhepatic

    spaces.

    a. Tendons

    b. Fibers

    c. Falciform ligament

    d. Ligaments

5. Name the ligament that is the left lateral extension of the greater omentum that connects the gastric greater curvature to the superior splenic hilum and forms a portion of the left lateral border of the lesser sac.

    a. the splenorenal ligament

    b. the gastrosplenic ligament

    c. the falciform ligament

    d. the gastrorenal ligament

6. This ligament forms the posterior portion of the left lateral border of the lesser sac and separates the lesser sac from the renosplenic recess.

    a. the gastrosplenic ligament

    b. the falciform ligament

    c. the splenorenal ligament

    d. the costophrenic ligament

7. Which lobe of the liver is a lesser sac structure?

    a. the medial segment of the left lobe

    b. the lateral segment of the left lobe

    c. the posterior segment of the right lobe

    d. the caudate lobe

8. Ascites will displace the bladder inferiorly but not posteriorly (true or false).

9. Inflammatory or malignant ascites would present with all of the following characteristics except:

    a. anechoic patterns

    b. clumping of bowel loops

    c. fine or coarse internal echoes

    d. thickening of interfaces

10. What lesion may mimic a gas-containing abscess?

    a. fibroid

    b. teratoma

    c. lipoma

    d. hemangioma

11. Differential diagnosis of a lesser-sac abscess should include all except:

    a. pseudocyst

    b. gastric outlet obstruction

    c. fluid-filled stomach

    d. pancreatic carcinoma

12. Subphrenic abscess collections may be easily differentiated from ascites (true or false).

13. A renal carbuncle is an abscess that forms outside the renal parenchyma (true or false).

14. A perinephric abscess is usually the result of a perforated renal abscess that leaks purulent material into the tissues adjacent to the kidney (true or false).

15. The most common site(s) for abdominal abscess formation is (are) the:

    a. appendix

    b. retrovesical space

    c. hepatic recesses and perihepatic spaces

    d. portal vein

16. The presence of a right subhepatic abscess generally implies previous contamination of the right subhepatic space (true or false).

17. The most common abdominal pathologic process that requires immediate surgery is:

    a. renal carbuncle

    b. acute appendicitis

    c. perirenal abscess

    d. cholangitis

18. _____ is an extrahepatic loculated collection of bile that may develop because of iatrogenic, traumatic, or spontaneous rupture of the biliary tree.

    a. Biloma

    b. Bilitis

    c. Cholangitis

    d. Choleductitis

19. An encapsulated collection of urine is:

   a. seroma

   b. nephroma

   c. uroma

   d. urinoma

20. The sandwich sign represents a mass infiltrating the mesenteric leaves and encasing the superior mesenteric artery (true or false).

Case Reviews

1. A 43-year-old female has had an increasing abdominal girth over the past 2 months. What are your findings (Figure 11-4)?

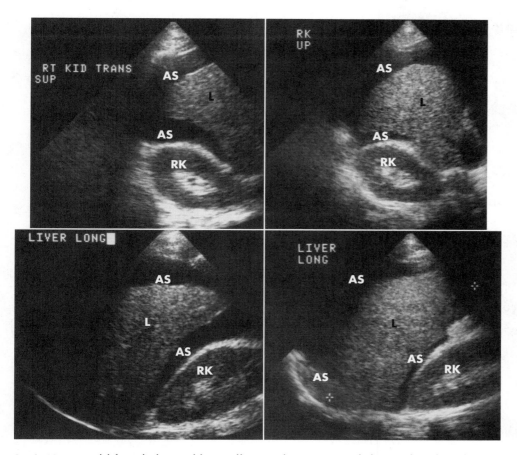

2. A 49-year-old female has ankle swelling and increasing abdominal girth. What are your findings (Figure 11-5)?

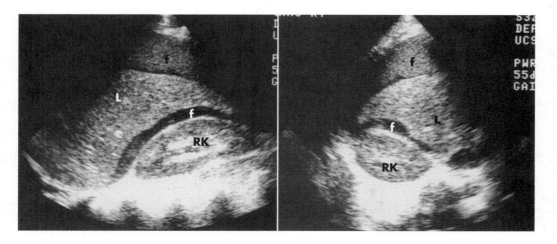

3. A 38-year-old female has right upper quadrant pain. What are your findings (Figure 11-6)?

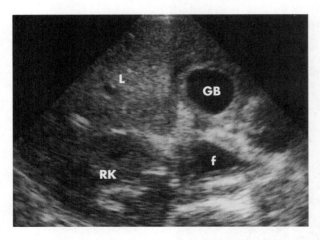

4. A 36-year-old female has severe right upper quadrant pain and fever. What are your findings (Figure 11-7)?

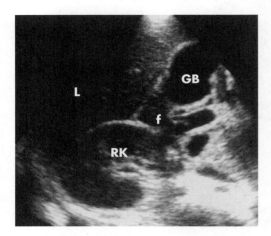

5. A 60-year-old male has shortness of breath. What are your findings (Figure 11-8)?

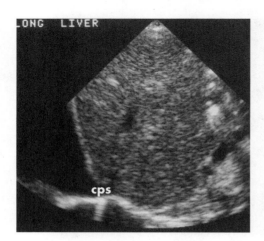

6. A 22-year-old male has right lower quadrant pain near McBurney's point. The patient has had a fever and vomiting for the past 3 days. Laboratory values show an increased white blood count. What are your findings (Figure 11-9)?

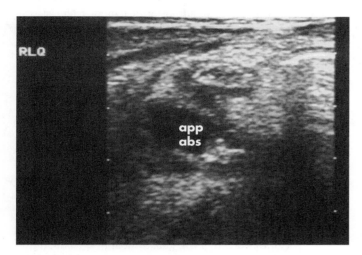

7. A 60-year-old male comes to the emergency department 2 days postcardiac catherization to the right groin. What are your findings (Figure 11-10)?

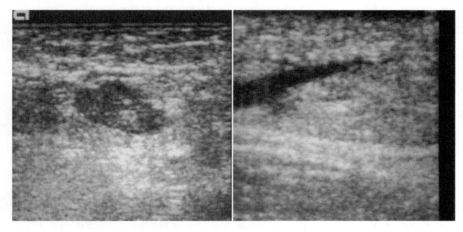

8. A 32-year-old male has abdominal pain and fever. What are your findings (Figure 11-11)?

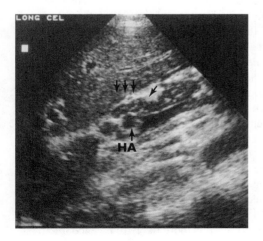

Answers to Review Exercise A

1. Higher frequency transducers should be used to image the abdominal wall. Comparison should be made of the muscular layers in the abdominal wall to look for asymmetry. The peritoneal cavity should be examined with a medium frequency transducer.

2. Because of the coronary ligament attachments, collections in the right posterior subphrenic space cannot extend between the bare area of the liver and the diaphragm. The right pleural space extends medially to the attachment of the right superior coronary ligament; pleural collections may appear apposed to the bare area. Pleural fluid will tend to distribute postero-medially.

3. Subcapsular liver and spleen collections are seen when inferior to the diaphragmatic reflection and conform to the shape of the organ capsule. Subcapsular collections to the liver will be confined to the falciform ligament and may extend medially to the attachment of the superior coronary ligament.

4. A mass is confirmed when anterior renal displacement or anterior displacement of dilated ureters can be documented. A mass interposed anteriorly or superiorly to the kidneys can be located either intraperitoneally or retroperitoneally. Fatty and collagenous connective tissues in the perirenal or anterior pararenal space produce echoes that are best demonstrated on sagittal scans. Retroperitoneal lesions displace the echoes ventrally and cranially; hepatic and subhepatic lesions produce inferior and posterior displacement. Anterior displacement of SMA and SMV, splenic vein, renal vein, and IVC excludes an intraperitoneal location. Large right-sided retroperitoneal masses rotate the intrahepatic portal veins to the left. The left portal vein may flow from right to left rather than the umbilical portion entering the liver in a postero-anterior direction. Right posterior hepatic masses of similar dimension produce minor displacement of the intrahepatic portal vein. Primary liver masses should move simultaneously with the liver.

5. Delineation of the undisrupted peritoneal line demarcates extraperitoneal from intraperitoneal locations. Demonstration of posterior or lateral bladder displacement suggests an extraperitoneal or retroperitoneal location.

6. a. subphrenic and subhepatic spaces
   b. falciform ligament
   c. ligamentum teres
   d. bare area
   e. gastrohepatic ligament, lesser sac
   f. lesser sac
   g. lesser omentum
   h. gastrosplenic ligament
   i. splenorenal ligament

7. Douglas' pouch may also be called the retrovesical space that is divided by the uterus into the anterior vesicouterine recess and posterior rectouterine sac.

8. Ascites displaces the distended urinary bladder inferiorly, but not posteriorly.

9. Serous ascites appears as echofree fluid regions indented and shaped by the organs and viscera it surrounds or between which it is interposed. The fluid first fills Douglas' pouch and then the lateral paravesical recesses, and then ascends to both paracolic gutters. The major flow of fluid from the pelvis is via the right paracolic gutter.

   In a patient who is supine, small volumes of fluid first appear around the inferior tip of the right lobe in the superior portion of the right flank and in the pelvic cul-de-sac, followed by a collection in the paracolic gutters, lateral and anterior to the liver.

   Small bowel loops will sink or float in surrounding ascitic fluid, depending on the relative gas content and amount the of fat in the mesentery. The middle portion of the transverse colon usually floats on top of the fluid because of gas content, whereas the ascending portions of colon, which are fixed retroperitoneally, remain in normal location with or without gas.

   Floating loops of small bowel, anchored posteriorly by mesentery and with fluid between the mesenteric folds, have a characteristic anterior convex fan shape or arcuate appearance.

10. Inflammatory or malignant ascites appears as fine or coarse internal echoes, loculation, or unusual distribution, matting or clumping of bowel loops, and thickening of interfaces between the fluid and neighboring structures.

11. An abdominal abscess has a cyst-like, fluid appearance to a solid composition. The sonographer may see well-defined debris, septa, gas (scattered air reflectors), and acoustic shadowing from debris within. The configuration depends on the anatomic compartment involved. An abscess tends to hold its shape and displace or indent neighboring structures unless it meets with resistant boundaries such as the liver capsule or sacral promontory.

12. The echo characteristics of hematomas are highly variable and are dependent on the age of the collection and on the transducer frequency. In the acute phase a hematoma may be echofree with increased through transmission. The subsequent organization of hemolyzed clot within hematomas results in generation of internal echoes.

    The shape is determined by its location. An intraperitoneal collection is ovoid or spherical and tends to displace rather than conform to adjacent structures. A lenticular configuration is more likely to be encountered in instances when hemorrhage dissects along well-defined tissue planes, i.e., splenic hematoma.

13. Extrahepatic loculated collections of bile may develop because of iatrogenic, traumatic, or spontaneous rupture of the biliary tree. A biloma is cystic in nature with sharp margins and with weak internal echoes, or a fluid-filled level.

14. Abdominal cysts may be embryologic, traumatic or acquired, neoplastic, or infective and degenerative.

    Mesenteric and omental cysts are uni-or multiloculated, with smooth walls and thin internal septations. A hemorrhage into the omental or mesenteric cysts may cause rapid distension and clinically mimic ascites.

15. A urinoma is an encapsulated collection of urine that may result from closed renal injury or surgical intervention, or may arise spontaneously secondary to an obstructing lesion.

    The extraperitoneal extravasation may be subscapular or perirenal; the latter collections are sometimes termed uriniferous pseudocysts. They may leak around the ureter, where perinephric fascia is weakest, or into the adjoining fascial planes and peritoneal cavity.

    Cystic masses are most often oriented inferomedially, with upward and lateral displacement of the lower pole of the kidney and medial displacement of the ureter.

    Ultrasound findings include anechoic or contain low-level echoes, sharp margins, and an elliptical shape. They may be indented by adjacent solid organs and have thin septa.

16. A uniformly thick, hypoechoic, band-shaped structure that follows the convexity of the anterior and lateral abdominal wall is the omental band. Lymphoma is a lobulated confluent hypoechoic mass surrounding a centrally positioned echogenic area. The sandwich sign is a mass infiltrating the mesenteric leaves and encasing the SMA.

17. Rectus sheath hematomas are acute or chronic collections of blood lying either within the rectus muscle or between the muscle and its sheath. A rectus sheath hematoma may be the result of direct trauma, pregnancy, degenerative muscle diseases, surgical injury, anti-coagulation therapy, steroids, or extreme exercise.

    Clinically the patient presents with acute, sharp, persistent nonradiating pain. Ultrasound shows a mass that is anechoic with scattered internal echoes.

18. A hernia may present as peristalsing bowel and may mimic other masses. It commonly originates near the junction of the linea semilunaris and arcuate line. The hernia penetrates both the transversus abdominal muscle and internal oblique muscle, expanding laterally in the space between two oblique muscles.

    The sonographer should scan obliquely between the anterior superior iliac spine and pubic crest and along the course of the inguinal ligament. The femoral artery and vein are seen anterior to the iliopubic junction.

    Masses arising in relation to femoral vessels and beneath the inguinal ligament include the femoral hernias, lipomas, soft tissue sarcomas, and lymph nodes.

    Abnormalities arising superior to femoral vessels and the inguinal ligament include direct and indirect inguinal hernias, ectopic testicles, and extension of femoral hernias.

Answers to Review Exercise B

1. a. subdiaphragmatic;
   b. Morison's pouch;
   c. subphrenic space;
   d. gutters;
   e. pelvis
2. a. surgery
   b. trauma
3. a. abscess
   b. biloma
   c. cyst
   d. cyst with necrosis
   e. hematoma
   f. pseudocyst
4. Draw a straight line between the umbilicus and the anterior-superior iliac spine, and then move medial 2″. It is associated with acute appendicitis.

5. a. right lower quadrant
   b. cul-de-sac
   c. liver-lung interface
   d. pelvis: evaluate ovaries and fallopian tubes
6. a. abscess
   b. hematoma
7. Morison's pouch is located in the subhepatic space, anterior to the right kidney and posterior to the right lobe of the liver.
8. Douglas' pouch is located posterior to the bladder; in females it is between the uterus and rectum; in males it is between the bladder and rectum.
9. In malignant ascites, the fluid may contain debris within. A high-frequency transducer should be used to inspect the anterior abdominal wall for metastasis; the bowel may appear matted.

10. a. urinoma
    b. lymphocele
    c. hematoma
11. A tuboovarian abscess has thick, shaggy walls and possible internal echoes. It is predominately cystic.
12. appendicitis
13. a. spontaneous
    b. traumatic
    c. iatrogenic
14. physician induced
15. The bowel is pushed centrally into the abdominal and pelvic cavities.
16. The patient should be upright. The sonographer should take care to localize anterior to the rib (away from vessels). Be sure to localize the collection at the time of the tap.

17. The patient should be rolled into a right lateral decubitus position.
18. a. realign the transducer with the needle
    b. adjust the focal zone to the tip of the needle
    c. jiggle the needle or stylet to see the tip
    d. inject a small amount of saline to image the tip
19. The sonographer should put a little fluid in the tube, watch for microbubbles in the fluid, and roll the patient.
20. If the pancreas is not well defined on conventional ultrasonography, the patient may be given 16 to 24 ounces of degassed water to outline the duodenum to see the pancreatic tail, body, and head. The patient should be scanned in a semi-upright position.

Answers to Self-Test

1. b	**8.** true	**15.** c
2. true	**9.** a	**16.** true
3. c	**10.** b	**17.** b
4. d	**11.** d	**18.** a
5. b	**12.** false	**19.** d
6. c	**13.** false	**20.** true
7. d	**14.** true	

Answers to Case Reviews

1. (Figure 11-4) Ascites may fill the peritoneal cavity. Small volumes of fluid in the supine position first appear around the inferior tip of the right lobe of the superior portion of the right flank. The fluid changes as the patient changes position, always moving to the most dependent portion of the body. The fluid is first seen in the paracolic gutters, then the posterior cul-de-sac, and then in Morison's pouch. *A,* Transverse: Liver *(L),* Right kidney *(RK),* Ascites *(As); B,* Transverse; *C,* Longitudinal with fluid in Morison's pouch; *D,* Longitudinal.
2. (Figure 11-5) Fine echoes within the ascitic fluid may represent debris, hemorrhage, bacteria, or tumor infiltration. *A,* Longitudinal: Liver *(L),* Right Kidney *(RK),* fluid *(f)* in Morison's pouch; *B,* Transverse.
3. (Figure 11-6) A fluid collection was seen in Morison's pouch in a patient with acute cholecystitis. Liver *(L),* Right Kidney *(RK),* fluid *(f),* gallbladder *(GB).*
4. (Figure 11-7) Abscess collections appear with varied echogenicity, shape, and borders. This scan was from a 36-year-old febrile patient who was in acute RUQ pain. Rupture of the gallbladder wall is seen *(f).*
5. (Figure 11-8) A large right pleural effusion was noted superior to the dome of the liver. The fluid fills the

costophrenic sulcus *(cps).* The patient should be instructed to breath slowly so the sonographer can watch the movement of the diaphragm.
6. (Figure 11-9) An ultrasound examination over the right lower quadrant showed an inflamed appendix that had ruptured. A complex mass represents an appendiceal abscess. *(app abs)* The appendix is shown anterior to the abscess as an enlarged structure with an echogenic inner layer surrounded by a thickened hypoechoic outer layer. With gentle compression, this mass did not compress.
7. (Figure 11-10) Hematomas may occur anywhere in the abdomen, superficial muscular area, groin, or extremities. New bleeds are primarily cystic, with some debris along the posterior border. As the blood organizes, the blood clots form, and thus the mass becomes more complex. This patient recently had a cardiac catheterization and developed a hematoma postcatherization.
8. (Figure 11-11) Nodes in the superior mesenteric/celiac axis area may cause the vessels to be compressed or elevated from their origin from the abdominal aorta. Multiple small nodes *(arrows)* are seen to encompass the hepatic artery *(HA).*

CHAPTER
12
Superficial Structures

The Thyroid

OBJECTIVES

At the completion of this section, students will show orally, in writing, or by demonstration that they will be able to:

1. Describe the various texture patterns and size of the normal thyroid.
2. Define the internal, surface, and relational anatomies of the thyroid.
3. Illustrate the cross-sectional anatomy of the thyroid and adjacent structures.
4. Describe congenital anomalies affecting the thyroid.
5. Select pertinent laboratory tests and other diagnostic procedures.
6. Differentiate between sonographic appearances by explaining the clinical significance of the pathologic processes as related to the thyroid in the following diseases:
   a. goiter
   b. hypothyroidism
   c. hyperthyroidism
   d. thyroid cysts
   e. adenoma
   f. thyroiditis
   g. malignant lesions of the thyroid and parathyroid
   h. primary hyperparathyroidism
   i. thyroglossal duct cyst
   j. branchial cleft cyst
   k. cystic hygroma
   l. abscess
   m. adenopathy
7. Create high-quality diagnostic scans demonstrating the appropriate anatomy in all planes pertinent to the thyroid.
8. Select the correct equipment settings appropriate to the individual body habitus.
9. Distinguish between the normal and abnormal sonographic appearances of the thyroid.

To further enhance learning, students should use marking pens to color the anatomic illustrations that follow.

NECK

FIGURE 12-1

Root of the Neck on the Right Side of the Body

The neck is divided into various triangles: the posterior triangle, the anterior triangle, and the submandibular triangle. The muscles of these triangles have already been discussed in the section on the muscular system.

The arteries of the posterior triangle consist of the subclavian artery and the thyrocervical trunk, which branches to form the inferior thyroid artery, the suprascapular artery, and the transversae colli artery (Figure 12-1).

The arteries of the anterior triangle consist of the common carotid artery. This artery is a major branch of the brachiocephalic artery on the right, or the arch of the aorta on the left. The common carotid further divides into the internal and external carotid arteries.

The internal jugular vein emerges from the skull at the jugular foramen, together with the vagus nerve, and close to the internal carotid artery, where it enters the carotid canal. Along with the internal and external carotid arteries, the internal jugular vein and vagus nerve descend in a fibrous envelope, the carotid sheath, to leave the anterior triangle by passing deep to the sternomastoid muscle.

The submandibular gland is a major salivary gland. It is palpable as a soft mass over the posterior portion of the mylohyoid muscle.

Midline Structures

The cartilaginous skeleton of the larynx and trachea forms a set of landmarks to which other structures of the midline of the neck can be related:

Hyoid bone: a horseshoe-shaped bone with a central body and greater and lesser horns.

Larynx: the skeleton of the larynx consists of a group of cartilaginous structures at the level of cervical vertebrae 3, 4, 5, and 6.

Thyroid cartilage: consists of two flat plates, or laminae, joined anteriorly in the midline. Each lamina has a superior and an inferior cornu and on its lateral surface, a raised oblique line.

Cricoid cartilage: has the shape of a signet ring, with the wide part posteriorly. It provides a posterior point of articulation for the inferior horn or the thyroid cartilage.

Pharynx: a tube that serves both respiratory and digestive functions. It extends inferiorly from posterior to the nose to the level of the cricoid cartilage.

Esophagus: the superior portion of the digestive tube. It commences at the level of the cricoid cartilage and passes posteriorly to the trachea on an inferior course to the thoracic inlet.

Recurrent laryngeal nerve: a branch of the vagus nerve running in the groove between the trachea and esophagus and entering the larynx from below. It supplies all of the muscles of the larynx except one.

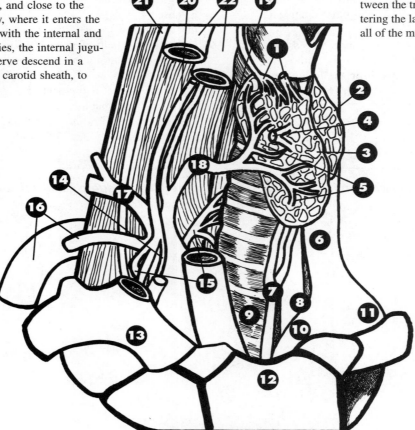

FIGURE 12-1, CONT'D.

1   superior thyroid artery and vein
2   thyroid gland, left lobe
3   thyroid gland, right lobe pulled anteriorly
4   middle thyroid vein
5   parathyroid glands
6   left internal jugular vein
7   inferior thyroid veins
8   left common carotid artery
9   trachea
10   left brachiocephalic vein
11   subclavian vein
12   suprasternal notch
13   subclavian, vertebral, and right brachiocephalic veins
14   cardiac branch of the vagus nerve
15   recurrent laryngeal nerve
16   subclavian and suprascapular arteries
17   transverse cervical artery
18   inferior thyroid artery
19   esophagus
20   vagus nerve and ascending cervical artery
21   phrenic nerve on the anterior scalene muscle
22   internal jugular vein and common carotid artery

FIGURE 12-2

Cross Section of the Neck at the Level of the 5th Cervical Vertebra

Thyroid Gland

The thyroid gland consists of a right and left lobe connected in the midline by an isthmus. Each lobe is bounded posterolaterally by the carotid artery and internal jugular vein and is lateral to the trachea (Figures 12-2 and 12-3). The sternocleidomastoid and strap muscles (sternothyroid, sternohyoid, and omohyoid) are situated anterolateral to the thyroid gland.

The right lobe is often the larger of the two lobes. The isthmus lies anterior to the trachea and may be variable in size. A triangular cephalic extension of the isthmus, the pyramidal lobe, is present in 15% to 30% of thyroid glands. When present, it is of varying size and is more commonly found on the left. A fibrous capsule encloses the gland and gives it a smooth contour.

Blood is supplied to the thyroid via four arteries. Two superior thyroid arteries arise from the external carotids and descend to the upper poles. Two inferior thyroid arteries arise from the thyrocervical trunk of the subclavian artery and ascend to the lower poles. The corresponding veins drain into the internal jugular vein.

Parathyroid Glands

The parathyroid glands are four small endocrine glands that secrete a hormone important in the metabolism of calcium. They are embedded in the posterior wall of the capsule of the thyroid gland.

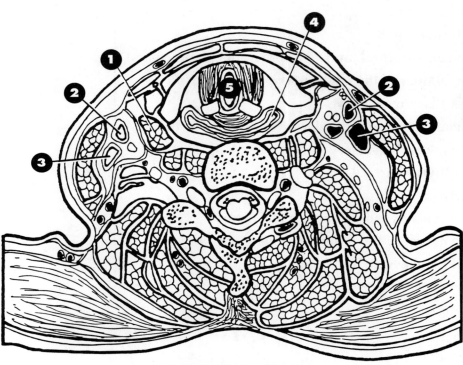

1	thyroid
2	carotid artery
3	jugular vein
4	pharynx
5	rima glottidis

FIGURE 12-3

Cross Section of the Neck at the Level of the 7th Cervical Vertebra

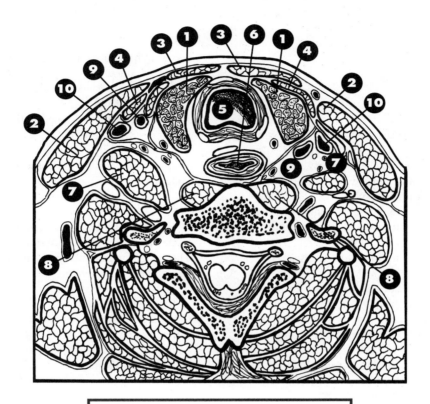

1	thyroid
2	sternocleidomastoid muscle
3	sternohyoid muscle
4	sternothyroid muscle
5	trachea
6	esophagus
7	scalenus anterior muscle
8	longus colli muscle
9	carotid artery
10	jugular vein

Thyroid Review Notes

THE ROLE OF ULTRASONOGRAPHY IN THYROID DISEASE

- Thyroid ultrasonography is used to determine the nature of a nodule:
  - single or multiple
  - solid or cystic
  - complex or calcified

THYROID ANATOMY

- The thyroid is located in the anterior neck at the level of the hyoid cartilage.
- The gland consists of a right lobe and left lobe, which are connected across the midline by the thyroid isthmus.
- The thyroid straddles the trachea anteriorly, and both lobes extend on either side and are bounded laterally by the carotid arteries and jugular veins.
- Both lobes are equal in size, and are found to be 5 cm to 6 cm in length and 2 cm in the anterior-posterior measurement.
- The isthmus, which lies anterior to the trachea, is variable in size.
- A pyramidal lobe, which extends superiorly from the isthmus, is present in 15% to 30% of thyroids.
- The normal thyroid parenchyma appears sonographically as a homogeneous gland of medium- to high-level echoes.
- Along the anterior surface of the thyroid gland lie the strap muscles, the sternothyroideus, the omohyoideus, and the sternohyoideus; these muscles are seen as thin sonolucent bands.
- The longus colli muscle is posterior and lateral to each thyroid lobe and appears as a hypoechoic triangular structure adjacent to the cervical vertebrae.
- Blood is supplied to the thyroid by four arteries.
  - Two superior thyroid arteries arise from the external carotids and descend to the upper poles.
  - Two inferior thyroid arteries arise from the thyrocervical trunk of the subclavian artery and ascend to the lower poles.
- Corresponding veins drain into the internal jugular veins.

PATHOLOGY

Common Causes of Thyroid Disorders

- The most common cause of thyroid disorders is iodine deficiency, which may lead to goiter formation and hypothyroidism.

Goiter of the Thyroid Gland

- Enlargement of the thyroid gland is termed *goiter.*
- Nodular hyperplasia, multinodular goiter, and adenomatous hyperplasia are some of the terms used to describe a goiter, which is the most common thyroid abnormality.

- On ultrasound examination, the goiterous gland is usually enlarged, nodular, and may be inhomogeneous.
- Goiters may be a result of hyperplasia or neoplasia, or may be an inflammatory process.

Hyperthyroidism

- Hyperthyroidism is a hypermetabolic state in which increased amounts of thyroid hormones are produced.
- The patient experiences weight loss, nervousness, and an increased heart rate.
- Hyperthyroidism associated with a diffuse hyperpastic goiter is termed *Graves' disease.*
  - The overactivity of Graves' disease is manifested sonographically by increased vascularity on color Doppler.

Hypothyroidism

- Hypothyroidism is a hypometabolic state resulting from inadequate secretion of thyroid hormones.
- The patient may experience lethargy, sluggish reactions, and a deep, husky voice.

Thyroid Cysts

- Cysts are thought to represent cystic degeneration of a follicular adenoma.
- Approximately 20% of solitary nodules are cystic.
- Blood or debris may be present within them.
- As with all simple cysts, the sonographic appearance of a simple thyroid cyst must have no internal echoes (be anechoic), must have sharp, well-defined walls, and distal acoustic enhancement.

Adenoma

- An adenoma is a benign thyroid neoplasm characterized by complete fibrous encapsulation.

Ultrasound Findings

- In appearance, adenomas range from echolucent to completely echodense, and commonly have a peripheral halo.
- Adenomas that contain echolucent areas are a result of cystic degeneration (probably from hemorrhage) and usually lack a well-rounded margin.
- Calcification, which is characteristically rimlike, can also be associated with adenomas.

Goiter

Diffuse Nontoxic Goiter (Colloid Goiter)

- Colloid goiter occurs as a compensatory enlargement of the thyroid gland because of thyroid hormone deficiency.
- The gland becomes diffusely and uniformly enlarged.

- In the first stage hyperplasia occurs; in the second stage, colloid involution occurs.
- Progression of this process leads to an asymmetric and multinodular gland.

Adenomatous Hyperplasia (Multinodular Goiter)

- Is one of the most common forms of thyroid disease.
- Nodularity of the gland can be the end stage of diffuse nontoxic goiter.
- This can be followed by focal scarring, focal areas of ischemia, necrosis, and cyst formation.
- Fibrosis or calcifications may also occur.
- Some of the nodules are poorly circumscribed; others appear to be encapsulated.
- Enlargement can involve one lobe to a greater extent than the other, which sometimes causes difficulty in breathing and swallowing.
- The multiple nodules of adenomatous hyperplasia may demonstrate halos and may have clear or nondiscrete borders.
- The solid portion of the lesions may have the same echotexture as the normal thyroid tissue.
- Calcifications and cystic areas may be present within the nodules.

Thyroiditis

- Thyroiditis causes swelling and tenderness of the thyroid.
- Thyroiditis is caused by infection or can be related to autoimmune abnormalities.
- On sonography, the gland appears enlarged and hypoechoic.
- The goiterous form of autoimmune thyroiditis is common and is called Hashimoto's thyroiditis.
- The thyroid in Hashimoto's thyroiditis is always diffusely abnormal on ultrasound examination, with decreased and inhomogeneous echogenicity.
- The gland may be normal or increased in size and may have an irregular surface.

Malignant Lesions

- Carcinoma of the thyroid is rare.
- A solitary nodule may be malignant in 10% to 25% of cases, but the risk of malignancy decreases with the presence of multiple nodules.
- A solitary thyroid nodule in the presence of cervical adenopathy on the same side suggests malignancy.

Ultrasound Findings

- The neoplasm can be of any size, can be single or multiple, and can appear as solid, partially cystic, or largely cystic masses.
- Calcifications are present in 50% to 80% of all types of thyroid carcinoma.

- Papillary thyroid cancer is the most common of the thyroid malignancies and is the predominant cause of thyroid cancer in children.
  - Metastatic cervical adenopathy will occur in 20% of patients with papillary thyroid cancer.
- Follicular carcinoma of the thyroid is usually a solitary mass of the thyroid.
  - An irregular, firm, nodular enlargement is characteristic of follicular carcinoma.
  - This type of thyroid cancer is more aggressive than papillary cancer.
- Medullary carcinoma accounts for 10% of thyroid cancers.
  - It presents as a hard, bulky mass that causes enlargement of a small portion of the gland and can involve the entire gland.
  - In patients with medullary thyroid carcinoma, thyroid lesions appear as punctuated, bright, echogenic foci within solid masses.
  - These masses correspond pathologically to deposits of calcium surrounded by amyloid.
- Anaplastic (undifferentiated) carcinoma is rare and makes up less than 10% of thyroid cancers.
  - It usually occurs after 50 years of age.
  - This lesion manifests as a hard, fixed mass with rapid growth.
  - Its growth is locally invasive into surrounding neck structures, and it usually causes death by compression and asphyxiation as a result of invasion of the trachea.

PARATHYROID ANATOMY

- The parathyroid glands are normally located on the posterior medial surface of the thyroid gland.
- Parathyroid glands have been found in different places other than normal, such as in the neck and in the mediastinum.
- The four parathyroid glands are paired.
- Two lie posterior to each superior pole of the thyroid, and the other two lie posterior to the inferior pole.
- Each gland is flat and disc-shaped.
- Enlarged glands (>5 mm) have a decreased echo texture and appear sonographically as elongated masses between the posterior longus coli muscle and the anterior thyroid lobe.

PHYSIOLOGY

- The parathyroid glands are the calcium-sensing organs in the body.
- They produce parathormone (PTH) and monitor the serum calcium feedback mechanism.
- When the serum calcium level increases, parathyroid activity decreases.
- PTH acts on bone, kidney, and intestine to enhance calcium absorption.

PATHOLOGY

Primary Hyperparathyroidism

- Primary hyperparathyroidism is a state of increased function of the parathyroid glands.
- Women have primary hyperparathyroidism two to three times more frequently than men, and it is particularly common after menopause.
- Primary hyperparathyroidism is characterized by hypercalcemia, hypercalciuria, and low serum levels of phosphate.
- Most patients are asymptomatic at the time of diagnosis and have no manifestations of hyperparathyroidism, such as nephrolitiniasis and osteopenia.
- Primary hyperparathyroidism occurs when increased amounts of PTH are produced by an adenoma, primary hyperplasia, or rarely, carcinoma located in the parathyroid gland.

Adenoma

- Adenoma is the most common cause of primary hyperparathyroidism.
- A solitary adenoma may involve any one of the four glands with equal frequency.
- Adenomas are benign and are usually less than 3 cm.
- The most common shape of a parathyroid adenoma is oval.
- Adenomas are encapsulated and have a discrete border.

Primary Hyperplasia

- Primary hyperplasia is hyperfunction of all parathyroid glands with no apparent cause.
- Only one gland may enlarge, with the remaining glands mildly affected, or all glands may be enlarged.
- In any case, the glands rarely reach greater than 1 cm in size.

Carcinoma

- Metastases to regional nodes or distant organs, capsular invasion, or local recurrence must be present for the diagnosis of cancer.
- Most cancers of the parathyroid glands are small, irregular, and rather firm masses.
- These cancerous masses sometimes adhere to surrounding structures.

Secondary Hyperparathyroidism

- Chronic hypocalcemia which may be caused by renal failure, vitamin D deficiency (rickets), or malabsorption syndromes, induces PTH secretion and leads to secondary hyperparathyroidism.
- The hyperfunction of the parathyroids is apparently a compensatory reaction; renal insufficiency and intestinal malabsorption cause hypocalcemia, which leads to stimulation of PTH.
- All four glands are usually affected.

MISCELLANEOUS NECK MASSES

Developmental Cysts

Thyroglossal Duct Cyst

- Thyroglossal duct cysts are congenital anomalies that occur in the midline of the neck anterior to the trachea.
- These cysts are fusiform or spherical masses and are rarely larger than 2 or 3 cm.
- A remnant of the tubular development of the thyroid gland may persist between the base of the tongue and the hyoid bone.
- This narrow hollow tract, which connects the thyroid lobes to the floor of the pharynx, normally atrophies in the adult.
- Failure to atrophy creates the potential for cystic masses to form anywhere along the tract.

Branchial Cleft Cyst

- A branchial cleft cyst is a cystic formation that is usually located laterally.
- During embryonic development, the branchial cleft is a slender tract extending from the pharyngeal cavity to an opening near the auricle or into the neck.
- A diverticulum may extend either laterally from the pharynx or medially from the neck.
- Although primarily cystic in appearance, these lesions may appear as solid components, usually of low-level echogenicity, particularly if they have become infected.

Cystic Hygroma

- A cystic hygroma results from congenital modification of the lymphatics.
- Cystic hygromas appear from the posterior occiput and are most frequently seen as large cystic masses on the lateral aspect of the neck.
- They can be multiseptated and multilocular.

Abscess

- Abscesses can arise in any location in the neck.
- Their sonographic appearance ranges from primarily fluid-filled to completely echogenic.
- Most commonly, they are masses of low-level echogenicity with rather irregular walls.
- Chronic abscesses may be particularly difficult to demonstrate because their indistinct margins blend with surrounding tissue.

Adenopathy

- Low-level echogenicity of well-circumscribed masses is the classical sonographic appearance of enlarged lymph nodes.
- Inflammatory processes may also exhibit a cystic nature.
- Differentiation between inflammatory and neoplastic processes is not always possible by sonographic criteria alone.

Review Exercise A • The Thyroid

1. What is the role of ultrasonography in thyroid disease? _____

_____

_____

_____

2. Describe the anatomy of the thyroid gland. _____

_____

_____

_____

3. What is the normal sonographic appearance of the thyroid gland? _____

_____

_____

_____

4. What is the normal technique used to examine the thyroid gland? _____

_____

_____

_____

5. What is the most common cause of thyroid disorders? _____

_____

6. What is a goiter of the thyroid gland? _____

_____

_____

7. What is hyperthyroidism? _____

_____

_____

8. What is hypothyroidism? _____

_____

_____

9. Discuss the occurrence of cysts in the thyroid gland and their ultrasound appearance. _____

_____

_____

10. What is the sonographic appearance of a thyroid adenoma? _____

_____

_____

11. Describe the sonographic appearance of a multinodular goiter. _____

_____

_____

12. What is the sonographic appearance of thyroiditis? _____

_____

13. What is the occurrence of cancer of the thyroid? What is the sonographic appearance? _____

_____

_____

_____

14. Describe the appearance of the parathyroid glands. _____

_____

_____

_____

15. Describe the sonographic technique used to image the parathyroid glands. _____

_____

_____

16. Briefly describe primary hyperparathyroidism. _____

_____

_____

17. What is the most common cause of primary hyperparathyroidism? _____

_____

_____

18. Describe the appearance of a thyroglossal duct cyst. _____

_____

_____

19. What is a branchial cleft cyst? _____

_____

_____

20. What is a cystic hygroma? Describe the sonographic appearance. _____

_____

_____

_____

21. Describe the sonographic appearance of an abscess in the neck. _____

_____

_____

22. What is the appearance of adenopathy in the neck? _____

_____

_____

Self-Test • The Thyroid

1. The thyroid is an endocrine gland that regulates metabolic function through the production of all of the following hormones except:

    a. thyroxine

    b. triiodothyronine

    c. thyrocalcitonin

    d. thyrodetonine

2. The thyroid gland consists of the following number of lobes:

    a. three

    b. four

    c. two

    d. six

3. The approximate dimensions of the thyroid gland are:

    a. 5 cm length, 3 cm width, 2 cm depth

    b. 4 cm length, 5 cm width, 2 cm depth

    c. 3 cm width, 5 cm length, 2 cm depth

    d. 6 cm length, 2 cm width, 3 cm depth

4. The lobes of the thyroid gland are connected by:

    a. ismal tissue

    b. isthmus

    c. island tissue

    d. parathyroid tissue

5. All of the following structures form neighboring structures for the thyroid gland except:

    a. superficial and deep fascia

    b. parotid muscle

    c. strap muscles

    d. sternocleidomastoid muscle

6. Sonographically the thyroid may be described as having characteristics of all of the following except:

    a. inhomogeneous echogenic pattern

    b. sternocleidomastoid, longus colli, and strap muscles are hypoechoic compared with thyroid tissue

    c. homogeneous texture of medium echogencity

    d. superior and inferior thyroid vessels are best imaged in sagittal plane

7. Characteristic ultrasound findings of a cyst of the thyroid gland include all except:

    a. cysts account for 20% of all cold thyroid nodules

    b. lesions are usually multiple

    c. vast majority result from hemorrhage or degenerative changes in an adenoma

    d. incidence of carcinoma in cystic lesions under 4 cm is less than 2%

8. The differential diagnosis for thyroiditis includes all except:

    a. goiter

    b. abscess

    c. hemorrhagic cyst

    d. multinodular goiter

9. Clinical signs of a thyroid goiter are:

    a. lymph node enlargement

    b. rapidly enlarging mass

    c. fainting

    d. thyroid enlargement

10. The most common benign tumor of the thyroid is:

    a. goiter

    b. Hashimoto's disease

    c. adenoma

    d. lymphoma

11. Characteristics of thyroid cancer include all except:

    a. central sonolucent halo

    b. most common endocrine malignancy

    c. found in women over 40 years of age

    d. rapid growth

12. Clinical findings in thyroid cancer include all except:

    a. lymph node enlargement

    b. rapidly growing mass

    c. pain

    d. palpitations

13. The best sonographic characteristic for a thyroid cancer is:

    a. well-defined borders

    b. more hyperechoic than normal thyroid tissue

    c. solid complex mass with heterogeneous echo pattern and irregular margins

    d. normal size lymph nodes

14. A strong association exists between lymphoma and Hashimoto's thyroiditis (true or false).

15. The most common feature of a thyroid adenoma is:

    a. diffuse echogenicity

    b. hemorrhage

    c. peripheral sonolucent halo

    d. inhomogeneity

16. The most frequent tumors to cause metastases to the thyroid are from:

    a. kidney, breast, lung, and melanoma

    b. breast, liver, and pancreas

    c. breast and colon

    d. kidney, lung, and liver

The Parathyroid Gland

17. The parathyroid glands produce a hormone that affects:

    a. liver, colon, and kidneys

    b. kidneys, bones, and gastrointestinal tract

    c. gastrointestinal tract, breast, and scrotum

    d. kidneys, heart, and colon

18. The sizes of the parathyroids are:

    a. 5 mm length, 3 mm width

    b. 4 mm length, 6 mm width

    c. 6 mm length, 1 mm width

    d. 6 mm length, 3 mm width

19. The parathyroid glands lie:

    a. between the posterior borders of the lateral lobes of the thyroid gland

    b. between the anterior borders of the lateral lobes of the thyroid gland

    c. between the anterior borders of the medial lobes of the thyroid gland

    d. between the posterior borders of the medial lobes of the thyroid gland

20. There are usually _____ parathyroid glands.

    a. two

    b. three

    c. four

    d. five

21. Sonographically, an enlarged parathyroid gland can be distinguished from a thyroid nodule by its oblong or teardrop shape and its typical location behind the thyroid (true or false).

22. A patient presents with osteoporosis. A hyperplastic parathyroid gland is seen on ultrasound examination. Your differential diagnosis would include all except:

    a. thyroid cyst

    b. hyperparathyroidism

    c. parathyroid adenoma

    d. parathyroid hyperplasia

23. The most common cause of hyperparathyroidism is:

   a. thyroid adenoma

   b. parathyroid adenoma

   c. parathyroid cyst

   d. parathyroid hemorrhagic cyst

24. A _____ presents as a palpable midline mass between the hyoid bone and the isthmus of the thyroid.

   a. thyroma

   b. parathyroid adenoma

   c. thyroglossal duct cyst

   d. carotid aneurysm

Case Reviews • The Thyroid

1. A 33-year-old female presents with a mass in her neck. What are your findings (Figure 12-4)?

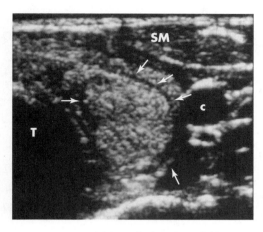

2. A 23-year-old female has had fullness in her neck for the past 6 months. What are your findings (Figure 12-5)?

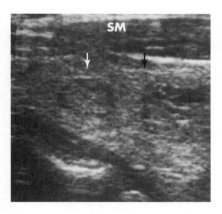

3. A 42-year-old female has had pain in her neck over the past few days. What are your findings (Figure 12-6)?

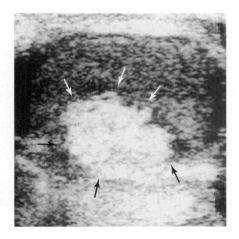

4. A 34-year-old female has a "solid" mass in her neck. What are your findings (Figure 12-7)?

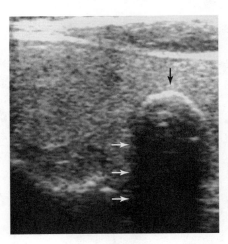

5. A 30-year-old female has abnormal thyroid laboratory values and an enlarged thyroid gland. What are your findings (Figure 12-8)?

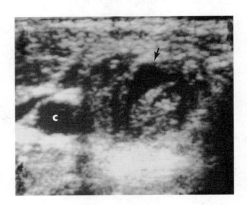

6. A 52-year-old female has a hard, palpable neck mass. What are your findings (Figure 12-9)?

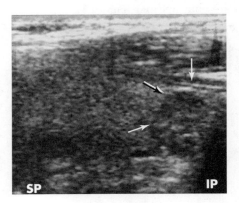

7. A 48-year-old female has a mass in the neck. What are your findings (Figure 12-10)?

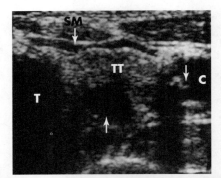

Answers to Review Exercise A

1. Ultrasonography is used to image the thyroid to determine whether a nodule is single or multiple, solid or cystic, and complex or calcified.

   The size and location of lesions are seen, as are any adjacent adenopathy.

2. The thyroid is located in the anterior neck at the level of the hyoid cartilage. The thyroid gland consists of a right lobe and a left lobe that are connected across the midline by the thyroid isthmus. The thyroid straddles the trachea anteriorly, and both lobes extend on either side and are bounded laterally by the carotid arteries and jugular veins. Both lobes are equal in size and are found to be 5 cm to 6 cm in length and 2 cm in the anterior-posterior measurement. The isthmus, which lies anterior to the trachea, is variable in size. A pyramidal lobe that extends superiorly from the isthmus is present in 15% to 30% of thyroids.

3. The normal thyroid parenchyma appears sonographically as a homogeneous gland of medium- to high-level echoes. Along the anterior surface of the thyroid gland lie the strap muscles, the sternothyroideus, the omohyoideus, and the sternohyoideus; these muscles are seen as thin sonolucent bands. The longus colli muscle is posterior and lateral to each thyroid lobe and appears as a hypoechoic triangular structure adjacent to the cervical vertebrae.

   Blood is supplied to the thyroid by four arteries. Two superior thyroid arteries arise from the external carotids and descend to the upper poles. Two inferior thyroid arteries arise from the thyrocervical trunk of the subclavian artery and ascend to the lower poles. Corresponding veins drain into the internal jugular veins.

4. The patient should be in the supine position, with the neck hyperextended. A high resolution linear 7.5 MHz to 10 MHz transducer should be used. Each lobe and the isthmus require careful scanning in both the longitudinal and transverse planes. The lateral, mid, and medial part of each lobe is examined in the longitudinal plane; and the upper, mid, and lower portions are examined in the transverse plane.

5. The most common cause of thyroid disorders is iodine deficiency, which may lead to goiter formation and hypothyroidism. In areas not deficient in iodine, autoimmune processes are believed to be the basis for most cases of thyroid disease, ranging from hyperthyroidism to hypothyroidism.

6. Enlargement of the thyroid gland is termed goiter. Nodular hyperplasia, multinodular goiter, and adenomatous hyperplasia are some of the terms used to describe a goiter, which is the most common thyroid abnormality. Goiters can be diffuse and symmetric, or they can be irregular and nodular. On ultrasound examination, the goiterous gland is usually enlarged, nodular, and may be inhomogeneous.

   Goiters may be a result of hyperplasia or neoplasia, or an inflammatory process. Normal thyroid function, hyperfunction, or hypofunction can also cause an enlargement of the gland.

7. Hyperthyroidism is a hypermetabolic state in which increased amounts of thyroid hormones are produced. The patient experiences weight loss, nervousness, and an increased heart rate. Expothalmos may develop when the condition is severe. Hyperthyroidism associated with a diffuse hyperplastic goiter is termed *Graves' disease.* The overactivity of Graves' disease is manifested sonographically by increased vascularity on color Doppler.

8. Hypothyroidism is a hypometabolic state resulting from inadequate secretion of thyroid hormones. Lethargy, sluggish reactions, and a deep, husky voice are physical manifestations.

9. Cysts are thought to represent cystic degeneration of a follicular adenoma. Approximately 20% of solitary nodules are cystic. Blood or debris may be present within them. As with all simple cysts, the sonographic appearance of a simple thyroid cyst must have no internal echoes (be anechoic), must have sharp, well-defined walls, and distal acoustic enhancement.

10. An adenoma is a benign thyroid neoplasm that is characterized by complete fibrous encapsulation. Adenomas have a broad spectrum of ultrasound appearances. They range from echolucent (no echoes) to completely echodense and commonly have a peripheral halo. The halo, or thin echolucent rim surrounding the lesion, may represent edema of the compressed normal thyroid tissue or the capsule of the adenoma. In a few instances, it may be blood around the lesion. Although the halo is a relatively consistent finding in adenomas, additional statistical information is necessary to establish its specificity.

    Adenomas that contain echolucent areas are a result of cystic degeneration (probably from hemorrhage) and usually lack a well-rounded margin. This lack of a discrete cystic margin is helpful in differentiation from a simple cyst. Calcification, which is characteristically rimlike, can also be associated with adenomas. Its acoustic shadow may preclude visualization posteriorly.

11. Diffuse nontoxic goiter (colloid goiter) occurs as a compensatory enlargement of the thyroid gland because of thyroid hormone deficiency. The gland becomes diffusely and uniformly enlarged. In the first stage hyperplasia occurs; in the second stage, colloid

involution occurs. Progression of this process leads to an asymmetric and multinodular gland.

Adenomatous hyperplasia (multinodular goiter) is one of the most common forms of thyroid disease. Nodularity of the gland can be the end stage of diffuse nontoxic goiter. This can be followed by focal scarring, focal areas of ischemia, and necrosis, and cyst formation. Fibrosis or calcifications may also occur. Some of the nodules are poorly circumscribed; others appear to be encapsulated. Enlargement can involve one lobe to a greater extent than the other, which sometimes causes difficulty in breathing and swallowing.

Lesions in multinodular goiter have many features of true adenomas. The multiple nodules of adenomatous hyperplasia may demonstrate halos and may have clear or nondiscrete borders.

The solid portion of the lesions may have the same echotexture as the normal thyroid tissue. Calcifications and cystic areas may be present within the nodules.

12. Thyroiditis causes swelling and tenderness of the thyroid. Thyroiditis is caused by infection or can be related to autoimmune abnormalities. By sonography, the gland appears enlarged and hypoechoic. There are many forms of thyroiditis. The goiterous form of autoimmune thyroiditis is common and is called Hashimoto's thyroiditis. The thyroid in Hashimoto's thyroiditis is always diffusely abnormal on ultrasound examination, with decreased and inhomogeneous echogenicity. The gland may be normal or increased in size and may have an irregular surface.

13. Carcinoma of the thyroid is rare. A solitary nodule may be malignant in 10% to 25% of cases, but the risk of malignancy decreases with the presence of multiple nodules. A solitary thyroid nodule in the presence of cervical adenopathy on the same side suggests malignancy.

The ultrasound appearance of thyroid cancer is highly variable. The neoplasm can be of any size, can be single or multiple, and can appear as solid, partially cystic, or largely cystic masses. Occasionally, thyroid cancer presents as a small solid nodule. Thyroid cancer is usually hypoechoic relative to a normal thyroid, but thyroid carcinomas with the same echo texture as normal thyroid have been reported. Calcifications are present in 50% to 80% of all types of thyroid carcinoma.

Papillary thyroid cancer is the most common of the thyroid malignancies and is the predominant cause of thyroid cancer in children. Metastatic cervical adenopathy will occur in 20% of patients with papillary thyroid cancer.

Follicular carcinoma of the thyroid is usually a solitary mass of the thyroid. An irregular, firm, nodular enlargement is characteristic. This type of thyroid cancer is more aggressive than papillary cancer.

Medullary carcinoma accounts for 10% of thyroid cancers. It presents as a hard, bulky mass that causes enlargement of a small portion of the gland and can involve the entire gland.

In patients with medullary thyroid carcinoma, thyroid lesions appear as punctuated, bright, echogenic foci within solid masses. These masses correspond pathologically to deposits of calcium surrounded by amyloid. Ultrasound is highly sensitive in detecting metastatic lymphadenopathy in these patients, so careful evaluation of the entire neck area surrounding the thyroid is important.

Anaplastic (undifferentiated) carcinoma is rare and makes up less than 10% of thyroid cancers. It usually occurs after 50 years of age. This lesion manifests as a hard, fixed mass with rapid growth. Its growth is locally invasive into surrounding neck structures, and it usually causes death by compression and asphyxiation as a result of invasion of the trachea.

Thyroid cancer is commonly isoechoic or hypoechoic on ultrasound examination. The interfaces of the lesion are often poorly defined, and a halo is rarely present. Cystic degeneration, if present, is minimal. Specks of calcium may also be noted but are seldom peripheral as with adenomas.

14. The parathyroid glands are normally located on the posterior medial surface of the thyroid gland. Most people have four paired parathyroid glands, but to have three to five parathyroid glands is not uncommon. Parathyroid glands have been found in different places other than normal, such as in the neck and in the mediastinum. Two lie posterior to each superior pole of the thyroid, and the other two lie posterior to the inferior pole.

Each gland is flat and disc-shaped. The echo texture is similar to that of the overlying thyroid gland. For this reason, the normal sized glands (less than 4 mm) are usually not seen by ultrasound, but occasionally a single one may be imaged and appear as a flat hypoechoic structure posterior to the thyroid and adjacent to it.

Enlarged glands (greater than 5 mm) have a decreased echo texture and appear sonographically as elongated masses between the posterior longus coli muscle and the anterior thyroid lobe.

15. For successful sonographic detection of parathyroid abnormalities, a high resolution (7.5 MHz to 10 MHz) transducer must be employed. The patient is placed in the supine position, with the neck slightly hyperextended. From the upper neck, just under the jaw, to the sternal notch, transverse and longitudinal planes must be examined and recorded. To detect any inferiorly located parathyroid glands, the patient is

asked to swallow to elevate the thyroid gland during real-time scanning. The normal parathyroid glands are seldom identified.

16. Primary hyperparathyroidism is a state of increased function of the parathyroid glands. Women have primary hyperparathyroidism two to three times more frequently than men, and it is particularly common after menopause. Primary hyperparathyroidism is characterized by hypercalcemia, hypercalciuria, and low serum levels of phosphate.

    Most patients are asymptomatic at the time of diagnosis and have no manifestations of hyperparathyroidism, such as nephrolitiniasis and osteopenia. Primary hyperparathyroidism occurs when increased amounts of PTH are produced by an adenoma, primary hyperplasia, or rarely, carcinoma located in the parathyroid gland.

17. In 80% of cases of primary hyperparathyroidism, adenoma is the most common cause. A solitary adenoma may involve any one of the four glands with equal frequency. Adenomas are benign and are usually less than 3 cm. The most common shape of a parathyroid adenoma is oval. The echogenicity of parathyroid adenomas is hypoechoic, and the vast majority are solid. Adenomas are encapsulated and will have a discrete border. Differentiation between adenomas and hyperplasia is difficult on histologic and morphologic grounds.

18. Thyroglossal duct cysts are congenital anomalies that occur in the midline of the neck anterior to the trachea. These cysts are fusiform or spherical masses and are rarely larger than 2 or 3 cm.

A remnant of the tubular development of the thyroid gland may persist between the base of the tongue and the hyoid bone. This narrow hollow tract, which connects the thyroid lobes to the floor of the pharynx, normally atrophies in the adult. Failure to atrophy creates the potential for cystic masses to form anywhere along the tract.

19. A branchial cleft cyst is a cystic formation that is usually located laterally. During embryonic development, the branchial cleft is a slender tract extending from the pharyngeal cavity to an opening near the auricle or into the neck.

    A diverticulum may extend either laterally from the pharynx or medially from the neck. These lesions are primarily cystic, although they may present with solid components, usually of low-level echogenicity, particularly if they have become infected.

20. A cystic hygroma results from a congenital modification of the lymphatics. The mass appears from the posterior occiput and is frequently seen as a large cystic mass on the lateral aspect of the neck. They can be multiseptated and multilocular.

21. An abscess can arise in any location in the neck. Its sonographic appearance ranges from primarily fluid-filled to completely echogenic. Most commonly, it is a collection of low-level echogenicity with irregular walls.

22. Low-level echogenicity of well-circumscribed masses is the classical sonographic appearance of enlarged lymph nodes. However, in some cases they appear echo free. Inflammatory processes may also exhibit a cystic nature.

Answers to Self-Test A

1. d	**9.** d	**17.** b
2. c	**10.** c	**18.** d
3. a	**11.** a	**19.** a
4. b	**12.** d	**20.** c
5. b	**13.** c	**21.** true
6. a	**14.** true	**22.** a
7. b	**15.** c	**23.** b
8. c	**16.** a	**24.** c

Answers to Case Reviews—The Thyroid

1. (Figure 12-4) Adenomas of the thyroid are the most common solid nodule. This mass may undergo cystic degeneration and rarely extends beyond the thyroid capsule. This figure shows a transverse scan of a large thyroid adenoma demonstrating a hypoechoic rim, or halo, which is typical of a thyroid adenoma. Strap muscle *(SM)*, Carotid *(C)*, Trachea *(T)*, Halo appearance *(arrows)*.

2. (Figure 12-5) This figure shows multiple adenomas, with hypoechoic cystic degeneration within each. The adenoma may have a broad spectrum of ultrasound patterns, ranging from sonolucent to complex to completely hyperechoic (if degeneration has occurred). Adenoma *(arrows)*, Strap muscle *(SM)*.

3. (Figure 12-6) It is typical for a thyroid adenoma to undergo degeneration. On ultrasound examination, the

appearance is very hyperechoic. This figure shows a longitudinal scan demonstrating a hemorrhagic adenoma. Adenoma *(arrows)*.

4. (Figure 12-7) Adenomas may degenerate and form a calcified rim, giving the appearance of a solid lesion. This figure shows a longitudinal scan demonstrating a calcified adenoma. Normal thyroid tissue *(T)*, Calcified adenoma *(arrows)*, Shadowing from the calcification *(double arrows)*.

5. (Figure 12-8) On ultrasound examination, a multinodular goiter demonstrating focal areas of ischemia and cystic areas is seen throughout the thyroid tissue. The differential of this disease is Hashimoto's disease, which is the most common inflammatory process of the thyroid gland. On ultrasound examination, the gland appears diffusely enlarged with a slightly inhomogeneous echo pattern, with many hypoechoic areas (nonfunctioning thyroid tissue). Carotid *(C)*, Cystic areas *(arrow)*.

6. (Figure 12-9) On ultrasound examination, the longitudinal scan of the thyroid showed a solid, hypoechoic lesion that was well circumscribed and caused enlargement of the inferior pole of the right lobe. This mass was removed and pathology confirmed medullary carcinoma. This type of tumor is slow growing, but does metastasize early. The prognosis is favorable with early intervention. Superior pole *(SP)*, Inferior pole *(IP)*, Medullary carcinoma lesion *(arrows)*.

7. (Figure 12-10) The ultrasound transverse scan showed a normal thyroid gland with an enlarged parathyroid gland. Strap muscles *(SM)*, Thyroid tissue *(TT)*, Trachea *(T)*, Parathyroid gland *(arrow)*, Carotid *(C)*, Coincidental plaque in carotid *(double arrow)*.

The Breast

OBJECTIVES

At the completion of this section, students will show orally, in writing, or by demonstration that they will be able to:

1. Describe the various texture patterns and size of the normal breast.
2. Define the internal, surface, and relational anatomy of the breast.
3. Illustrate the cross-sectional anatomy of the breast and adjacent structures.
4. Describe congenital anomalies affecting the breast.
5. Select pertinent laboratory tests and other diagnostic procedures.
6. Differentiate between sonographic appearances by explaining the clinical significance of the pathologic processes as related to the breast in the following diseases:
   a. simple cyst
   b. complex cyst
   c. galactocele
   d. fibroadenoma
   e. lipoma
   f. solitary papilloma
   g. intracystic papilloma
   h. intraductal carcinoma
   i. cystosarcoma phyllodes
   j. ductal carcinoma
   k. medullary carcinoma
   l. metastatic carcinoma
7. Create high-quality diagnostic scans demonstrating the appropriate anatomy in all planes pertinent to the breast.
8. Select the correct equipment settings appropriate to the individual body habitus.
9. Distinguish between the normal and abnormal sonographic appearances of the breast.

To further enhance learning, students should use marking pens to color the anatomic illustrations that follow.

FEMALE BREAST

FIGURE 12-11

Cross Section of the Female Breast

The breast is a differentiated apocrine sweat gland. Its function is to secrete milk during lactation. Its parenchymal elements are the lobes, ducts, lobules, and acini (Figure 12-11). Because the mammary gland is a skin derivative, the stromal elements include dense connective tissue, loose connective tissue, and fat. The age and functional state of the breast dictate the amount and arrangement of the various parenchymal and stromal elements.

The breast is composed of 15 to 20 lobes. Each lobe contains the parenchymal elements of the breast. The ducts extend from the lobes through the breast parenchyma to converge in a single papilla (the nipple), which is surrounded by the areola. The ducts are covered with a connective tissue layer that varies in thickness and density. The normal duct usually measures approximately 2 mm in diameter.

The entire breast is enveloped in a duplication of superficial pectoral fascia (Figure 12-12). The posterior part of the fascia is connected to the pectoral musculature, which is the anterior part of the skin by thin connective septa. The anterior and posterior fascial planes are connected by curvilinear connective tissue septa known as Cooper's ligaments. The connective tissue septa envelope the lobules and lobes of the breast and become the interlobular and interlobar connective tissues that surround the fat lobules and parenchyma of the breast.

There are three well-defined layers in the breast: the subcutaneous, mammary, and retromammary. The subcutaneous layer is bounded superficially by the dermis and deeply by the superficial connective tissue plane. The principal component of the layer is fat lobules enclosed by connective tissue septa. The mammary layer is composed of breast parenchyma and is found between the superficial and deep connective tissue layers. Fat is seen to be interspersed in a lobular fashion throughout the entire breast parenchyma. The retromammary layer consists of fat lobules that are separated anteriorly from the mammary layer by the deep connective tissue plane and posteriorly by the fascia over the pectoralis major muscle.

During pregnancy the ducts and parenchymal elements of the breast expand to such a degree that the mammary layer constitutes almost the entire breast. The subcutaneous fat layer and the retromammary layer become squeezed together during this period.

The major portion of the breast contained within the superficial fascia of the anterior thoracic wall is situated between the second or third rib superiorly, the sixth or seventh costal cartilage inferiorly, and the sternal border medially. The greatest amount of glandular tissue is located in the upper outer quadrant of the breast, which explains why tumors are most frequently found here.

The major pectoral muscle lies posterior to the retromammary layer. The minor pectoral muscle lies superolaterally posterior to it. The pectoralis minor courses from its origin in the rib cage to the point where it inserts into the coracoid process. The lower border of the pectoralis major muscle forms the anterior border of the axilla. Breast tissue can extend into this region and is referred to as the axillary tail, or tail of Spence.

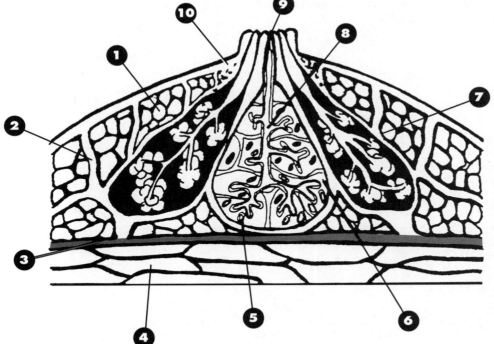

1	**subcutaneous fat**	**6**	**interlobular connective tissue**
2	**Cooper's ligaments**	**7**	**superficial fascia**
3	**retromammary layer (gray)**	**8**	**lactiferous duct**
4	**pectoralis major muscle**	**9**	**ampulla**
5	**acinus**	**10**	**Montgomery's gland**

FIGURE 12-12

Structure of the Female Breast as Seen from Above

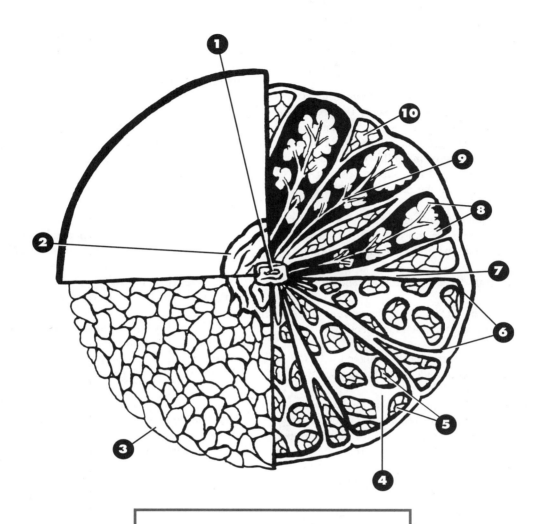

1	nipple
2	areola
3	subcutaneous fat
4	interlobular connective tissue
5	lobules
6	lobe
7	Cooper's ligaments
8	acini
9	lactiferous ducts
10	mammary fat

Breast Review Notes

HISTORY OF BREAST SONOGRAPHY

- Initial studies on ultrasound breast examination were carried out by Wild and Reid, and Howry and Bliss during the early 1950s.
- This research became overshadowed by mammography research as a potential tool for accurate breast screening.
- During the 1960's a small number of individual investigators throughout the world began to study the possibility of ultrasound visualization for breast examination.
- The early techniques that were used to couple the sound to the breast included many of the following methods:
  - A water bag with the patient in a supine position
  - Direct water coupling with the patient in a prone position
  - Direct water coupling with subjects in a supine position
  - Compression of the breast against a plastic window coupled to a water tank with the patient in a sitting position
  - A direct-contact transducer (which most laboratories use today)
- Most of these researchers tried to use the current ultrasound instrumentation with application specifically to the breast.
- Many of the transducers were poorly designed with too low of a frequency to record adequate diagnostic information for the clinician to interpret.
- The critical factors in developing such a transducer for breast imaging required a high frequency transducer (at least 5, 7.5, or 10 MHz), with a near focus, good lateral resolution, and good grey scale differentiation.
- In the late 1970's, Jellins et al suggested that ultrasound visualization should be the initial imaging examination for symptomatic patients under 30 years of age.
- This reasoning was based on the following facts: (1) a large number of women of that age have dense breasts, which are not well imaged by mammography; (2) ionizing radiation should be avoided in younger subjects; (3) if a mass is found, ultrasonography can determine whether it is cystic or solid; and (4) if the mass is benign, ultrasonography can be used to follow the patient's progress.
- These investigators diagnosed cystic structures with a 98% accuracy and detected cysts as small as 2 mm in diameter.
- Further investigation revealed that compression of the breast tissue improved the resolution in some of the patients who were more difficult to image.

SONOGRAPHIC ANATOMY OF THE BREAST

- Ultrasonography has the ability to distinguish soft tissue layers within the breast parenchyma.

- There can be considerable variation in the image depending on the ratio of the parenchymal to stromal elements in the area of the breast that is being imaged.
- The parenchyma includes the lactiferous ducts and alveoli of the breast as well as the intralobular connective tissue, and the stromal or supporting tissues can be divided into fat and dense connective tissue.
- In a normal premenstrual breast, the following areas are clearly demonstrated:
  - Subcutaneous fat
  - Fibroglandular tissue
  - Lactiferous ducts
  - Retromammary space
  - Muscle layers
  - Ribs
- The principle of ultrasonography relies on the fact that the amplitude of the echo generated by ultrasound reflections at an interface depends on the difference in acoustic impedance between the two tissues; fat/dense connective tissue is strongly echogenic as compared to the fat/parenchymal interfaces or dense connective tissue/parenchymal interfaces.
- Ultrasonography demonstrates that fatty tissue has a relatively low acoustic impedance and sparse low-level echoes in contrast to the high-level intensity echoes of fibrous tissue, which have a relatively high acoustic impedance.
- The proportions of parenchymal and stromal elements vary considerably within the breast, and therefore, careful interpretation of the images must consider this aspect of anatomy.

Skin

- The skin is imaged as a thick echogenic line of tissue.
- The thickness of this line depends on the degree of compression, either by the hand-held transducer or the plastic membrane of the water bath.

Subcutaneous Fat

- The subcutaneous fat lies deep in relation to the skin.
- The amount of fat varies tremendously with age and parity of the patient.
- Usually in the young woman there is little or no subcutaneous fat; the amount normally increases with age and parity.
- Multiple distinct fat lobules are often identified, separated by highly echogenic connective tissue ligaments **(Cooper's ligaments).**
- The orderly orientation of fat lobules is often best seen when scanning is being performed in the longitudinal plane, generally because of the lie of fat lobules and connective tissue ligaments.

- Sometimes these dense supporting ligaments cause attenuation shadowing, thereby making it difficult to image the posterior structures with ultrasonography.
- Moving the transducer with a slight angulation usually allows the sonographer to avoid the shadowing and image the structures beyond this ligament.

Fibroglandular Layer

- The fibroglandular (parenchymal) layer lies below the subcutaneous fatty layer.
- Separating these two layers is the highly echogenic band of tissue that represents the superficial fascia.
- The parenchymal layer consists of the ducts and alveoli, including the intralobular connective tissue.
- Some of the dense intralobular connective tissue, which is part of the stromal tissue component, may be difficult to differentiate from the remainder of the parenchyma because of similar imaging characteristics.
- The deep fascia is located deep to the fibroglandular tissue. The deep fascia has an appearance similar to that of the superficial fascia.

Retromammary Layer

- The retromammary layer lies between the deep connective tissue plane and the fascia of the underlying muscle.
- This layer predominantly contains fat lobules, which are smaller than those found in the subcutaneous layer.
- Connective tissue ligaments are not usually seen in this layer because they are thinner than those in the subcutaneous layer.

Pectoralis Muscles

- The pectoralis major and minor muscles are usually easily demonstrated, depending on the area of the breast that is being scanned.
- They are imaged as structures of relatively low echogenicity running deep in the breast above the ribs and parallel to the skin.
- The structures are more prominent in small-breasted women and may be quite large in athletic individuals.
- The muscles are best imaged in the transverse plane.

Ribs

- The ribs form the ventral aspect of the thoracic cage, over which the breasts lie.
- They are composed laterally of bone and medially of cartilage.
- When ultrasound scans are performed over the lateral aspect of the breast, the ribs are seen as highly attenuating structures interspaced by the intercostal muscles.
- Medially, the cartilage is visualized as oval masses with sparse internal echoes.
- The deep connective tissue plane and muscle groups that lie superficial to these structures must be identified

so the solid reflections from the ribs are not mistaken as breast lesions.

Nipple and Areola

- The nipple and areola are slightly more attenuatied than the rest of the breast.
- These structures show attenuation shadowing of the ultrasound beam, in part because of the dense connective tissue within the nipple itself and in part because of the columns of connective tissue surrounding the lactiferous ducts.

Lactiferous Ducts

- The lactiferous ducts are easily seen on most scans, especially when they are dilated.
- A typical breast is composed of 15 to 20 lobules, which are drained by a network of ducts.
- These ducts are branched in the peripheral parts of the breast and join in the subareolar region to form approximately 15 to 20 ducts that drain onto the surface of the nipple.
- The diameter of the ducts is therefore slightly larger in the subareolar region than in the periphery of the breast.
- The lactiferous ducts are usually collapsed in the nonlactating breast. At the sinus level in the subareolar region the ducts may have a potential diameter of 8 mm.
- In the periphery of the breast, a diameter of 2 to 4 mm is normal in the lactating breast.
- Surrounding the subareolar ducts are varying amounts of fibrosis, which accentuate the degree of nipple shadowing observed.

Breast Parenchymal Patterns

- In the young, nonlactating breast, the tissue is primarily composed of fibroglandular tissue, with little or no subcutaneous fat.
- With increasing age and parity, fat is deposited in both the subcutaneous and retromammary layers.
- During pregnancy there is a substantial increase in glandular tissue in the breast.
- The resultant image on ultrasound examination demonstrates a finely granular echo pattern with little subcutaneous fat.
- The subcutaneous and retromammary fat layers are compressed by the glandular tissue and are decreased in size.
- Late in pregnancy and during lactation, the lactiferous ducts increase in size and number, with resultant duct dilation throughout most of the breast tissue.
- Cyclic breast changes may occur with each menstrual cycle.
- Ultrasonography may image mild duct dilation during the period between ovulation and menstruation.
- In most normal women, no significant changes are noted.

- The postmenopausal breast demonstrates varying amounts of fibrous tissue interspersed among predominantly fatty tissue.
- With increasing age there is normal regression of the glandular tissue, with subsequent replacement by fat.
- Breast sonography is used as the initial method for evaluating the following symptomatic patients:
  - the young patient less than 30 years of age
  - the pregnant patient
  - follow-up of patients with fibrocystic disease (3 to 6 month intervals)
- Breast sonography is used as a complementary examination to mammography in the following situations:
  - evaluating areas of dense breast tissue on mammography
  - evaluating mass composition as demonstrated on mammography

PATHOLOGY OF BREAST DISEASE
- Most common pathologic lesions of the female breast are, in order of decreasing frequency:
  - Fibrocystic disease
  - Carcinoma
  - Fibroadenoma
  - Intraductal papilloma
  - Duct ectasia
- Benign lesions are the most common breast lesion.

Symptoms of Breast Masses
- Symptoms of breast masses may include pain, palpable mass, spontaneous or induced nipple discharge, skin dimpling, ulceration, and nipple retraction.
- With a benign mass, the patient may experience pain, mass, nipple discharge.
- With a malignant mass, the patient may experience skin dimpling or ulceration and nipple retraction.

Characteristic Signs of Breast Masses
- Contour or margin: smooth, irregular, spiculated
- Shape: round, oval, tubular, lobulated
- Internal echo pattern: anechoic or echogenic
- Boundary echoes: strong, weak, absent
- Attenuation effects: acoustic enhancement or shadowing
- Distal echoes: strong, intermediate, weak, absent
- Disruption of architecture

Benign Disease
Cystic Disease
- Common in women 35 to 55 years of age.
- Symptoms: pain, recent lump, tenderness; may change with cycle.
- Smooth, sharp, well-defined borders; lateral edge shadowing; anechoic wave pattern; posterior enhancement.

Fibrocystic Disease
- Fibrocystic disease is a result of cyclic dysplasia.
- Symptoms of this condition may include pain, nodularity, dominant mass, and occasional nipple discharge.
- May have dilation of ducts.
- Although fibrocystic disease is a benign condition, the affected patient is five times more at risk of developing breast cancer than patients with other benign conditions.
- Fibrocystic disease is characterized by an average amount of subcutaneous fat. Areas of fibrous stroma appear brighter than the parenchyma. There are small to large cysts throughout breast.

Fibroadenoma
- A fibroadenoma is the most common benign breast tumor.
- It may be unilateral or bilateral.
- Growth of a fibroadenoma is stimulated by estrogen.
- A fibroadenoma is characterized by smooth or lobulated borders, a strong anterior wall, low-level homogeneous internal echoes, and it may have calcification.

Lipoma
- A lipoma is composed of fatty tissue.
- Lipomas are most often found in middle age to menopausal women.
- A lipoma is difficult to see in a fatty breast. It appears as low-level echoes with posterior enhancement and smooth walls.

Abscess
- An abscess may be single or multiple.
- Acute abscesses have a poorly defined border, whereas mature abscesses are well encapsulated with sharp borders.
- Clinically, the patient may have pain, swelling, and reddening of skin; he or she may be febrile and have swollen axillary nodes.
- On ultrasound examination, the sonographer will see a diffuse mottled appearance of the breast, a dense breast, generally irregular borders, posterior enhancement, low-level internal echoes.

Cystosarcoma Phyllodes
- Cystosarcoma phyllodes is an uncommon breast neoplasm.
- It is found in women who are in their fifties, and it is usually unilateral.
- On ultrasound examination, a cystosarcoma has irregular borders, is very large in size, has a weak posterior margin, disruption of architecture, has anechoic or low-level wave patterns.

Intraductal Papilloma

- Intraductal papilloma occurs most frequently in women who are 40 to 50 years of age.
- Nipple discharge comes from a single duct.
- Papillomas are usually small, multiple, and multicentric.
- Trauma may rupture the stalk, filling the duct with blood or serum.

Malignant Disease

- Malignant cells grow along a line of least resistance, such as in fatty tissue.
- In fibrotic tissue, most cancer growth occurs along the borders.
- Lymphatics and blood vessels are frequently used as pathways for new tumor development.
- Most cancer arises in the ducts.

- Cancer of the breast is of two types: sarcoma and carcinoma.
- Sarcoma refers to breast tumors that arise from the supportive or connective tissues. It grows rapidly and invades fibrous tissue.
- Carcinoma refers to breast tumors that arise from the epithelium in the ductal and glandular tissue, and it usually has tentacles.
- Other malignant diseases affecting the breast are a result of systemic neoplasms, such as leukemia or lymphoma.
- Cancer may be classified as infiltrating or noninfiltrating.
- Ultrasound findings include irregular spiculated contour or margin; round or lobulated mass; weak, nonuniform internal echoes; intermediate anterior and absent or weak posterior boundary echoes; increased attenuation.

Review Exercise B • Breast Sonography

1. Who were the pioneers of breast ultrasonography? Why was their work not used? _____

    _____

    _____

2. Describe the early techniques used to image the breast. _____

    _____

    _____

    _____

    _____

3. Why was ultrasonography proposed as the initial screening examination for symptomatic patients under 30 years

    of age? _____

    _____

    _____

4. What are the three transducer design parameters for a single focus transducer to image the breast? _____

    _____

    _____

    _____

5. Discuss the ultrasound anatomy of the breast. _____

    _____

    _____

    _____

    _____

    _____

6. What is the problem with fatty lobules in the breast? _____

    _____

    _____

    _____

    _____

7. Describe the sonographic appearance of subcutaneous fat. _____

    _____

    _____

    _____

    _____

8. Describe the fibroglandular layer of the breast. _____

    _____

    _____

    _____

9. What is the significance of imaging the retromammary layer and pectoralis muscles of the breast? _____

_____

_____

_____

_____

10. How can the lactiferous ducts be identified on ultrasonography? _____

_____

_____

_____

11. Describe the breast parenchymal patterns as seen on ultrasound examination. _____

_____

_____

_____

_____

_____

_____

_____

12. When should breast ultrasonography be used? _____

_____

_____

_____

_____

_____

Review Exercise C • Breast Imaging

TABLE 12-1 Differential Diagnosis of Breast Masses: Imaging Characteristics
Complete the Following Chart:

Mass	Wall	Internal Echo	Attenuation/Enhancement
Benign Masses (Adjacent tissues are basically normal, except for the compressed tissue sign)			
Simple cyst			
Galactocele			
Scar tissue			
Fibroadenoma			
Lipoma			
Solitary papilloma			
Intracystic papilloma			

TABLE 12-1, CONT'D. Differential Diagnosis of Breast Masses: Imaging Characteristics

Complete the Following Chart:

Mass	Wall	Internal Echo	Attenuation/Enhancement
Malignant Masses			
Intraductal carcinoma			
Cystosarcoma phyllodes			
Ductal carcinoma (scirrhous)			
Ductal carcinoma (multilobular)			
Medullary carcinoma			
Metastatic carcinoma (from opposite breast)			
Metastatic carcinoma (from distant source)			

Self-Test B • The Breast

1. The breast is anatomically divided into four zones. Which is incorrect?

   a. skin, nipple, subareolar

   b. pectoralis major

   c. subcutaneous region

   d. parenchyma

   e. retromammary region

2. The size of the lobar collecting ducts are:

   a. 1 cm

   b. 1 mm

   c. 3 mm

   d. 2 mm

3. Fat, Cooper's ligaments, connective tissue, blood vessels, nerves, and lymphatics are found in which layer or zone?

   a. the retromammary region

   b. the parenchyma

   c. the subcutaneous layer

   d. the subareolar area

4. The _____ is mostly glandular tissue, while the peripheral part is adipose tissue rimmed by _____ .

   a. central layer, superficial fascia

   b. outer layer, connective tissue

   c. peripheral layer, Cooper's ligaments

   d. retromammary layer, nerves

5. Sonographically, the breast may be characterized by:

   a. a homogeneous parenchymal pattern

   b. an inhomogeneous parenchymal pattern

   c. a highly echogenic parenchymal pattern

   d. dense internal echoes

6. Cooper's ligaments are best characterized as:

   a. low reflectivity in the retromammary layer

   b. high reflectivity in the retromammary layer

   c. echogenic line interfaces in the subcutaneous layer

   d. homogeneous reflections in the parenchyma

7. The retromammary layer is sonographically imaged as:

   a. hyperechoic

   b. dense

   c. hypoechoic

   d. high reflectivity

8. The most important signs to look for in determining a cystic lesion of the breast include all except:

   a. well-defined borders

   b. good through transmission

   c. anechoic

   d. disruption of architecture

9. Clinical findings of lumpy, painful, tender breasts that vary with monthly cycles usually represents:

   a. carcinoma

   b. fibrocystic disease

   c. cyst

   d. adenoma

10. The characteristic findings of a papilloma of the breast include all except:

    a. well-circumscribed solid mass with microcalcifications

    b. sonolucent cystic lesions with medium level encapsulated component

    c. single or multiple

    d. no disruption of architecture

11. The most common solid benign tumor of the breast is:

    a. fibrocystic disease

    b. fibroadenoma

    c. papilloma

    d. lipoma

12. Fibroadenomas may change in size with the menstrual cycle (true or false).

13. The most characteristic finding of a fibroadenoma is:

    a. a well-defined border

    b. uniform, low-level homogeneous echoes

    c. increased through transmission

    d. disruption of architecture

14. A cystic enlargement of a distal duct filled with milk is called a:

    a. lactoadenoma

    b. lactoma

    c. galactocele

    d. lactiferoma

15. The most common malignant neoplasm of the breast in women is a:

    a. lymphoma

    b. adenocarcinoma

    c. mucinous carcinoma

    d. cystosarcoma phyllodes

16. Characteristic findings of breast carcinoma include all except:

 a. attenuation of sound

 b. irregular margins

 c. strong posterior margin

 d. inhomogeneous low-level internal echo pattern with calcifications

17. Skin dimpling may be caused by:

 a. old age

 b. retraction of tissue secondary to tumor infiltration

 c. enlarged ducts

 d. thrombosis of arterial vessels

18. The most common clinical sign of breast carcinoma is:

 a. skin dimpling

 b. skin discoloration

 c. palpable lump

 d. pain

19. Breast ultrasonography is a useful screening tool for women over forty (true or false).

20. A breast lesion that presents with well-defined borders, low-level internal echoes, and good through transmission most likely represents:

 a. a hemorrhagic cyst

 b. a simple cyst

 c. fibroadenoma

 d. cystosarcoma phyllodes

Case Reviews • The Breast

1. A young female has a palpable breast lesion. What are your findings (Figure 12-13)?

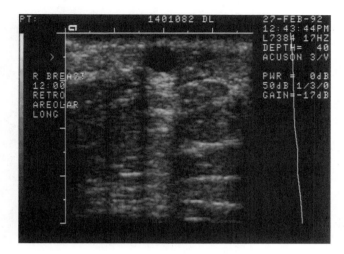

2. A young woman has cyclic pain in her breasts. What are your findings (Figure 12-14)?

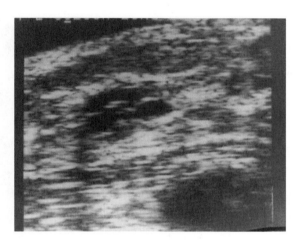

3. A 23-year-old female has tender, painful areas over the breast after a recent cyst aspiration. What are your findings (Figure 12-15)?

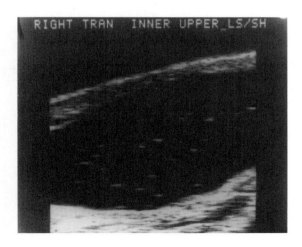

4. A 32-year-old female has a breast mass. What are your findings (Figure 12-16)?

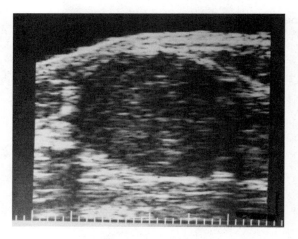

5. A 42-year-old female has a solid breast mass on palpation. What are your findings (Figure 12-17)?

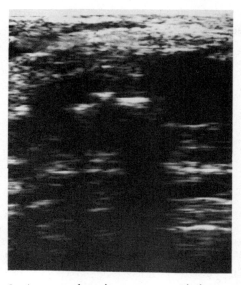

6. A young female presents with fever, pain, and swelling in her breast. What are your findings (Figure 12-18)?

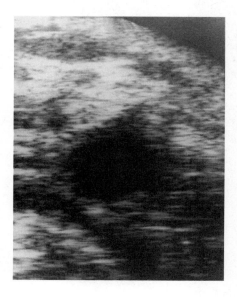

7. A young female has a solid breast mass on palpation. What are your findings (Figure 12-19)?

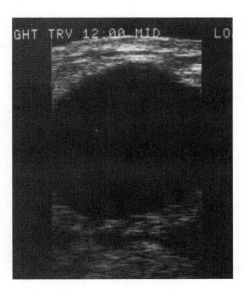

8. A 53-year-old female has an abnormal mammogram. What are your findings (Figure 12-20)?

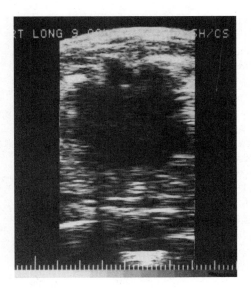

Answers to Review Exercise B

1. Initial studies on ultrasound breast examination were carried out by Wild and Reid, and Howry and Bliss during the early 1950s. This research became overshadowed by the mammography research as a potential tool for accurate breast screening.

2. During the 1960s a small number of individual investigators throughout the world began to study the possibility of ultrasound visualization for breast examination. Interestingly enough, the early techniques used to couple the sound to the breast included many of the following methods: a water bag with the patient in a supine position, direct water coupling with the patient in a prone position, direct water coupling with subjects in a supine position, compression of the breast against a plastic window coupled to a water tank with the patient in a sitting position, and a direct-contact transducer (which most laboratories use today).

   Most of these researchers tried to use the current ultrasound instrumentation with application specifically to the breast. Therefore, many of the transducers were poorly designed with too low of a frequency to record adequate diagnostic information for the clinician to interpret. The critical factors in developing such as transducer for breast imaging required a high frequency transducer (at least 5, 7.5, or 10 MHz), with a near focus, good lateral resolution, and good gray scale differentiation.

   Furthermore, investigators tried to use ultrasonography as a massive screening tool that would be effective for all ages. To do this, equipment was developed that "automatically" scanned the breast tissue. This equipment could be moved at small millimeter increments in a transverse or longitudinal plane, or could be rotated about 1 point in a circular plane.

   In the 1970's, the Japanese applied color ultrasonography and C-mode (coronal) to examine the breast. With this development came improved gray scale and range resolution of the breast tissue.

   In the mid-seventies, the Australian group developed the large diameter, long focal length transducers to scan the breasts as they floated in a waterbath. With this improved image capability, further investigation by these investigators produced the Octoson equipment. This employed eight large diameter transducers mounted within a water bath. The patient would lie supine across the open tank, with her breasts suspended within the open tank. Higher frequency transducers were employed with varying focal length. Problems were still encountered in the region deep to the nipple areola and the outer edges of the breast where total reflection of the sound beam occurred.

3. In the late 1970's Jellins and his colleagues from Australia suggested that ultrasound visualization should be the initial imaging examination for symptomatic patients under 30 years of age.

   This reasoning was based on the following facts: (1) a large number of women of that age have dense breasts, which are not well imaged by mammography; (2) ionizing radiation should be avoided in younger subjects; (3) if a mass is found, ultrasonography can determine whether it is cystic or solid; and (4) if the mass is benign, ultrasonography can be used to follow the patient's progress.

   These investigators diagnosed cystic structures with a 98% accuracy and detected cysts as small as 2 mm in diameter.

4. For single-focus transducers, only three transducer design parameters control range, lateral resolution, and depth of field: (1) the diameter; (2) the focal length; and (3) the frequency.

5. Ultrasonography has the ability to distinguish soft tissue layers within the breast parenchyma. There can be considerable variation in the image depending on the ratio of the parenchymal to stromal elements in the area of the breast that is being imaged. The parenchymal elements include the lactiferous ducts and alveoli of the breast as well as the intralobular connective tissue, and the stromal or supporting tissues can be divided into fat and dense connective tissue.

   In a normal premenstrual breast, the following areas are clearly demonstrated: subcutaneous fat, fibroglandular tissue, lactiferous ducts, retromammary space, muscle layers, and ribs.

6. The principle of ultrasonography relies on the fact that the amplitude of the echo generated by ultrasound reflections at an interface depend on the difference in acoustic impedance between the two tissues; fat/dense connective tissue is strongly echogenic as compared to the fat/parenchymal interfaces or dense connective tissue/parenchymal interfaces.

   Ultrasonography demonstrates that fatty tissue has a relatively low acoustic impedance and sparse low-level echoes in contrast to the high-level intensity echoes of fibrous tissue, which has a relatively high acoustic impedance. The proportions of parenchymal and stromal elements vary considerably within the breast, and therefore, careful interpretation of the images must consider this aspect of anatomy.

7. The subcutaneous fat lies deep in relation to the skin. The amount of fat varies tremendously with age and parity of the patient. Usually in the young woman there is little or no subcutaneous fat; the amount normally increases with age and parity. Multiple distinct fat

lobules are often identified, separated by highly echogenic connective tissue ligaments (Cooper's ligaments).

The orderly orientation of fat lobules is often best seen when scanning is being performed in the longitudinal plane (generally because of the line of fat lobules and connective tissue ligaments). Sometimes these dense supporting ligaments cause attenuation shadowing, making it difficult to image the posterior structures with ultrasonography. Moving the transducer with a slight angulation usually allows one to avoid the shadowing and image the structures beyond this ligament.

8. The fibroglandular (parenchymal) layer lies below the subcutaneous fatty layer. Separating these two layers is the highly echogenic band of tissue that represents the superficial fascia. The parenchymal layer consists of the ducts and alveoli, including the intralobular connective tissue. Some of the dense intralobular connective tissue, which is part of the stromal tissue component, may be difficult to differentiate from the remainder of the parenchyma because of similar imaging characteristics. The deep fascia is located deep to the fibroglandular tissue. The deep fascia has an appearance similar to that of the superficial fascia.

9. The retromammary layer lies between the deep connective tissue plane and the fascia of the underlying muscle. This layer predominantly contains fat lobules that are smaller than those found in the subcutaneous layer. Connective tissue ligaments are not usually seen in this layer because they are thinner than in the subcutaneous layer.

The pectoralis major and minor muscles are usually easily demonstrated depending on the area of the breast that is being scanned. They are imaged as structures of relatively low echogenicity running deep in the breast above the ribs and parallel to the skin. The structures are more prominent in small-breasted women and may be quite large in athletic individuals. The muscles are best imaged in the transverse plane.

10. The lactiferous ducts are easily seen on most scans, especially when they are dilated. A typical breast is composed of 15 to 20 lobules that are drained by a network of ducts. These ducts are branched in the peripheral parts of the breast and join in the subareolar region to form approximately 15 to 20 ducts that drain onto the surface of the nipple. The diameter of the ducts is therefore slightly larger in the subareolar region than in the periphery of the breast.

The lactiferous ducts are usually collapsed in the nonlactating breast; at the sinus level in the subareolar region the ducts may have a potential diameter of 8 mm. In the periphery of the breast, a diameter of 2 to 4 mm is normal in the lactating breast. Surrounding the subareolar ducts are varying amounts of fibrosis, which accentuate the degree of nipple shadowing observed.

11. In the young, nonlactating breast, the tissue is primarily composed of fibroglandular tissue with little or no subcutaneous fat. With increasing age and parity, fat is deposited in both the subcutaneous and retromammary layers.

During pregnancy there is a substantial increase in glandular tissue in the breast. The resultant image on ultrasound examination demonstrates a finely granular echo pattern with little subcutaneous fat. The subcutaneous and retromammary fat layers are compressed by the glandular tissue and are decreased in size. Late in pregnancy and during lactation, the lactiferous ducts increase in size and number, with resultant duct dilation throughout most of the breast tissue.

Cyclic breast changes may occur with each menstrual cycle. Ultrasonography may image mild duct dilation during the period between ovulation and menstruation. In most normal women, no significant changes are noted.

The postmenopausal breast demonstrates varying amounts of fibrous tissue interspersed among predominantly fatty tissue. With increasing age there is normal regression of the glandular tissue, with subsequent replacement by fat.

12. Breast sonography is used as the initial method for evaluating the young patient less than 30 years and the pregnant patient, and to follow-up patients with fibrocystic disease (3 to 6 month intervals).

Breast sonography is used as a complementary examination to mammography in evaluating areas of dense breast tissue on mammography and evaluating mass composition as demonstrated on mammography.

Answers to Review Exercise C

TABLE 12-1 Differential Diagnosis of Breast Masses: Imaging Characteristics

Mass	Wall	Internal Echo	Attenuation/ Enhancement
Benign Masses (Adjacent tissues are basically normal, except for the compressed tissue sign)			
Simple cyst	Smooth	None	Posterior enhancement (usually)
Galactocele	Smooth	Sparse, low level	Same as simple cyst
Scar tissue	Jagged	Highly echogenic	Slight to marked attenuation
Fibroadenoma	Smooth	Uniform	None visible or slight attenuation
Lipoma	Smooth	Sparse, low level	Same as fibroadenoma
Solitary papilloma	Smooth	Uniform	Same as fibroadenoma
Intracystic papilloma	Smooth or jagged	Nonuniform	None visible or slight attenuation from area on wall where tumor is attached
Malignant Masses			
Intraductal carcinoma	(Duct dilation with thickened Cooper's ligaments)		
Cystosarcoma phyllodes	Smooth in part	Uniform with cystic spaces	Moderate to marked attenuation
Ductal carcinoma (scirrhous)	Jagged	Nonhomogeneous	Marked to moderate attenuation
	(Adjacent reactive fibrosis in adjacent tissues)		
Ductal carcinoma (multilobular)	Partially smooth but jagged	Nonhomogeneous	Moderate attenuation
	(Adjacent reactive fibrosis in adjacent tissues)		
Medullary carcinoma	Jagged, but less than scirrhous	Nonhomogeneous	Slight attenuation to posterior enhancement
Metastatic carcinoma (from opposite breast)	Jagged if mass is present	Nonhomogeneous	Moderate to marked attenuation
	(Diffuse disruption of architecture and skin edema)		
Metastatic carcinoma (from distant source)	Smooth in part	Nonhomogeneous	Slight to no attenuation
	(Mild architecture changes to normal)		

Answers to Self-Test B

1. b	**8.** d	**15.** b
2. d	**9.** b	**16.** c
3. c	**10.** d	**17.** b
4. a	**11.** b	**18.** c
5. b	**12.** false	**19.** false
6. c	**13.** b	**20.** a
7. c	**14.** c	

Answers to Case Reviews—The Breast

1. (Figure 12-13) A simple cyst is seen within the breast. The borders are well defined, the mass is hypoechoic with good through transmission, and the walls are thin. Generally the cysts are round or oval in shape with no distortion in surrounding architecture.

2. (Figure 12-14) Three small cysts are seen within the breast parenchyma. It is difficult to image cysts in women with multicystic disease of the breast because the cystic lesions change size with ovulation.

3. (Figure 12-15) This figure shows a huge cyst with hemorrhagic particles within. This lesion is usually the result of trauma or occurs postaspiration. The appearance of the mass changes over time according to the stage of organization of the hemorrhage.

4. (Figure 12-16) A large fibroadenoma was seen within the breast. These are benign lesions and quite common in the breast. They usually appear homogeneous with very low-level echoes within. They are round or oval in shape, with well defined borders, although some may appear lobulated or may calcify.

5. (Figure 12-17) A fibroadenoma with calcifications was seen within the breast. The calcifications shadowed when the ultrasound beam was directly perpendicular.

6. (Figure 12-18) This figure shows an abscess with ill-defined borders. The clinical story is really the clue in defining an abscess from a carcinoma of the breast. An abscess usually has ill-defined borders with irregular margins, although an abscess may also appear with well-circumscribed borders and good through transmission, depending on the amount of debris within the mass.

7. (Figure 12-19) Ultrasonography of the breast showed a huge, solid-looking lesion that appeared to be well marginated, but was more attenuating than a fibroadenoma. Cystosarcomaphyllodes was found at surgery.

8. (Figure 12-20) A large, irregular-shaped mass was seen within the breast parenchyma. The mass appeared solid and hypoechoic with no through transmission. This mass was an infiltrating ductal carcinoma of the breast at surgery.

The Scrotum

OBJECTIVES

At the completion of this section, students will show orally, in writing, or by demonstration that they will be able to:

1. Describe the various texture patterns and size of the normal scrotum.
2. Define the internal, surface, and relational anatomy of the scrotum.
3. Illustrate the cross-sectional anatomy of the scrotum and adjacent structures.
4. Describe congenital anomalies affecting the scrotum.
5. Select pertinent laboratory tests and other diagnostic procedures.
6. Differentiate between sonographic appearances by explaining the clinical significance of the pathologic processes as related to the scrotum in the following diseases:
   a. primary testicular cancer
   b. benign testicular lesions
   c. microlithiasis
   d. extratesticular processes
   e. infections
   f. varicocele
   g. hydrocele
   h. epididymal cysts
   i. hernia
   j. trauma
7. Create high-quality diagnostic scans demonstrating the appropriate anatomy in all planes pertinent to the pancreas.
8. Select the correct equipment settings appropriate to the individual body habitus.
9. Distinguish between the normal and abnormal sonographic appearances of the scrotum.

To further enhance learning, students should use marking pens to color the anatomic illustrations that follow.

PELVIC VISCERA IN THE MALE

FIGURE 12-21

Contact Surfaces of the Abdominal Viscera as Seen from the Left

The posterior pelvic cavity is occupied by the rectum, colon, and ileum (Figure 12-21). The anterior parts are occupied by the bladder, ureter, vasa deferentia, seminal vesicles, prostate, and prostate urethra (Figure 12-22).

The visceral pelvic fascia covers and supports the pelvic viscera. It is continuous, with the fascia covering the levator ani and coccygeus muscles, and with the parietal pelvic fascia on the pelvic walls.

Bladder

The urinary bladder lies posterior to the pubic bones. The empty bladder is pyramidal and has an apex, a base, a neck, and superior and inferolateral surfaces.

The superolateral angles of the base are joined by the ureters, and the inferior angle gives rise to the urethra. The vasa deferentia separate the seminal vesicles at the posterior surface of the bladder.

Ureter

The ureter crosses the pelvic inlet anterior to the bifurcation of the common iliac artery. At the ischial spine it turns forward and medially and enters the lateral upper angle of the bladder. Near its termination, the vas deferens crosses it.

Vas Deferens

The vas deferens arises from the deep inguinal ring and passes the inferior epigastric artery. It crosses the ureter near the ischial spine, then runs posterior to the bladder. The terminal end is dilated to form the ampulla of the vas deferens. The inferior end of the ampulla narrows and joins the duct of the seminal vesicle to form the ejaculatory duct.

Prostate

The prostate is a fibromuscular and glandular organ that surrounds the prostatic urethra. It lies between the neck of the bladder and the urogenital diaphragm. It is surrounded by a fibrous capsule, which in turn is surrounded by a fibrous sheath (part of the visceral layer of the pelvic fascia).

The arterial supply to the prostate is from the inferior vesical and middle rectal arteries. The veins drain into the internal iliac veins.

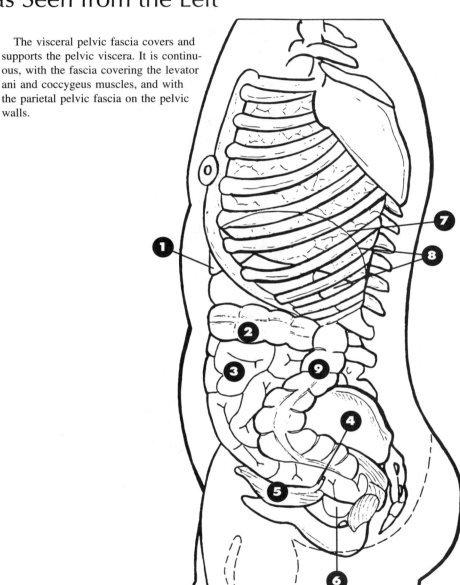

1	liver	6	prostate
2	transverse colon	7	diaphragm
3	intestine	8	spleen
4	ureter	9	descending colon
5	bladder		

FIGURE 12-22
Coronal Section of the Male Pelvis

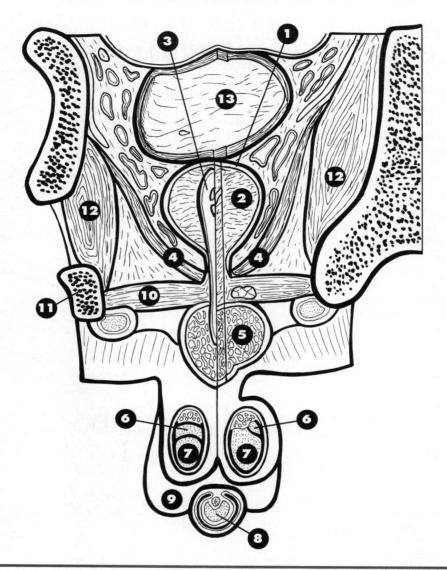

1 **ejaculatory duct**	8 **corpus cavernosum penis**
2 **prostate**	9 **scrotum**
3 **urethra**	10 **tranverse perineal muscle**
4 **levator ani muscle**	11 **pubis**
5 **bulbous corpus cavernosum**	12 **obturator internus muscle**
6 **epididymis**	13 **urinary bladder**
7 **testis**	

FIGURE 12-23
Perineal Muscles and Floor of the Pelvis

Male Urogenital Triangle

Superficial Perineal Pouch

The superficial perineal pouch contains structures that form the root of the penis and their surrounding muscles. The root of the penis is made up of three masses of erectile tissue: the bulb of the penis and the right and left crura. The bulb is in the midline and is attached to the urogenital diaphragm. The urethra traverses it. The outer surface is covered by the bulbocavernous muscles. The crura are attached to the pubic arch and covered by the ischiocavernous muscles. The bulb projects forward into the body of the penis to form the corpus spongiosum. The two crura converge in the posterior body to form the corposa cavernosa. The superficial transverse perineal muscles lie in the posterior superficial perineal pouch. They serve to maintain the perineal body in the center of the perineum.

Several muscles are attached to the perineal body (Figure 12-23):
1) the external and sphincter
2) the bulbospongiosus
3) the superficial transverse perineal

The perineal branch of the pudendal nerve terminates in the superficial perineal pouch.

Deep Perineal Pouch

The deep perineal pouch contains the membranous part of the urethra, the sphincter urethrae, the bulbourethral glands, the deep transverse perineal muscles, the internal pudendal vessels, and the dorsal nerves of the penis.

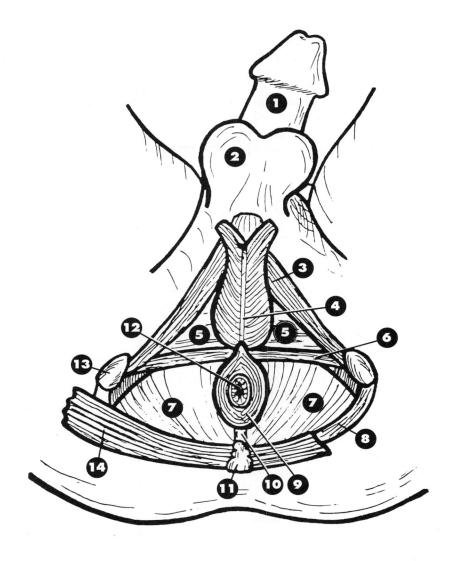

1	penis	8	sacrotuberous ligament
2	scrotum	9	sphincter ani externus muscle
3	ischiocavernosus muscle	10	anococcygeal ligament
4	bulbospongiosus muscle	11	coccyx
5	urogenital diaphragm	12	anus
6	transverse perineal muscle	13	ischial tuberosity
7	levator ani muscle	14	gluteus maximus muscle

Scrotum Review Notes

NORMAL ANATOMY

- The scrotum is a pendent sac that is divided into two lateral compartments by a septum, called the median raphe.
- Each compartment contains a testicle, an epididymus, a vas deferens, and a spermatic cord.
- The scrotal sac is lined internally by the parietal layer of the tunica vaginalis.
- The visceral layer of the tunica vaginalis surrounds the testicle, except for a small area posteriorly, which is termed the *bare area.*
- Blood vessels, lymphatics, nerves, and spermatic ducts travel through the bare area.

The Testes

- The testes are the two male reproductive glands.
- Each testicle is ovoid in shape and measures approximately 2 cm to 3 cm in diameter and 3 cm to 5 cm in length.
- The testicular parenchyma is encased within a thick fibrous capsule known as the tunica albuginea.

Tunica Albuginea

- The tunica albuginea is surrounded by the parietal layer of the tunica vaginalis.
- The tunica albuginea inserts into the posterior aspect of the testicle, where the efferent ductules and blood vessels enter to form a vertical septum called the mediastinum.
- Each testicle is made up of several hundred lobules.

Seminiferous Tubules

- Each lobule is made up of one or several very tortuous tubules called seminiferous tubules.
- The seminiferous tubules converge at the mediastinum and form the rete testis.
- The tubules of the rete testis then empty into the efferent ducts.

Epididymis

- The efferent ducts empty into the epididymis.
- The epididymis lies along the posterolateral aspect of the testis and is made up of a head, body, and tail.
- Its size is 6 cm to 7 cm, and it contains more than 6 meters of coiled tubule.
- The epididymal head, which is also called the globus major, is located over the upper pole of the testicle.
- It is round or triangular in shape and measures approximately 6 mm to 15 mm in width.
- A small protuberance may arise from the epididymal head, known as the appendix of the epididymis.
- The body courses along the posterolateral surface of the testicle to the tail, located under the lower pole of the testicle.

Vas Deferens

- Beginning with the body and ending at the tail of the epididymis, the vas deferens is formed from these structures.
- The vas deferens ascends medially and cephalad and carries semen.
- The vas deferens continues cephalad until reaching an ampulla just proximal to the prostate and adjacent to the seminal vesicles.

Blood Supply

- The majority of the blood supplied to the testis comes from the testicular artery, which arises directly from the aorta.
- The vas deferens and epididymis receive blood from the deferential artery, which is a branch of the vesical artery.
- The peritesticular tissue is supplied by the cremasteric artery, which is a branch of the inferior epigastric artery.
- Both the deferential and cremasteric arteries anastomose with the testicular artery.
- The testicle is drained by a network of veins that arise from the mediastinum to form the pampiniform plexus, which is located within the spermatic cord.
- The pampiniform plexus converges into three veins, the testicular, the deferential, and the cremasteric vein.
- The right testicular vein drains directly into the vena cava and the left drains into the left renal vein.

CONGENITAL ANOMALIES
Undescended Testicle

- The testes are formed in the retroperitoneum of a male fetus.
- The testes then descend into the scrotum via the inguinal canal shortly before birth or early within the neonatal period.
- A deficiency of gonadotropin hormonal stimulation or physical factors such as adhesions or anatomic maldevelopments can interrupt the descent of the testes.
- The undescended testicle is ovoid in shape and is smaller and more hypoechoic than normal testicles.
- If surgery is not performed at an early age, the testis becomes atrophic and is at a high risk for cancer.

MALIGNANT TESTICULAR TUMORS
Primary Testicular Cancer

- Primary testicular cancer occurs in young men who are between the ages of 15 and 34. Acute scrotal pain occurs in 10% to 50% of the cases.
- Ninety-five percent of primary testicular neoplasms are of germ-cell origin.

Seminoma

- Seminoma is the most common germinal tumor and peaks in the fourth decade of life.

- Seminomas spread via the lymphatics and are very radiosensitive.
- Seminomas have the best prognosis.

Embryonal Cell Tumors
- Embryonal cell tumors are less common and more aggressive and lethal than seminomas.
- The 20- to 30-year age group is most susceptible.
- Embryonal cell tumors spread through the blood and via the lymph nodes.

Ultrasound Findings
- Malignant testicular tumors appear on ultrasound examination as well-defined masses and are hypoechoic, although they can be heterogeneous.
- Seminomas tend to be more homogeneous and hypoechoic than other germ cell tumors.

Yolk Sac Tumors
- Yolk sac tumors are the most common germ cell testicular tumors of infancy and childhood.

Choriocarcinoma
- Choriocarcinoma is a rare primary malignancy of the testicle.
- Choriocarcinoma occurs only as a small nodule and often without testicular enlargement.
- The mass may have cystic areas that are caused by hemorrhage and necrosis.

Germ Cell Tumors
- Germ cell tumors are associated with an elevated HCG and AFP.
- Tumors larger than 1.5 cm are usually hypervascular and tend to have disorganized blood flow.
- Tumors of the sex cord stroma include *Leydig cell tumors* and *certoli cell tumors.*
- Leydig cell tumors and certoli cell tumors occur less commonly than germ cell tumors and appear sonographically as an inhomogeneous testis.

Benign Testicular Lesions
- Benign intratesticular lesions are rare.
- These lesions are testicular cysts that have well-rounded borders; anechoic lesions with posterior enhancement are also rare.
- An echo-poor or complex abnormality within the testis could be an abscess, orchitis, torsion, or a benign or malignant tumor.

Microlithiasis
- Two or three calcifications in the testicle are common, although multiple tiny calcifications throughout the testes have been found and termed *microlithiasis.*
- Microlithiasis has been seen in normal patients, but it is associated with tumors, sterility, and cryptorchidism.
- Sonographically, microlithiasis appears as multiple echogenic nonshadowing areas throughout the testis, and these calcifications may obscure other pathology.

EXTRATESTICULAR PROCESSES
Torsion
- The testicle is attached to the scrotum at the bare area.
- If the bare area is small, a small remnant stalk of tunica vaginalis allows the testicle to be mobile.
- Torsion occurs when the testicle revolves one or more times on this short stalk, which obstructs blood flow to the testicle and results in severe pain.
- Torsion is more common in males less than 25 years of age, with a peak incidence at 13 years of age.
- Once torsion occurs, the testicle becomes congested and edematous because of the veins in the twisted cord.
- Pressure within the testicle then begins to build up because of arterial obstruction, which leads to testicular ischemia.
- It is important to correctly diagnose this abnormality early because necrosis of the torsed testicle will occur within 24 hours.

Ultrasound Findings
- A torsed testicle appears normal in the first 4 hours of torsion.
- Although the real-time appearance of the testes is normal, color and pulsed Doppler appearances are abnormal.
- There is an absence of flow in the testicle and the epididymus.
- After 4 hours, the torsed testicle appears enlarged and hypoechoic.
- The testicle may have some inhomogenous appearances as a result of hemorrhage.
- Other findings include enlargement of the epididymus, a reactive hydrocele, and scrotal wall thickening.

INFECTIONS
- With epididymitis, the scrotum becomes swollen and tender.
- In most cases, epididymitis is unilateral.
- The patient has a fever and painful urination.
- Infection usually begins in the epididymus and will then spread to the testicle.
- Sonographically, acute epididymitis usually shows enlargement of the epididymal head, with decreased echogenicity secondary to edema.
- A reactive hydrocele may be present.
- Color Doppler findings include an increased amount of flow in and around the epididymus.
- If an abscess has formed, complex cystic areas may be identified in the epididymus.

Orchitis

- Infection that has spread to the testicle is termed *orchitis*.
- The testicle may appear normal or enlarged in size.
- The echogenicity may be decreased or heterogeneous.
- Reactive hydroceles and skin thickening are associated with orchitis.
- With color Doppler, the testicle will have increased blood flow.
- The ultrasound appearance of chronic orchitis appears as layers of heterogeneous testicular parenchyma.
- Focal orchitis occurs without involvement of the epididymus and has the same appearance as a neoplasm.
- Focal orchitis cannot be distinguished from a neoplasm although clinical symptoms such as fever and an increased white blood count strongly suggest an infectious process.

VARICOCELE

- A varicocele is the abnormal dilation and tortuosity of the veins in the pampiniform plexus of the spermatic cord.
- Varicoceles are more common on the left side, but do occur bilaterally.
- The right internal spermatic vein drains directly into the IVC, whereas the left internal spermatic vein drains into the left renal vein at a 90-degree angle.
  - This angle prevents the formation of a valve.
  - As a result, 99% of varicoceles are left-sided and only 1% are bilateral.
- Varicoceles may cause infertility because they are associated with low sperm counts and decreased mobility.
- Varicoceles appear sonographically as an extratesticular collection of tortuous tubular structures.

HYDROCELE

- A hydrocele is a collection of fluid between the visceral and parietal layers of the tunica vaginalis.
- Hydroceles can be congenital, idiopathic, or acquired.
- Acquired hydroceles are a result of infarction, inflammation, neoplasm, or trauma.

- Hydroceles appear on ultrasound examination as anechoic fluid in the scrotum surrounding the testicle and epididymus.
- Occasionally, small particles and septations are seen in the fluid.

EPIDIDYMAL CYSTS

- Spermatoceles are benign cysts consisting of nonviable sperm.
- They are commonly located in the head of the epididymus but have been found in the body and tail.
- Septations have been seen, and spermatoceles can be singular or multiple.
- On ultrasound examination, a spermatocele appears as a cyst, anechoic with posterior enhancement, and rounded, well-defined walls.
- A spermatocele cannot be differentiated from a simple epididymal cyst.
- Epididymal cysts are composed of clear serous fluid, not sperm.
- They are much less common than spermatoceles.

HERNIA

- Scrotal hernia occurs when a section of bowel herniates through a patent processus vaginalis into the scrotum.
- The patient with a scrotal hernia has scrotal enlargement.
- Ultrasonography helps to make the diagnosis of hernia by demonstrating peristalsing loops of bowel in the scrotum.

TRAUMA

- Testicular parenchymal injury or hemorrhage can alter the normal homogeneous appearance of the testicle.
- Hematomas in the epididymus or scrotal wall have variable sonographic appearances.
- Like hematomas in other parts of the body, the appearance is different, depending on the age of the hematoma.
- The first appearance of a hematoma will be hypoechoic.
- As the hematoma ages, its appearance becomes more echogenic.

Review Exercise D • The Scrotum

1. Describe the indications for an ultrasound examination of the scrotum. _____

_____

_____

_____

_____

2. Discuss the normal anatomy of the scrotum. _____

_____

_____

_____

_____

_____

_____

3. What is the vascular supply to the testes? _____

_____

_____

_____

4. Discuss the ultrasound technique used to image the normal scrotum. _____

_____

_____

_____

_____

5. Describe the development and descent of the normal testes. _____

_____

_____

_____

_____

_____

6. At what age does primary testicular cancer occur? What symptoms are usually present? _____

_____

_____

_____

7. How can sonography aid in the diagnosis of testicular cancer? _____

_____

_____

_____

_____

8. What is the most common germinal tumor found in the scrotum? _____

_____

_____

_____

9. What is the frequency and pathway of embryonal cell tumors in the scrotum? _____

_____

_____

10. Describe the ultrasound appearance of malignant testicular tumors. _____

_____

_____

11. What abnormal laboratory values are associated with germ cell tumors? _____

_____

_____

12. Discuss the vascular pattern of malignant testicular tumors. _____

_____

_____

_____

13. Discuss the occurrence and ultrasound appearance of benign testicular lesions. _____

_____

_____

_____

14. What is the significance of calcification within the testicle? _____

_____

_____

_____

15. Discuss the occurrence and significance of testicular torsion. _____

_____

_____

_____

16. Describe the signs and symptoms of epididymitis. _____

_____

_____

_____

17. What is the sonographic appearance of epididymitis? _____

_____

_____

_____

18. What is the definition of orchitis? What is the ultrasound experience? _____

_____

_____

_____

19. What is a varicocele? Describe the ultrasound appearance. _____

_____

_____

_____

_____

20. Describe a hydrocele and the ultrasound appearance. _____

_____

_____

_____

_____

21. Define epididymal cysts and describe their ultrasound appearance. _____

_____

_____

_____

_____

22. What is the significance of a hernia? What is the ultrasound appearance? _____

_____

_____

_____

_____

23. What role does ultrasonography play in the evaluation of a patient with scrotal trauma? _____

_____

_____

_____

_____

Self-Test C • The Scrotum

1. The scrotum contains:

   a. testes, spermatic cord, and prostate

   b. testes, mediastinum, and epididymis

   c. testes, epididymis, and spermatic cord

   d. testes and spermatic cord

2. The testes are covered by a fibrous capsule formed by the:

   a. tunica albuginea

   b. Cowper's fascia

   c. cremaster muscle

   d. dartos muscle

3. The testes measure:

   a. 6 cm length, 3 cm A-P, 3 cm width

   b. 4 cm length, 3 cm A-P, 2 cm width

   c. 2 cm length, 5 cm A-P, 5 cm width

   d. 4 cm length, 3 cm A-P, 3 cm width

4. Sonographic characteristics of the testes includes:

   a. an inhomogenous pattern with dense internal echoes

   b. a homogeneous pattern with low-level internal echoes

   c. a homogeneous pattern with medium-level echoes

   d. an inhomogeneous pattern with medium-level echoes

5. A linear stripe of variable thickness and echogenicity running through the testis in a craniocaudal direction represents the:

   a. Cowper's fascia

   b. mediastinum testis

   c. epithelial layer

   d. dartos muscle

6. The epididymis is located:

   a. anterior and inferior to the testis

   b. anterior and superior to the testis

   c. posterior and inferior to the testis

   d. posterior and superior to the testis

7. The epididymis is usually a lower echogenicity than the testis (true or false).

8. Which fact about an undescended testis is false?

   a. the testis originates in the retroperitoneum at the level of the fetal kidney

   b. all undescended testes are found in the inguinal canal

   c. there is a 40% to 50% association with testicular malignancy

   d. there is an increased incidence of infertility

9. The differential diagnosis for an undescended testis includes all except:

    a. lymph node

    b. collapsed bowel

    c. retroperitoneal neoplasm

    d. hernia

10. A hydrocele is an abnormal collection of serous fluid in the potential space between the two layers of the tunica vaginalis (true or false).

11. The hydrocele fluid usually accumulates in the posteromedial aspect of the scrotum (true or false).

12. Common causes of a secondary hydrocele include all except:

    a. trauma

    b. undescended testes

    c. infection

    d. neoplasm

13. Which of the following statements is false regarding varicocele?

    a. varicoceles refer to dilated, serpiginous, and elongated veins of the pampiniform plexus

    b. they are more common on the right side

    c. primary varicoceles result from incompetent valves in the spermatic vein

    d. secondary varicoceles develop from compression of the spermatic vein

14. A spermatocele usually lies:

    a. in the head of the epididymis, superior to the testis

    b. in the body of the epididymis, posterior to the testis

    c. in the tail of the epididymis, inferior to the testis

    d. in the body of the epididymis, lateral to the testis

15. A common problem that is viral in origin that affects some adolescent and middle age men is:

    a. an epididymal cyst

    b. epididymitis

    c. a spermatocele

    d. testiculitis

16. A problem that may occur secondary to an acute systemic infection is:

    a. epididymitis

    b. a hydrocele

    c. orchitis

    d. a spermatocele

17. Clinical findings of acute scrotal pain during rest are suggestive of:

    a. orchitis

    b. epididymitis

    c. a neoplasm

    d. torsion

18. Most testicular tumors are of germ cell origin (true or false).

19. The most common neoplasm associated with undescended testes is:

    a. seminoma

    b. lymphoma

    c. adenocarcinoma

    d. teratocarcinoma

20. Characteristic sonographic findings of torsion include all except:

    a. enlargement of the testis

    b. hypoechoic parenchyma

    c. hyperechoic parenchyma

    d. hydrocele

21. Sonographic patterns of testicular neoplasms include all except:

    a. focal and well-defined homogeneous hypoechoic region

    b. diffuse and ill-defined region of decreased echogenicity

    c. complex mass with internal anechoic and echogenic areas

    d. anechoic pattern with increased transmission

22. The differential diagnosis of a testicular neoplasm may include all except:

    a. abscess

    b. infarction

    c. orchitis

    d. hemorrhage

Case Reviews • The Scrotum

1. A 42-year-old male has had firm testicular swelling for the last 2 months. What are your findings (Figure 12-24)?

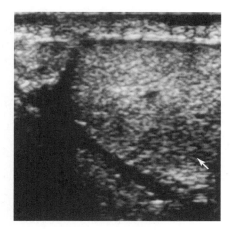

2. A young male with vague scrotal pain was referred for an ultrasound examination. What are your findings (Figure 12-25)?

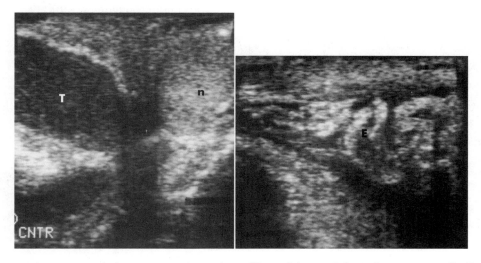

3. A young male has acute pain and swelling of the testicle. What are your findings (Figure 12-26)?

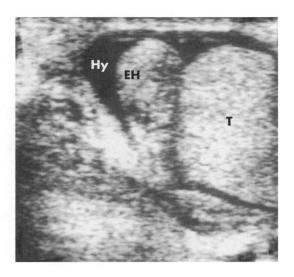

4. A 23-year-old male has fever, malaise, and acute swelling of the scrotum. What are your findings (Figure 12-27)?

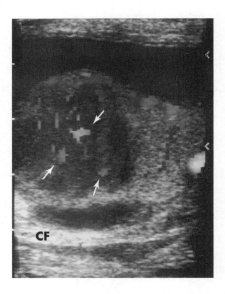

5. An elderly male presents with a "heavy" sensation in his left scrotum. What are your findings (Figure 12-28)?

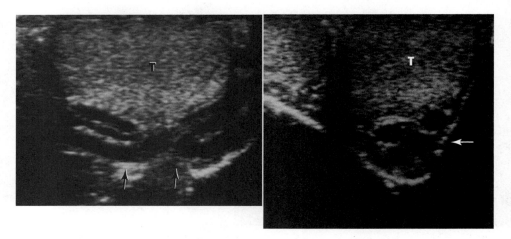

6. A 6-year-old male has a swollen scrotum. What are your findings (Figure 12-29)?

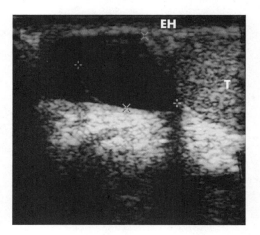

7. A 62-year-old male has groin pain. What are your findings (Figure 12-30)?

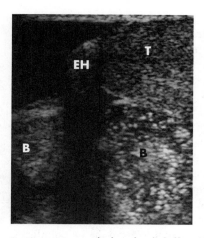

8. A young male has had dull pain and scrotal swelling over the past several months. What are your findings (Figure 12-31)?

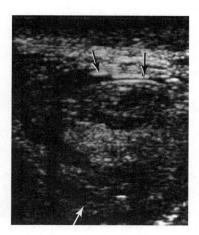

Answers to Review Exercise D

1. Sonography is useful for evaluating testicular size, differentiating between intratesticular or extratesticular abnormalities causing scrotal enlargement or a palpable mass, finding an occult (concealed) neoplasm, evaluating the condition of the testicle in cases of trauma or infection, determining the presence or absence of a varicocele in an infertility workup, and locating an undescended testis.

2. The scrotum is a pendant sac that is divided into two lateral compartments by a septum, called the median raphe. Each compartment contains a testicle, an epididymus, a vas deferens, and a spermatic cord. The scrotal sac is lined internally by the parietal layer of the tunica vaginalis.

   The visceral layer of the tunica vaginalis surrounds the testicle, except for a small area posteriorly, which is termed the *bare area*. At this site, the testicle is against the scrotal wall, thereby preventing torsion. Blood vessels, lymphatics, nerves, and spermatic ducts travel through the bare area.

   The testes are the two male reproductive glands. Each testicle is ovoid in shape and measures approximately 2 cm to 3 cm in diameter and 3 cm to 5 cm in length. The testicular parenchyma is encased within a thick fibrous capsule known as the tunica albuginea. The tunica albuginea is surrounded by the parietal layer of the tunica vaginalis. The tunica albuginea inserts into the posterior aspect of the testicle, where the efferent ductules and blood vessels enter to form a vertical septum called the mediastinum.

   Each testicle is made up of several hundred lobules. Each lobule is made up of one or several very tortuous tubules called seminiferous tubules. The seminiferous tubules converge at the mediastinum and form the rete testis. The mediastinum appears as an echogenic line going through the testicle. The tubules of the rete testis then empty into the efferent ducts. The efferent ducts continue on to empty into the epididymis.

   The epididymis lies along the posterolateral aspect of the testis and is made up of a head, body, and tail. Its overall size is 6 cm to 7 cm, and it contains more than 6 meters of coiled tubule. The epididymal head, which is also called the globus major, is located over the upper pole of the testicle. It is round or triangular in shape and measures approximately 6 mm to 15 mm in width. A small protuberance may arise from the epididymal head, known as the appendix of the epididymis. The body courses along the posterolateral surface of the testicle to the tail, located under the lower pole of the testicle.

   Beginning with the body and ending at the tail of the epididymis, the vas deferens is formed from these structures. The vas deferens ascends medially and cephalad, and carries semen. The vas deferens continues cephalad until reaching an ampulla just proximal to the prostate and adjacent to the seminal vesicles.

3. The majority of the blood supplied to the testis comes from the testicular artery, which arises directly from the aorta. The vas deferens and epididymis receive blood from the deferential artery, which is a branch of the vesical (bladder) artery. The peritesticular tissue is supplied by the cremasteric artery, which is a branch of the inferior epigastric artery. Both the deferential and cremasteric arteries anastomose with the testicular artery.

   The testicle is drained by a network of veins that arise from the mediastinum to form the pampiniform plexus, which is located within the spermatic cord. The pampiniform plexus converges into three veins: the testicular, the deferential, and the cremasteric vein. The right testicular vein drains directly into the vena cava, and the left drains into the left renal vein.

4. To optimally visualize the scrotum, a high resolution, real-time 7.5 MHz to 10 MHz linear transducer should be used. Instrumentation that is capable of demonstrating flow with color and spectral Doppler is extremely helpful to demonstrate flow in normal and abnormal conditions. The Doppler settings should be set for low volume, low velocity flow to optimize the visualization of the small testicular arteries. Color Doppler is also helpful in locating a vessel for further evaluation by pulsed Doppler.

   To prepare for the scan, the patient should be placed in the supine position. The sonographer should avoid a cold room to reduce testicular retraction and skin thickening. The penis should be gently drawn up toward the patient's lower abdomen and covered with a towel. A second towel can then be placed under the scrotum for support during imaging.

   Both testicles should be scanned completely, in both the longitudinal and transverse planes. The longitudinal plane should indicate the lateral, mid, and medial portions of the testicle. A separate image of the epididymal head in relation to the superior portion of the testicle should be obtained. Upper, mid, and lower transverse planes should also be evaluated. An image comparing the echogenicity and size of both testes should be included in the examination.

   The epididymal head and body, and the tail, if possible, should be evaluated. The tail is small and is therefore difficult to distinguish. The spermatic cord area should be scanned from the inguinal canal to the scrotum.

5. The testes are formed in the retroperitoneum of a male fetus. The testes then descend into the scrotum

via the inguinal canal shortly before birth or early within the neonatal period. A deficiency of gonadotropin hormonal stimulation or physical factors such as adhesions or anatomic maldevelopments can interrupt the descent of the testes.

Eighty percent of undescended testes will be found in the inguinal canal, and may occasionally be found intraabdominally or in the femoral area. Undescended testes in the inguinal canal can be demonstrated with ultrasonography. The undescended testicle is ovoid in shape and is smaller and more hypoechoic than normal testicles.

6. Primary testicular cancer occurs in young men between the ages of 15 and 34. Acute scrotal pain occurs in 10% to 50% of the cases.

7. Sonography can determine if a mass is intratesticular or extratesticular. This is important because most intratesticular masses are malignant, and most extratesticular masses are benign. Although testicular masses can be well described and differentiated by using ultrasonography, the ultrasound examination cannot confirm absolutely that a mass is malignant.

In general, testicular tumors are divided into germ cell and sexcord stromal tumors. Ninety-five percent of all testicular tumors are of germ cell origin.

8. Seminoma is the most common germinal tumor and peaks in the fourth decade of life. Seminomas spread via the lymphatics and are very radiosensitive. Seminomas have the best prognosis of all the scrotal tumors.

9. Embryonal cell tumors are less common, but are much more aggressive and lethal than seminomas. The 20- to 30-year age group is most susceptible. Embryonal cell tumors spread through the blood and via the lymph nodes.

10. Malignant testicular tumors appear on ultrasound examination as well-defined masses and are hypoechoic, although they can be heterogeneous. Seminomas tend to be more homogeneous and hypoechoic than other germ cell tumors. There can also be many focal areas.

11. Germ cell tumors are associated with an elevated HCG and AFP.

12. Tumors larger than 1.5 cm are usually hypervascular and tend to have disorganized blood flow.

13. Benign intratesticular lesions are rare. Anechoic testicular cysts with well-rounded borders and posterior enhancement are also rare. The differential of an echo-poor or complex abnormality within the testis could be an abscess, orchitis, torsion, or a benign or malignant tumor.

14. Two or three calcifications in the testicle may be common, although multiple tiny calcifications throughout the testes have been termed *microlithiasis*. Microlithiasis has been seen in normal patients, but it is also associated with tumors, sterility, and cryptorchidism.

Sonographically, microlithiasis appears as multiple echogenic nonshadowing areas throughout the testis. The sonographer must be careful not to have these calcifications obscure other pathology.

15. The testicle is attached to the scrotum at the bare area. If the bare area is small, a small remnant stalk of tunica vaginalis allows the testicle to be mobile. Torsion occurs when the testicle revolves one or more times on this short stalk, which obstructs blood flow to the testicle and results in severe pain. Torsion is more common in males less than 25 years of age, with a peak incidence at 13 years of age.

Once torsion occurs, the testicle becomes congested and edematous because of the veins in the twisted cord. Pressure within the testicle then begins to build up because of arterial obstruction, which leads to testicular ischemia. It is important to correctly diagnose this abnormality early because necrosis of the torsed testicle will occur within 24 hours.

The ultrasound image is normal in the first 4 hours of torsion. Although the real-time appearance of the testes is normal at this time, color and pulsed Doppler appearances are abnormal. There is an absence of flow in the testicle and the epididymus.

After 4 hours, the torsed testicle appears enlarged and hypoechoic. The testicle may have some inhomogenity of the parenchyma secondary to hemorrhage. Other findings include enlargement of the epididymus, reactive hydrocele, and scrotal wall thickening. As in the early phase of torsion, Doppler demonstrates absence of flow within the testicle and epididymus.

16. In patients with epididymitis, the scrotum becomes swollen and tender. In most cases, it is unilateral. The patient has a fever and painful urination. Infection usually begins in the epididymus and spreads to the testicle. Severe infection can lead to an abscess in the epididymus or testicle.

17. Sonographically, acute epididymitis usually shows enlargement of the epididymal head, with decreased echogenicity secondary to edema. A reactive hydrocele may be present. Color Doppler findings show an increased amount of flow in and around the epididymus. If an abscess has formed, complex cystic areas may be identified in the epididymus.

18. Infection that has spread to the testicle is termed *orchitis*. With orchitis, the testicle may appear normal or enlarged in size. The echogenicity may be decreased or heterogeneous. Reactive hydroceles and skin thickening are associated with orchitis. With color Doppler, the testicle will have increased blood flow. The ultrasound appearance of chronic orchitis appears as layers of heterogeneous testicular parenchyma.

Focal orchitis occurs without involvement of the epididymus and has the same appearance as a neoplasm. Focal orchitis cannot be distinguished from a neoplasm, although clinical symptoms such as fever and an increased white blood count strongly suggest an infectious process.

19. A varicocele is the abnormal dilation and tortuosity of the veins in the pampiniform plexus of the spermatic cord. Varicoceles are more common on the left side, but do occur bilaterally. The right internal spermatic vein drains directly into the inferior vena cava, whereas the left internal spermatic vein drains into the left renal vein at a 90-degree angle. This angle prevents the formation of a valve. As a result, 99% of varicoceles are left-sided, and only 1% are bilateral. Varicoceles may cause infertility because they are associated with low sperm counts and decreased mobility.

    Varicoceles appear sonographically as an extratesticular collection of tortuous tubular structures. By having the patient stand or perform the Valsalva maneuver, the size of the varicoceles may increase, making them more obvious. Blood flow is present and can even be reversed, but failure to detect flow cannot exclude diagnosis of a varicocele.

20. A hydrocele is a collection of fluid between the visceral and parietal layers of the tunica vaginalis. A hydrocele can be congenital, idiopathic, or acquired. The size of hydroceles varies from just a few cubic centimeters to as much as a liter. Acquired hydroceles are a result of infarction, inflammation, neoplasm, or trauma. Hydroceles appear on ultrasound examination as anechoic fluid in the scrotum surrounding the tes-

ticle and epididymus. Occasionally, small particles and septations are seen in the fluid.

21. Spermatoceles are benign cysts consisting of nonviable sperm. They are commonly located in the head of the epididymus but have been found in the body and tail. Septations have been seen, and spermatoceles can be singular or multiple. On ultrasound examination, a spermatocele appears as a cyst, anechoic with posterior enhancement, and rounded, well-defined walls.

    A spermatocele cannot be differentiated from a simple epididymal cyst. Epididymal cysts are composed of clear serous fluid, not sperm. They are much less common than spermatoceles.

22. A scrotal hernia occurs when a section of bowel herniates through a patent processus vaginalis into the scrotum. The patient with a hernia has scrotal enlargement. Ultrasonography helps to make the diagnosis of hernia by demonstrating peristalsing loops of bowel in the scrotum.

23. In cases of scrotal trauma, ultrasonography can be helpful in evaluating the extent of the injury. Testicular parenchymal injury or hemorrhage can alter the normal homogeneous appearance of the testicle. Hematomas in the epididymus or scrotal wall have variable sonographic appearances. Like hematomas in other parts of the body, the appearance is different depending on the age of the hematoma. The first appearance of a hematoma will be hypoechoic. As the hematoma ages, its appearance becomes more echogenic.

Answers to Self-Test C

1. c	**9.** d	**16.** c
2. a	**10.** true	**17.** d
3. d	**11.** false	**18.** true
4. c	**12.** b	**19.** a
5. b	**13.** b	**20.** c
6. d	**14.** a	**21.** d
7. false	**15.** b	**22.** c
8. b		

Answers to Case Reviews—The Scrotum

1. (Figure 12-24) Ultrasonography of the testicle shows a diffuse mass containing multiple, well-defined tumors with decreased echogenicity, demonstrating a seminoma. A seminoma *(S)* is the most common primary neoplasm. Metastasis is uncommon, and the prognosis is good. The lesion presents as a hypoechoic mass within the testis. The mass is well delineated with smooth, well-defined borders.

2. (Figure 12-25) This is a transverse sonogram of the testicle containing multiple bright echoes caused by tiny calcifications demonstrating microlithiasis. No other lesions were noted.

3. (Figure 12-26) This transverse sonogram of both testicles shows asymmetry of the testes in echogenicity and size. The torsed testicle *(T)* is hypoechoic and enlarged. Normal testicle *(N)*.

4. (Figure 12-26) This is a longitudinal sonogram of epididymitis, demonstrating an enlarged heterogeneous epididymis with a reactive hydrocele. The testis may appear normal, but has focal hypoechoic areas within, as a result of focalized orchitis. Increased flow in the epididymis is seen with color Doppler. Hydrocele *(Hy)*, Epididymal head *(EH)*, Testicle *(T)*.

5. (Figure 12-28) This shows longitudinal scans of a dilated vein of the left pampiniform plexus representing a varicocele *(arrow)*. The varicocele occurs more commonly on the left side, as a result of the angle of the left spermatic vein emptying into the left renal vein. The veins appear as tubular, hypoechoic structures, superior and posterior to the testicle. Color Doppler demonstrates venous flow within the vericocele. Testicle *(T)*.

6. (Figure 12-29) A large spermatocele is shown in the epididymis. These collections usually arise near the head of the epididymis. They appear as a sonolucent, loculated lesion, and are indistinguishable from a hydrocele on ultrasound examination. Epididymal head *(EH)*, Testicle *(T)*.

7. (Figure 12-30) The most common cause of inguinal swelling is a scrotal hernia. This occurs when herniation of the bowel occurs into the scrotal sac. The sonographer should watch the fluid collection to detect the presence of peristalsis within the hernia. A hydrocele may also be present. Epididymal head *(EH)*, Testicle *(T)*, Peristalsing bowel *(B)*.

8. (Figure 12-31) This figure shows chronic orchitis. This transverse scan demonstrates the layering effect of a chronic condition of orchitis.

Practice Registry Examination

1. A vertical plane that bisects the body into right and left halves is the:

   a. sagittal plane

   b. median plane

   c. coronal plane

   d. lateral plane

2. Any plane parallel to the median plane is the:

   a. coronal plane

   b. transverse plane

   c. lateral plane

   d. sagittal plane

3. Any vertical plane at right angles to the median plane is the:

   a. sagittal plane

   b. coronal plane

   c. transverse plane

   d. median plane

4. Any plane at right angles to both the median and coronal planes is the:

   a. transverse plane

   b. coronal plane

   c. sagittal plane

   d. median plane

5. The location that is toward the front of the body.

   a. dorsal

   b. coronal

   c. anterior

   d. cranial

6. The location that is at the back of the body or in back of another structure.

   a. ventral

   b. anterior

   c. superior

   d. posterior

7. The location that is farther from the midline or to the side of the body.

   a. lateral

   b. dorsal

   c. ventral

   d. distal

8. The location that is closer to the point of origin or closer to the body.

   a. distal

   b. proximal

   c. superior

   d. inferior

9. The location that is away from the point of origin or away from the body.

   a. Proximal

   b. Inferior

   c. Superior

   d. Distal

10. The location that is toward the head.

    a. caudal

    b. ventral

    c. cranial

    d. inferior

11. The _____ is a serous membrane lining the walls of the abdominal cavity and clothing the abdominal viscera.

    a. pericardium

    b. omentum

    c. greater sac

    d. peritoneum

12. The accumulation of fluid in the peritoneal cavity is called:

    a. ascites

    b. pericardial effusion

    c. pleural effusion

    d. fluid retention

13. All the following statements about the lesser sac are true except:

    a. the lesser sac is an extensive peritoneal pouch located behind the lesser omentum and stomach

    b. it extends upward to the diaphragm and inferior between the layers of the greater omentum

    c. it attaches the stomach to another viscus organ

    d. the right margin of the lesser sac opens into the greater sac through the epiploic foramen

14. The right posterior subphrenic space lies between the right lobe of the liver, the right kidney, and the right colic flexure. This is called:

    a. Douglas' pouch

    b. peritoneal recess

    c. renal gutter

    d. Morison's pouch

15. When scanning an obese patient for an abdominal ultrasound, you discover you are not able to image the posterior aspect of the right lobe of the liver. As a sonographer you would do all of the following except:

    a. roll the patient into a right posterior oblique

    b. roll the patient into a left posterior oblique

    c. use a lower frequency transducer

    d. adjust the TGC and overall gain of the system

16. The arterial and venous system differ in the composition of their three layers. This difference is seen in the:

    a. tunica intima

    b. tunica moderator

    c. tunica media

    d. tunica adventitia

17. The valve that separates the inferior vena cava from the right atrium is the:

    a. diaphragmatic valve

    b. Windsor's valve

    c. Heister's valve

    d. eustachian valve

18. All of the following structures are tributaries of the inferior vena cava except:

    a. portal vein

    b. right testicular vein

    c. inferior phrenic vein

    d. right adrenal vein

19. The Valsalva maneuver is useful to delineate a vein from an artery because it causes the vein to:

    a. pulsate with respiration

    b. dilate at the end of valsalva

    c. cause spontaneous contrast within the vessel

    d. collapse

20. This vessel courses along the upper border of the head of the pancreas, behind the posterior layer of the peritoneal omental bursa, to the upper margin of the superior part of the duodenum.

    a. left hepatic artery

    b. right hepatic artery

    c. common hepatic artery

    d. left gastric artery

21. The distribution of the superior mesenteric artery is to the:

    a. distal stomach

    b. proximal half of the colon and the small intestine

    c. distal half of the colon and small intestine.

    d. transverse colon, descending colon, and rectum

22. The course of the right renal artery is:

    a. anterior to the inferior vena cava

    b. superior to the kidney

    c. posterior to the inferior vena cava

    d. anterior to the portal vein

23. These vessels are the largest tributary of the inferior vena cava. They originate in the liver and drain into the IVC at the level of the diaphragm.

    a. portal veins

    b. superior mesenteric veins

    c. hepatic veins

    d. phrenic veins

24. All the following statements regarding the portal veins are true except:

    a. they increase in caliber as they approach the porta hepatis

    b. their walls are brighter

    c. they increase in caliber as they approach the diaphragm

    d. they course transversely through the liver

25. The most common cause of an aortic aneurysm is:

    a. arteriosclerosis

    b. cystic medial necrosis

    c. hypertension

    d. syphilis

26. When examining a patient for an abdominal aneurysm, all the following considerations should be made except:

    a. the relationship of the aneurysm to the renal arteries

    b. the extension into the iliac arteries

    c. the measurement of the aneurysm in A-P, length, and width dimensions

    d. the change in respiratory variation

27. The normal dimensions of the aorta, the aortic bifurcation, and the iliac arteries are:

    a. 3,2,1 cm

    b. 4,3,2 cm

    c. 3,3,2 cm

    d. 3,1,1 cm

28. The development of excruciating chest pain in a patient with a known abdominal aneurysm is thought to represent:

    a. an aortic rupture

    b. a dissection of the aorta

    c. a myocardial infarction

    d. a hypertensive event

29. Other lesions that may simulate an abdominal aneurysm include all except:

    a. retroperitoneal mass

    b. horseshoe kidney

    c. arteriovenous fistula

    d. pancreatic carcinoma

30. A patient who experiences leg edema, lower back and pelvic pain, and gastrointestinal complaints most likely has:

    a. complete thrombosis of the inferior vena cava

    b. dissection of the aorta

    c. arteriovenous fistula

    d. thrombosis of the common femoral vein

31. In patients who develop portal venous hypertension, the portal blood flow becomes

    _____ instead of

    _____ .

    a. hepatopetal, hepatofugal

    b. hepatofugal, hepatopetal

    c. hepatopetal, hepatofluge

    d. hepatofugal, hepatopudal

32. Examples of high resistive vessels include all except:

    a. external carotid

    b. internal carotid

    c. iliac artery

    d. brachial artery

33. Examples of low resistive vessels include all except:

    a. hepatic artery

    b. renal artery

    c. external carotid

    d. superior mesenteric artery

34. The normal Doppler velocity pattern of the inferior vena cava is:

    a. biphasic

    b. triphasic

    c. cyclical

    d. resistive

35. Periportal collateral circulation in patients with chronic portal vein obstruction is:

    a. portal venous hypertension

    b. Budd-Chiari syndrome

    c. cavernous transformation

    d. arteriovenous fistula

36. On ultrasound examination, if a patient has splenic varices, the following will occur:

   a. splenic flow will be hepatopetal

   b. splenic flow will be hepatofugal

   c. splenic flow will be hepatopetal but portal flow will be hepatofugal

   d. splenic flow will cease

37. Hepatic veins course between the hepatic lobes and segments (true or false).

38. One of the following statements is false:

   a. the right lobe of the liver is divided into anterior and posterior segments

   b. the left lobe is divided into medial and lateral segments

   c. the quadrate lobe is part of the medial segment of the left lobe

   d. the caudate lobe is part of the posterior segment of the right lobe

Match the following terms:

a. RHV

b. IVC fossa

c. LHV

d. RPV (anterior)

e. LPV (initial)

f. ligamentum teres

39. _____ separates the caudate lobe from the medial and lateral segments of the left lobe.

40. _____ separates the right and left hepatic lobes.

41. _____ divides the anterior and posterior segments of the right hepatic lobe and courses between the anterior and posterior branches of the RPV.

42. _____ separates the caudate lobe posteriorly from the medial segment of the left lobe anteriorly.

43. _____ divides the medial and lateral segments of the left lobe.

44. _____ courses centrally in the anterior segment of the right hepatic lobe.

45. Viral hepatitis is a disease in which the virus attacks the liver cells and damages or destroys them. This is considered:

   a. hepatocellular disease

   b. metabolic disease

   c. obstructive disease

   d. destructive disease

46. Elevation of serum bilirubin results in:

   a. hepatitis

   b. obstructive disease

   c. jaundice

   d. cirrhosis

47. Aspartate aminotransferase is an enzyme that is present in tissues that have a high rate of metabolic activity. If this value is elevated, it may represent all but the following disease states:

   a. acute hepatitis

   b. cirrhosis

   c. infectious mononucleosis

   d. chronic cholelithiasis

48. The laboratory value that is a good indicator of obstruction is:

   a. alkaline phosphatase

   b. lactic acid dehydrogenase

   c. aspartate aminotransferase

   d. prothrombin time

49. A sonogram of the liver shows increased echogenicity with increased attenuation and decreased vascular borders. This most likely represents:

   a. hepatitis

   b. fatty liver

   c. glycogen storage disease

   d. chronic granulomatous disease

50. Which statement is false regarding the sonographic findings in cirrhosis of the liver?

   a. coarsening of the liver parenchyma

   b. nodularity of the liver border

   c. hepatosplenomegaly with ascites

   d. increased transmission beyond the portal vein radicles

51. An extrahepatic mass on sonography may show the following characteristics except:

    a. internal invagination or discontinuity of the liver capsule

    b. displacement of the hepatic vascular radicles

    c. formation of a triangular fat wedge

    d. anterior displacement of the right kidney

52. Of patients with polycystic liver disease, what percent will also have polycystic renal disease?

    a. 10% to 30%

    b. 50% to 60%

    c. 20% to 40%

    d. 60% to 75%

53. Which statement is false regarding polycystic liver disease?

    a. it is easy to distinguish a neoplastic growth in the liver

    b. cysts within the porta hepatis may enlarge and cause biliary obstruction

    c. cysts are multiple throughout the liver

    d. the cysts are small, usually 2 cm to 3 cm in size

54. Bacteria may gain access to the liver through several routes. These include all of the following except:

    a. the biliary tree

    b. the portal vein

    c. the gastrointestinal tract

    d. the hepatic artery

55. Clinical signs of a hepatic pyogenic abscess include all except:

    a. leuokocytosis

    b. hematuria

    c. elevated liver function tests

    d. anemia

56. In patients with hepatic candidiasis, other areas that may be infected include all except:

    a. kidneys

    b. brain

    c. spleen

    d. heart

57. A patient without previous history of hepatic disease comes to the hospital with gastrointestinal symptoms of abdominal pain, diarrhea, leukocytosis, and low fever. The most likely diagnosis for this is:

    a. echinococcal cyst

    b. chronic granulomatous disease

    c. necrotic tumor

    d. amebic abscess

58. The sonographic finding of a "water-lily" sign is usually seen in which disease on ultrasound examination?

    a. echinococcal cyst

    b. candidiasis

    c. polycystic liver disease

    d. necrotic tumor

59. One of the following statements is not true regarding a malignancy:

    a. the mass is uncontrolled

    b. the mass is prone to metastasize to distant structures via the bloodstream and lymph nodes

    c. a neoplasm is a new growth of tissue

    d. the mass does not invade surrounding structures

60. An echogenic mass found in the subcapsular hepatic parenchyma in an asymptomatic patient most likely represents:

    a. a cavernous hemangioma

    b. an adenoma

    c. a focal nodular hyperplasia

    d. granulomatous disease

61. The common lesion found in women that has been related to oral contraceptive use is:

    a. cavernous hemangioma

    b. Von Gierke's disease

    c. liver cell adenoma

    d. cystadenoma

62. Hepatocellular carcinoma is a tumor of the liver that is commonly found in men with a previous history of:

    a. Von Gierke's disease

    b. hemachromatosis

    c. focal nodular hyperplasia

    d. cirrhosis

63. The primary sites of metastastic disease of the liver originate from all except the:

    a. colon

    b. pancreas

    c. breast

    d. lung

64. The liver is the third most common organ injured in the abdomen after the:

    a. spleen and kidney

    b. spleen and pancreas

    c. kidney and pancreas

    d. spleen and gallbladder

65. The most important vascular structure to image after a liver transplant is:

    a. aorta

    b. superior mesenteric artery

    c. hepatic artery

    d. gastroduodenal artery

66. When the normal venous channels in the liver become obstructed, what happens?

    a. the blood flows hepatopedally to the liver

    b. collateral circulation develops

    c. the flow becomes less resistive

    d. the systolic velocity of the flow is reversed.

67. Budd-Chiari syndrome represents:

    a. obstructive flow to the hepatic veins

    b. obstructive flow to the portal veins

    c. obstructive flow to the superior mesenteric vein

    d. obstructive flow to the umbilical vein

68. When there is thrombosis of the right, middle, and left hepatic veins, the _____ lobe becomes enlarged.

    a. right

    b. left

    c. caudate

    d. quadrate

69. In a patient who is 50 years of age, the normal common duct has a diameter of:

    a. 4 mm

    b. 6 mm

    c. 8 mm

    d. 10 mm

70. The common bile duct is joined by the main pancreatic duct, and together they open through:

    a. Sphincter of Oddi

    b. Wirsung's ampulla

    c. Vater's ampulla

    d. Santorini's ampulla

71. The common duct moves after it descends behind the duodenum and enters the pancreas.

    a. posterior

    b. superior

    c. lateral

    d. medial

72. The normal location of the liver is:

    a. occupies the left hypochondrium, epigastrium, and umbilical area

    b. occupies the right hypochondrium, part of epigastrium and umbilical area

    c. occupies the epigastrium, umbilical, and mid-hypochondrium area

    d. occupies the upper abdominal cavity

73. The _____ lobe is situated on the posterior surface of the right lobe, bounded by the porta; on the right, by the fossa for the IVC, and on the left by the fossa for the ductus venosus.

    a. left   c. quadrate

    b. caudate   d. right

74. The portal vein is formed by the junction of the:

    a. superior mesenteric artery and IVC

    b. splenic vein and splenic artery

    c. superior mesenteric vein and splenic vein

    d. hepatic vein and splenic vein

75. A 34-year-old patient comes to the hospital with a palpable mass, hepatomegaly, and has normal liver function tests. The ultrasound demonstrated a normal hepatic parenchyma except for a central mass that was smooth-walled, anechoic, and showed good through transmission. The most likely diagnosis would be:

    a. abscess of the liver

    b. dilated gallbladder

    c. hepatoma

    d. liver cyst

76. Clinical signs of jaundice, ascites, spider angiomate of the face, and palmar erythema may represent:

    a. metastases

    b. diabetes

    c. cirrhosis

    d. biliary abscess

77. The inferior vena cava runs _____ through the retroperitoneal space and posterior to the liver

    a. horizontally

    b. vertically

    c. transversely

    d. obliquely

78. Which vascular structures are useful for the localization of the pancreas?

    a. common bile duct, portal vein, splenic vein, aorta

    b. superior mesenteric artery and vein, splenic vein, splenic artery, left renal vein, aorta, and IVC

    c. right and left hepatic veins, splenic vein, aorta, portal vein

    d. common bile duct, right renal vein, splenic vein, and portal vein

79. The superior border of the body of the pancreas is usually outlined by which vessel?

    a. splenic vein

    b. portal vein

    c. splenic artery

    d. superior mesenteric artery

80. Primary acute cholecystitis is characterized by:

    a. gallstones

    b. an enlarged anechoic gallbladder with a hypoechoic rim, and no response to fatty meal

    c. posterior shadowing

    d. nonvisualization

81. A common cause of obstruction to the distal common duct is all of the following except:

    a. impacted gallstones

    b. carcinoma of the pancreatic head

    c. biliary papillomatosis

    d. stricture of the common bile duct

82. A choledochal cyst is:

    a. a necrotic tumor of the biliary system

    b. a gallbladder containing inspissated bile

    c. a dilatation of the extrahepatic biliary tree

    d. carcinoma of the duodenum

83. One differential between a retroperitoneal mass and an abscess is:

    a. abscesses always appear cystic, and masses do not

    b. abscesses tend to fill available space between organs, and masses displace organs

    c. abscesses can never appear as complex echo patterns

    d. abscesses are hyperechoic, and masses are hypoechoic

84. The characteristics of a fluid-filled lesion include all except:

    a. well-defined, sharp posterior border

    b. anechoic, even at high gain

    c. diminished through transmission

    d. increased through transmission

85. The characteristics of solid lesions include all except:

    a. anechoic, even at high gain

    b. fine to coarse internal echoes

    c. poorly defined posterior border

    d. normal or diminished through transmission

86. Which of the following structures are retroperitoneal?

    a. liver

    b. pancreas

    c. gallbladder

    d. spleen

87. A renal transplant lies:

    a. in the renal fossa, taking the place of the kidney that has been removed

    b. in the RUQ

    c. posterior in the pelvis

    d. along the iliac wing

88. One of the following statements is false regarding ascites:

    a. it extends more superior on the right than the left

    b. it may push the liver medially

    c. it commonly collects anterior to the bladder

    d. it may collect within the pelvis behind the bladder and/or uterus

89. Examination of the right kidney confirms the presence of a mass seen on the IVP. The wall of the mass is somewhat irregular and little increased transmission is present. At high gain the mass does not fill in with echoes. This mass most likely represents:

    a. an uncomplicated renal cyst

    b. a lobulated renal cyst

    c. a splenic cyst

    d. a necrotic tumor

90. During the ultrasound examination of a patient with known pancreatitis, you suspect that the anteriorly located fluid collection in the LUQ actually represents a fluid-filled stomach rather than a pseudocyst. Which procedure would you not do?

    a. drain the nasogastric tube that the patient already has in place

    b. roll the patient onto his left side for 10 to 15 minutes to help drain the stomach

    c. roll the patient onto his right side to drain the stomach

    d. sit the patient upright and give the patient 16 oz. of water

91. The characteristics of a fluid-filled lesion include all except:

    a. sharp posterior border

    b. poorly defined posterior border

    c. sonolucent even at high gain

    d. increased through transmission

92. The characteristics of a solid lesion include:

    a. diffuse fine internal echoes

    b. poorly defined posterior border

    c. increased through transmission

    d. normal or diminished through transmission

93. All of the following structures are retroperitoneal except:

    a. kidneys

    b. pancreas

    c. lymph nodes

    d. spleen

94. Ascites is all except:

    a. characteristically extends more superior on the right than the left

    b. may push the liver medially

    c. may collect within the pelvis behind the bladder and/or uterus

    d. commonly collects anterior to the bladder

95. Scans of the abdomen and kidneys demonstrate a large solid mass superior to the right kidney. The mass appears to elevate the inferior vena cava anteriorly. The origin of this mass is most likely:

    a. biliary

    b. adrenal

    c. aorta

    d. pancreas

96. Sagittal scans of the patient's right hemidiaphragm on inspiration and expiration show no motion. In addition, there appears to be a separation of the liver from the diaphragm. This probably represents:

   a. normal respiration

   b. subphrenic abscess

   c. aneurysm

   d. pseudocyst

97. Entities that produce increased transmission of sound include:

   a. calcified pancreatic pseudocyst, fluid-filled stomach, fluid-filled transverse colon

   b. hepatoma, renal cyst, gas-filled transverse colon

   c. gallbladder, ascitic fluid, urinary bladder

   d. pancreas, gallbladder, urinary bladder

98. A rib artifact:

   a. is caused by not using enough air-free gel when scanning

   b. is produced by a slow reverberation of the sound wave between the transducer face and the patient's rib

   c. is produced by a rapid reverberation of the sound wave between the transducer face and the patient's rib

   d. is the result of a faulty crystal within the transducer

99. Nonshadowing, low-amplitude echoes in a dependent gallbladder are most characteristic of:

   a. cholelithiasis

   b. porcelain gallbladder

   c. cholecystitis

   d. sludge

100. The ligamentum venosum lies between the:

   a. medial and lateral segments of the left lobe of the liver

   b. anterior and posterior segments of the right lobe of the liver

   c. caudate lobe and the left lobe of the liver

   d. anterior and posterior segments of the left lobe of the liver

101. The ligamentum teres is:

   a. the obliterated umbilical vein of the fetus

   b. the falciform ligament in the adult

   c. the obliterated ductus venosus of the fetus

   d. the division of right and left lobes of the liver

102. Which area(s) other than the left upper quadrant should be scanned when ruling out a ruptured spleen?

   a. right upper quadrant

   b. psoas muscles

   c. RUQ, psoas muscles, Douglas' pouch

   d. Douglas' pouch, psoas muscles

103. The renal sinus is comprised of the:

   a. renal artery and vein, renal pelvis

   b. renal artery and vein, ureter, arcuate artery

   c. renal artery and vein, renal pelvis, pelvic fat

   d. renal artery and vein, ureter

104. The echogenic area around the kidney includes all of the following except:

   a. renal capsule

   b. perirenal fat

   c. retroperitoneal fat

   d. Bowman's capsule

105. Which of the following lab tests, when elevated, would be an indication of renal obstruction?

   a. BUN and creatinine

   b. ALT and amylase

   c. amylase and creatinine

   d. BUN and amylase

106. A sonographic examination of a patient with renal cell carcinoma should include:

   a. inferior vena cava and liver

   b. liver and renal artery

   c. inferior vena cava, renal veins, liver, and kidneys

   d. inferior vena cava, renal veins and arteries, kidneys

107. All of the following may be complications of renal transplants except:

    a. perinephric abscess

    b. lymphocele

    c. urinoma

    d. nephrolithiasis

108. Hydronephrosis may be caused by any of the following except:

    a. prostate cancer

    b. nephrolithiasis

    c. retroperitoneal fibrosis

    d. acute glomerulonephritis

109. In the presence of a large adrenal mass, the kidneys may be displaced:

    a. anterior, medial, and inferior

    b. posterior, lateral, and inferior

    c. anterior, lateral, and superior

    d. posterior, medial, and inferior

110. Which of the following primary tumors may likely metastasize to the adrenal glands?

    a. leukemia and bronchogenic carcinoma

    b. breast carcinoma and leukemia

    c. pheochromocytoma and breast carcinoma

    d. bronchogenic carcinoma and breast carcinoma

111. A type of primary adrenal tumor is:

    a. pheochromocytoma

    b. hypernephroma

    c. blastocytoma

    d. seminoma

112. On a routine abdominal ultrasound examination, a patient is found to have bilateral Grade II hydronephrosis. Which of the following is the most likely cause of renal obstruction?

    a. ruptured appendix

    b. ascites in the cul-de-sac

    c. enlarged prostate gland

    d. hepatomegaly

113. Klatzkin's tumor is located:

    a. near the sphincter of Oddi

    b. junction of the cystic and common hepatic ducts

    c. junction of Vater's ampulla and the common duct

    d. confluence of the right and left hepatic ducts

114. What is the correct order of anatomy from anterior to posterior?

    a. pancreas, SMA, aorta, left renal vein

    b. pancreas, SMA, left renal vein, aorta

    c. SMA, pancreas, left renal vein, aorta

    d. SMA, pancreas, aorta, left renal vein

115. What is the correct order of anatomy from anterior to posterior?

    a. pancreas, SMV, right renal artery, IVC

    b. SMV, pancreas, right renal artery, IVC

    c. liver, SMA, IVC, aorta

    d. pancreas, SMV, IVC, right renal artery

116. Which of the following structures is located most anterior?

    a. IVC

    b. gastroduodenal artery

    c. common bile duct

    d. right renal artery

117. Multicystic dysplastic kidneys may be difficult to differentiate on ultrasonography because of:

    a. infantile polycystic renal disease

    b. hydronephrosis

    c. choledochal cyst

    d. renal agenesis

118. A young child with a status of post- left nephrectomy for a Wilm's tumor, is referred to ultrasonography. Which area(s) are likely sites for metastases?

    a. right kidney, liver

    b. right kidney, liver, spleen

    c. right kidney, liver, IVC

    d. right kidney, liver, spleen, ovaries, and IVC

119. A choledochal cyst is:

    a. an acquired disease of the bile duct as a result of a stone obstruction

    b. an acquired disease of the gallbladder as a result of stone obstruction

    c. a congenital abnormality of the common bile duct

    d. a congenital defect of the gallbladder

120. Unilateral renal agenesis is:

    a. associated with congenital anomalies of the biliary system

    b. associated with congenital anomalies of the skeletal system

    c. has no association with congenital anomalies

    d. associated with congenital anomalies of the uterus

121. Name the bright linear reflector that is a reliable indicator for the location of the gallbladder.

    a. main lobar fissure

    b. intersegmental fissure

    c. right interhepatic fissure

    d. biliary fissure

122. Inflammation of the gallbladder is a chronic illness. This is called:

    a. cholelithiasis

    b. choledocolithiasis

    c. cholecystitis

    d. choledocolosis

123. What is the false statement regarding gallbladder sludge?

    a. may be thick or inspissated bile

    b. may be found in the bile duct

    c. is gravity-dependent

    d. always changes immediately with patient position

124. All of the following may cause gallbladder wall hypertrophy except:

    a. hepatoma

    b. ascites

    c. AIDS

    d. cholecystitis

125. False positive findings of cholelithiasis include all except:

    a. polyp

    b. very small stones

    c. adenomyosis

    d. sludge ball

126. The following conditions may show no evidence of cholelithiasis except:

    a. contracted gallbladder

    b. sludge

    c. gallstone in fundal cap

    d. WES

127. Choledochal cysts may be associated with:

    a. gallstones, pancreatitis, biloma

    b. cirrhosis, pancreatitis, hepatoma

    c. gallstones, pancreatitis, cirrhosis

    d. cirrhosis, ascites

128. A patient whose status is postcholecystectomy presents with diffuse shadowing throughout the liver parenchyma. This most likely represents:

    a. multiple stones in the hepatic ducts

    b. air within the hepatic ducts

    c. obstruction of the hepatic duct

    d. neoplastic growth within the hepatic ducts

129. A hyperplastic change in the gallbladder wall is most representative of:

    a. cholesterol polyp

    b. adenomyomatosis

    c. gallbladder carcinoma

    d. biliary dyskinesia

130. Patients with this disease have an increased incidence of carcinoma of the gallbladder:

    a. biliary stricture

    b. cholesterol polyp

    c. gangrenous cholecystitis

    d. porcelain gallbladder

131. All of the following statements regarding the gallbladder are true except:

    a. carcinoma of the gallbladder is very rare

    b. a small tumor in the neck is always seen with ultrasonography

    c. the tumor infiltrates the gallbladder locally or diffusely and causes thickening and rigidity of the wall

    d. the adjacent liver is often invaded by direct continuity extending through tissue spaces

132. All of the following statements regarding dilated ducts are true except:

    a. they are never found in the absence of jaundice

    b. biliary obstruction may involve one hepatic duct

    c. early obstruction may be secondary to carcinoma

    d. gallstones may cause intermittent obstruction

133. Differential diagnosis for a choledochal cyst would include all except:

    a. hepatic cyst

    b. pancreatic pseudocyst

    c. hepatic artery aneurysm

    d. abdominal aortic aneurysm

134. Clinical signs and laboratory values in a patient with cholelithiasis would include all except:

    a. RUQ pain radiating to the shoulder

    b. ascites

    c. positive Murphy's sign

    d. nausea and vomiting

135. The laboratory values that are the most effective in diagnosing pancreatitis are:

    a. amylase and lipase

    b. alkaline phosphatase and amylase

    c. lipase and bilirubin

    d. amylase and glucose

136. A young patient has cystic fibrosis and RUQ pain. You would expect to find:

    a. small cysts throughout the liver

    b. cholelithiasis and small pancreatic cysts

    c. small pancreatic cysts and hydronephrosis

    d. hepatosplenomegaly

137. The most common cause of pancreatitis is:

    a. cirrhosis

    b. pseudocyst

    c. biliary tract disease

    d. trauma

138. One of the following statements is false regarding pancreatitis:

    a. the secretions migrate to the surface of the gland

    b. the fluid breaks through the pancreatic connective tissue layer and peritoneum to enter the lesser sac

    c. the juice enters the posterior pararenal space

    d. collections of fluid in the peripancreatic area generally retrain communication with the pancreas

139. Clinical signs of acute pancreatitis include all except:

    a. moderate to severe epigastric pain radiating to the back

    b. positive Murphy's sign

    c. abdomen is distended with ileus

    d. fever and leukocytosis is present

140. Hemorrhagic pancreatitis is a rapid progression of acute pancreatitis. Further necrosis of the blood vessels results in the development of hemorrhagic areas referred to as:

    a. Grey Turner's sign

    b. Murphy's sign

    c. silhouette sign

    d. sandwich sign

141. An area of diffuse inflammatory edema of soft tissues that may proceed to necrosis and suppuration is called a:

    a. hemorrhage

    b. retroperitoneal fibrosis

    c. phlegmon

    d. necrotic tumor

142. Chronic pancreatitis may occur with all of the following findings except:

    a. irregular borders and dilated duct

    b. ductal lithiasis

    c. small, atrophic gland

    d. enlarged, edematous gland

143. One of the following statements is false regarding pancreatic pseudocysts:

    a. the cyst has a lining epithelium

    b. it develops through the lesser omentum

    c. the walls form in the potential available space

    d. commonly found in the lesser sac

144. The most common primary tumor of the pancreas is:

    a. cystadenocarcinoma

    b. pancreaticocarcinoma

    c. cystadenoma

    d. adenocarcinoma

145. The most frequent finding for a tumor in the head of the pancreas is:

    a. hydrops, ductal dilatation, jaundice

    b. ductal dilation, normal gallbladder

    c. intrahepatic ductal dilatation with jaundice

    d. ductal dilation, compression of the IVC with tumor infiltration

146. A line drawn from the right anterior superior iliac spine to the umbilicus is known as:

    a. Murphy's sign

    b. Grey Turner's sign

    c. McBurney's point

    d. veriformis line

147. One of the following statements is false regarding gastric carcinoma:

    a. it is the sixth leading cause of death

    b. one half of the tumors occur in the pylorus

    c. target or pseudokidney sign is seen on ultrasound examination

    d. gastric wall is normal

148. Clinical signs of acute appendicitus include all except:

    a. LUQ pain and rebound tenderness

    b. nausea and vomiting, diarrhea

    c. leukocytosis and RLQ pain

    d. anorexia and LLQ pain

149. Ultrasound findings in appendicitis include all except:

    a. increased wall thickness

    b. sandwich sign

    c. target sign

    d. hypoechoic ring with lack of peristalsis

150. Common pitfalls in the diagnosis of a renal mass may be caused by all except:

    a. extrarenal pelvis

    b. prominent Bertin's column

    c. dromedary hump

    d. junctional parenchymal defect

151. The most common fusion anomaly of the kidney is:

    a. crossed renal ectopia

    b. horseshoe kidney

    c. duplex kidney

    d. pelvic kidney

152. Impairment of renal function and increased protein catabolism result in:

    a. BUN decrease

    b. BUN elevation

    c. urea increase

    d. hematuria

153. Clinical findings in a patient with a suspected renal abscess include all but:

    a. fever, flank pain

    b. increased BUN

    c. pyuria

    d. decreased BUN

154. The mass found in the renal hilum that doesn't communicate with the renal collecting system is a:

    a. simple renal cyst

    b. parapelvic cyst

    c. renal carbuncle

    d. duplicated system

155. Cysts associated with multiple renal neoplasms include diseases such as:

    a. polycystic renal disease and acquired cysts of dialysis

    b. multicystic renal disease and medullary sponge kidney

    c. tuberous sclerosis and Von Hippel-Lindau

    d. medullary sponge kidney and tuberous sclerosis

156. Large echogenic kidneys that progress to renal failure and intrauterine demise are more likely to represent:

    a. autosomal-dominant polycystic disease

    b. autosomal-recessive polycystic disease

    c. medullary sponge kidney

    d. multicystic dysplastic kidney

157. One of the following statements is false regarding multicystic disease:

    a. occurs unilateral

    b. kidneys are enlarged in neonates and are small in adults

    c. contralateral ureteropelvic obstruction may be present

    d. occurs bilateral

158. A 60-year-old male presents with left flank pain and hematuria. The ultrasound examination of the kidneys shows a complex mass with some areas of calcification on the left kidney. You should also evaluate the:

    a. inferior vena cava for tumor involvement

    b. spleen

    c. pancreatic bed

    d. stomach

159. The most common primaries that cause metastases to the kidney include all except:

    a. melanoma

    b. lungs

    c. cervix

    d. liver

160. One of the following statements is false regarding Wilm's tumor:

    a. Venous obstruction may result with findings of leg edema, varicocele, or Budd-Chiari syndrome

    b. Tumor may spread beyond the renal capsule and invade the venous channel with tumor cells extending into the inferior vena cava and right atrium

    c. Tumor is always unilateral

    d. Tumor may metastasize into the lungs

161. A tumor comprised of fat cells that appears hyperechoic on ultrasound examination is most likely:

    a. hemangioma

    b. sinus lipomatosis

    c. angiomyolipoma

    d. adenoma

162. If a patient has hydronephrosis, the sonographer should also look in the following areas:

    a. bladder to search for ureteral jets

    b. uteropelvic junction to search for stones

    c. bladder to search for dilation of the ureters

    d. renal cortex to look for atrophy

163. Increased echogenicity of the renal parenchyma may be seen in patients with all except:

    a. lupus nephritis

    b. AIDS

    c. sickle cell nephropathy

    d. papillary necrosis

164. Massive dilation of the renal pelvis with loss of renal parenchyma is representative of:

    a. grade III hydronephrosis

    b. grade I hydronephrosis

    c. sinus lipomatosis

    d. prominent renal pelvis

165. Nonobstructive hydronephrosis may be caused from each of the following such problems except:

    a. pregnancy

    b. reflux

    c. bladder carcinoma

    d. infection

166. False positive interpretation of hydronephrosis may be attributed to all except:

    a. parapelvic cysts

    b. congenital megacalices

    c. papillary necrosis

    d. ureteral stone

167. A patient has an irregular mass, somewhat triangular in appearance along the periphery of the renal border. This most likely represents a:

    a. renal infection

    b. renal infarction

    c. pyonephrosis

    d. acute tubular necrosis

168. Acute tubular necrosis usually appears on ultrasound examination as:

    a. bilateral renal enlargement, with hyperechoic pyramids

    b. normal renal size, with hypoechoic pyramids

    c. enlarged kidneys with anechoic pyramids

    d. small kidneys with hyperechoic pyramids

169. The most common finding in a patient with nephrocalcinosis is:

    a. hypoechoic renal parenchyma

    b. echogenic pyramids with shadowing

    c. enlarged, hypoechoic pyramids

    d. small pyramids with isoechoic borders

170. The following patterns have been found in rejection except:

    a. enlargement and decreased echogenicity of the pyramids

    b. increased echogenicity of the pyramids

    c. hyperechoic cortex

    d. patchy sonolucent areas involving the cortex and medulla

171. A common cause of acute renal transplant failure is:

    a. acute tubular necrosis

    b. graft rupture

    c. renal vein thrombosis

    d. obstruction

172. The most common cause of focal splenic lesions is:

    a. splenic cyst

    b. splenic trauma

    c. splenic infarct

    d. splenic abscess

173. A patient has left upper quadrant pain, left shoulder pain, left flank pain, and is hypotensive after a boating accident. These symptoms most likely represent:

    a. splenic infarct

    b. splenic abscess

    c. splenic tumor

    d. splenic rupture

174. What structure crosses anterior to the crus and posterior to the inferior vena cava at the level of the right kidney?

    a. ligament of the diaphragm

    b. left renal vein

    c. right renal artery

    d. right adrenal gland

175. Enlarged nodes may be found in all but:

    a. mantle of nodes in the paraspinal location

    b. anterior displacement of the aorta secondary to enlarged nodes

    c. mesenteric sandwich sign

    d. draping renal sign

176. The anterior and posterior fascial planes are connected by curvilinear connective tissue septas known as:

    a. Cooper's ligaments

    b. faliciform ligaments

    c. mammorary ligaments

    d. retrofascial ligaments

177. The mammary layer is also known as:

a. subcutaneous fat layer

b. retrofascilar tissue layer

c. glandular breast tissue

d. retromammary layer

178. A breast mass that shows uniform homogeneous internal echoes, smooth border, and no through transmission in a young women is most likely:

a. fibrocystic disease

b. fibroadenoma

c. hemorrhagic cyst

d. cystosarcoma phyllodes

179. Distinguishing features of a solid mass within the breast include all except:

a. irregular spiculated contour or margin

b. round or lobulated

c. nonuniform internal echoes

d. good through transmission

180. The lateral group of muscles that are located near the thyroid gland include all except:

a. sternothyroideus

b. longus colli

c. sternocleidomastoid

d. sternohyoideus

181. Characteristics of a thyroid adenoma include all but:

a. irregular border with increased through transmission

b. echolucent to echo dense

c. halo surrounding the lesion

d. complete fibrous encapsulation

182. Epididymitis on ultrasound examination appears as:

a. dilation and tortuosity of the veins

b. fluid between the visceral and parietal layers of the tunica vaginalis

c. microcalcifications throughout the scrotum

d. enlargement of the epididymal head with decreased echogenicity

183. This occurs when two or more reflectors are encountered in the sound beam path:

a. refraction

b. attenuation

c. reverberation

d. acoustic speckle

184. This occurs when the sound wave bends or changes direction when traveling from one medium to another:

a. attenuation

b. refraction

c. reverberation

d. multipath

185. This occurs when acoustic energy is emitted by the transducer in some direction other than the main axis, usually at the edges or side of the beam:

a. side lobes

b. refraction

c. electronic noise

d. range ambiguity

186. This occurs when the sound beam encounters a strong reflector in its path, causing a second image to be produced on the other side of the strong reflector:

a. attenuation

b. mirror image

c. reverberation

d. multipath

187. This appears as tissue texture close to the transducer, but is not true tissue:

a. reverberation

b. acoustic speckle

c. multipath

d. range ambiguity

188. This occurs when the sound beam takes one path to an object and a different path back to the transducer:

a. range ambiguity

b. mirror image

c. multipath

d. aliasing

189. This occurs when sound travels a medium with a lower attenuation rate than the surrounding tissue:

a. enhancement

b. acoustic speckle

c. reverberation

d. range ambiguity

190. This occurs when the transducer sends out a pulse before the reflection from a previous pulse is received:

a. enhancement

b. range ambiguity

c. electronic noise

d. aliasing

191. This occurs when interference from 60-cycle or AC electrical currents is picked up by the imaging screen:

a. aliasing

b. electronic noise

c. acoustic speckle

d. side lobes

192. All of the following techniques can be used to eliminate aliasing except:

a. increase the PRF

b. shift the Doppler baseline

c. increase the transducer frequency

d. decrease the transducer frequency

193. Low-level echoes along the anterior wall of the urinary bladder are most likely:

a. refraction

b. acoustic speckle

c. mirror image

d. side lobes

194. When the liver is shown superior to the diaphragm on a sagittal scan, this most position likely represents:

a. reverberation

b. acoustic speckle

c. mirror image

d. side lobes

195. Blurring of echoes in the far field of the liver parenchyma represent:

a. incorrect focusing

b. transducer frequency too high

c. decreased gain settings

d. electronic noise

196. Low-level echoes within the bladder that are difficult to reproduce represent:

a. insufficient gain

b. incorrect depth

c. reverberation

d. noise

197. Inhomogeneous hepatic parenchyma may be caused by:

a. banding, incorrect TGC

b. increased gain

c. incorrect focusing

d. electronic noise

198. Linear-spaced bright echoes in the liver parenchyma are most likely from:

a. reverberations

b. incorrect focusing

c. reflection

d. mirror image

Answers—Mock Registry Review Examination

1. b	**53.** a	**105.** a
2. d	**54.** c	**106.** c
3. b	**55.** b	**107.** d
4. a	**56.** c	**108.** d
5. c	**57.** d	**109.** b
6. d	**58.** a	**110.** d
7. a	**59.** d	**111.** a
8. b	**60.** a	**112.** c
9. d	**61.** c	**113.** d
10. c	**62.** d	**114.** b
11. d	**63.** b	**115.** d
12. a	**64.** a	**116.** b
13. c	**65.** c	**117.** b
14. d	**66.** b	**118.** c
15. a	**67.** a	**119.** c
16. c	**68.** c	**120.** d
17. d	**69.** b	**121.** a
18. a	**70.** c	**122.** c
19. b	**71.** a	**123.** d
20. c	**72.** b	**124.** a
21. b	**73.** b	**125.** b
22. c	**74.** c	**126.** d
23. c	**75.** d	**127.** c
24. c	**76.** c	**128.** b
25. a	**77.** a	**129.** b
26. d	**78.** b	**130.** d
27. a	**79.** c	**131.** b
28. b	**80.** b	**132.** a
29. c	**81.** c	**133.** d
30. a	**82.** c	**134.** b
31. b	**83.** b	**135.** a
32. b	**84.** c	**136.** b
33. c	**85.** a	**137.** c
34. b	**86.** b	**138.** c
35. c	**87.** d	**139.** b
36. t	**88.** c	**140.** a
37. b	**89.** d	**141.** c
38. d	**90.** b	**142.** d
39. f	**91.** b	**143.** a
40. b	**92.** c	**144.** d
41. a	**93.** d	**145.** a
42. e	**94.** d	**146.** c
43. c	**95.** b	**147.** d
44. d	**96.** b	**148.** c
45. a	**97.** c	**149.** b
46. c	**98.** c	**150.** a
47. d	**99.** d	**151.** b
48. a	**100.** c	**152.** b
49. b	**101.** a	**153.** d
50. d	**102.** c	**154.** b
51. b	**103.** c	**155.** c
52. b	**104.** d	**156.** b

157. d	**171.** a	**185.** a
158. a	**172.** c	**186.** b
159. d	**173.** d	**187.** b
160. c	**174.** c	**188.** c
161. c	**175.** d	**189.** a
162. a	**176.** a	**190.** b
163. d	**177.** c	**191.** b
164. a	**178.** b	**192.** c
165. c	**179.** d	**193.** b
166. d	**180.** b	**194.** c
167. b	**181.** a	**195.** a
168. a	**182.** d	**196.** d
169. b	**183.** c	**197.** a
170. b	**184.** b	**198.** a

References

Anderson PD: *Clinical anatomy and physiology for allied health sciences,* Philadelphia, 1976, Saunders.

Bejar R, Coen R: Normal cranial ultrasonography in neonates. In James HE, Anas NG, Perkin RM (eds): *Brain insults in infants and children: pathophysiology and management,* Orlando, 1985, Grune & Stratton.

Brown B, Filly R, Callen P: Ultrasonographic anatomy of the caudate lobe, *J Clin Ultrasound Med* 1:189–192, June–July 1982.

Crafts RC: *A textbook of human anatomy,* ed 2, New York, 1979, John Wiley & Sons.

Hagen-Ansert SL: *Textbook of diagnostic ultrasonography,* ed 2; resolution ultrasonography of superficial structures (Schorzman L), Breast (Ezo L, Hagen-Ansert SL), Ultrasound evaluation of the neonatal skull (Appareti K et al); St Louis, 1983, Mosby.

Hollinshead WH: *Textbook of anatomy,* 3rd ed, Philadelphia, 1982, Harper & Row.

Introduction to medical sciences for clinical practice, Unit XIII: Obstetrics. Chicago, 1977, Yearbook.

Kapit W, Elson LM: *The anatomy coloring book,* New York, 1977, Harper & Row.

Lyons EA: *A color atlas of sectional anatomy,* St Louis, 1978, Mosby.

Marks W, Filly R, Callen P: Ultrasound anatomy of the liver: a review with new applications, *J Clin Ultrasound* 7:137–146, April 1979.

Moore KL: *The developing human,* Philadelphia, 1973, Saunders.

Netter FH: *The CIBA collection of medical illustrations,* vol 3, Summit, NJ, 1977, CIBA.

Netter FH: *The CIBA collection of medical illustrations,* vol 5, Summit, NJ, 1974, CIBA.

Pernkopf E: *Atlas of topographical and applied human anatomy,* vol 2, Philadelphia, 1964, Saunders.

Rumack CM, Johnson ML: *Perinatal and infant brain imaging,* Chicago, 1984, Year Book.

Sahn DJ, Anderson F: *Two-dimensional anatomy of the heart,* New York, 1982, John Wiley & Sons.

Snell RS: *Clinical anatomy for medical students,* Boston, 1973, Little, Brown & Co.

Thompson JS: *Core textbook of anatomy,* Philadelphia, 1977, Lippincott.